Inderbir Singh's

Textbook of
HUMAN NEUROANATOMY

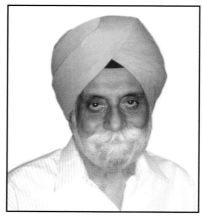

Late Professor Inderbir Singh
(1930–2014)

Tribute to a Legend

Professor Inderbir Singh, a legendary anatomist, is renowned for being a pillar in the education of generations of medical graduates across the globe. He was one of the greatest teachers of his time. He was a passionate writer who poured his soul into his work. His eagle's eye for details and meticulous way of writing made his books immensely popular amongst students. He managed his lifetime to become enmeshed in millions of hearts. He was conferred the title of Professor Emeritus by Maharshi Dayanand University, Rohtak.

On 12th May, 2014, he was awarded posthumously with Emeritus Teacher Award *by* National Board of Examination *for making invaluable contribution in teaching of Anatomy.* This award is given to honour legends who have made tremendous contribution in the field of medical education. He was a visionary for his time, and the legacies he left behind are his various textbooks on *Gross Anatomy*, *Histology*, *Neuroanatomy* and *Embryology*. Although his mortal frame is not present amongst us, his genius will live on forever.

Inderbir Singh's

Textbook of
HUMAN NEUROANATOMY

(Fundamental and Clinical)

──── **Tenth Edition** ────

Editors

PRITHA S BHUIYAN
MBBS MS (Anatomy) PGDME
Professor and Head
Department of Anatomy
Seth GS Medical College & KEM Hospital
Mumbai, Maharashtra, India

LAKSHMI RAJGOPAL
MS (General Surgery) DNB MNAMS (Anatomy)
Professor (Additional)
Department of Anatomy
Seth GS Medical College & KEM Hospital
Mumbai, Maharashtra, India

K SHYAMKISHORE
MS (Anatomy)
Professor (Additional)
Department of Anatomy
Seth GS Medical College & KEM Hospital
Mumbai, Maharashtra, India

The Health Sciences Publisher
New Delhi | London | Panama

Jaypee Brothers Medical Publishers (P) Ltd

Headquarters

Jaypee Brothers Medical Publishers (P) Ltd
4838/24, Ansari Road, Daryaganj
New Delhi 110 002, India
Phone: +91-11-43574357
Fax: +91-11-43574314
Email: jaypee@jaypeebrothers.com

Overseas Offices

J.P. Medical Ltd
83 Victoria Street, London
SW1H 0HW (UK)
Phone: +44 20 3170 8910
Fax: +44 (0)20 3008 6180
Email: info@jpmedpub.com

Jaypee Brothers Medical Publishers (P) Ltd
17/1-B Babar Road, Block-B, Shaymali
Mohammadpur, Dhaka-1207
Bangladesh
Mobile: +08801912003485
Email: jaypeedhaka@gmail.com

Jaypee-Highlights Medical Publishers Inc
City of Knowledge, Bld. 235, 2nd Floor, Clayton
Panama City, Panama
Phone: +1 507-301-0496
Fax: +1 507-301-0499
Email: cservice@jphmedical.com

Jaypee Brothers Medical Publishers (P) Ltd
Bhotahity, Kathmandu
Nepal
Phone: +977-9741283608
Email: kathmandu@jaypeebrothers.com

Website: www.jaypeebrothers.com
Website: www.jaypeedigital.com

Textbook of Human Neuroanatomy

First Edition	: 1997	Seventh Edition	: 2006
Reprint	: 2008	Eighth Edition	: 2009
Reprint	: 2010	Revised & Updated Eighth Edition	: 2013
Ninth Edition	: 2014	Tenth Edition	: **2018**

ISBN: 978-93-5270-148-3

Printed at: Ajanta Offset & Packagings Ltd., Faridabad, Haryana.

Preface to the Tenth Edition

The method of teaching Anatomy especially Neuroanatomy has undergone a vast change over the past decade. Medical students are needed not only to know the facts about the nervous system, but should also know how to apply that knowledge to 'localize' the neurological lesion which means they should correctly identify the 'site' and 'side' of lesion. This is possible only with a thorough knowledge of Neuroanatomy. So in this book, we have strived to provide the readers with ample opportunities to exercise their grey cells and practise this 'localization'.

We are thankful to all the comments, criticisms and feedback received for the ninth edition. These gave us a direction to revamp and modify the current edition to fulfill the requirements of undergraduate students.

The current edition has been refined to suit the needs of undergraduate students. This has been achieved by reducing the total number of chapters to 16 from the previous edition's 20. This edition will also help the undergraduate medical students to achieve the required competencies of understanding and describing the gross anatomy of central and peripheral nervous systems and correlating the anatomical basis of clinical manifestations.

The language has been very simplified so that all students can understand the subject better. New dissection photographs which are of high resolution have been added as eight plates at the beginning of the book. These are in black background and have been labelled to help students identify various parts of the brain not just during brain prosection studies, but even revise later outside of dissection hall or at home. More line diagrams, tables and new flowcharts have been added to facilitate easy understanding. Anatomical basis of a lot of neurological conditions have been highlighted in coloured boxes.

A new addition to this edition is that each chapter has a section on "Clinical Cases" which will stimulate the students to apply what they have learnt in the chapter and find a solution to the problem. This will enhance their clinical problem-solving skills and help them to hone their competencies as per the evolving 'Competency-based curriculum'. Each chapter also has short and long answer questions collated from various university examinations and these will help the students to do self-assessment and to practise for their examinations.

We would whole heartedly like to thank Mr Jitendar P Vij (Group Chairman), Mr Ankit Vij (Group President) of Jaypee Brothers Medical Publishers (P) Ltd, New Delhi, India for his useful and innovative suggestion to include photographs of brain specimens in black background which, we are sure, will be welcome by the students. We would also like to thank the whole editorial team at Jaypee Brothers especially Mr Sabarish Menon (Commissioning editor), for the constant support and coordination, Mr Ankush Sharma (Designer), for refining the diagrams and Mr Deep Dogra (Operator), for type-setting and formatting.

We are grateful to the staff members of Department of Anatomy, Seth GS Medical College & KEM Hospital especially Dr Praveen Iyer for the support, Mr Prashant Jadhav and Mrs Jyoti Kerkar for the technical support given.
We are thankful to Dr Avinash Supe, Dean, Seth GS Medical College & KEM Hospital and Director (Medical Education & Major Hospitals) for his encouragement to our academic activities.

Last, but not the least, we would like to express our heartfelt gratitude to our family members for bearing with our preoccupation with the completion of the book.

We hope this edition will be used extensively not only by undergraduate medical and paramedical students but also by postgraduates and medical teachers.

Pritha S Bhuiyan, Lakshmi Rajgopal, K Shyamkishore

Preface to the Ninth Edition

Professor Inderbir Singh has been a doyen in the field of Anatomy, and he has been looked upon as a guide and mentor by many students and teachers. So, it is indeed a great honour for us to edit the ninth edition of 'Inderbir Singh's Textbook of Human Neuroanatomy (Fundamental and Clinical). While editing, this book has provided us an opportunity to revisit neuroanatomy, we have enjoyed this relook thoroughly.

To highlight what the students should learn from each chapter, 'Specific Learning Objectives' have been added. A comprehensive rearrangement of chapters has been done to make it easy for the students to understand the subject. Important clinical conditions are given as 'Clinical Correlation' in Boxes. Validated 'Multiple Choice Questions' have been added at the end of each chapter for self-assessment. New diagrams and photographs of dissected and plastinated specimens have been incorporated to make it reader friendly. New tables and flowcharts have been inserted for making comprehension of neuroanatomy easy. The chapter on 'Imaging Techniques of the Central Nervous System' is updated completely keeping in mind the emerging trends in newer imaging techniques.

We are grateful to the Dean, Seth GS Medical College and KEM Hospital, for giving us the permission to edit this book. We are also thankful to Dr HD Deshmukh, Professor and Head, Department of Radiology, for providing us CT scans and MRI scans. Our special acknowledgement to Mr Prashant Jadhav for helping us with the photography. Our special thanks to all our students for making us take up this challenging task despite our academic and administrative responsibilities. We thank our family members for their continued support.

We hope that this edition will be useful to the students and teachers interested in neuroanatomy, and we welcome feedback from the readers to improve future editions.

Pritha S Bhuiyan, Lakshmi Rajgopal, K Shyamkishore

Contents

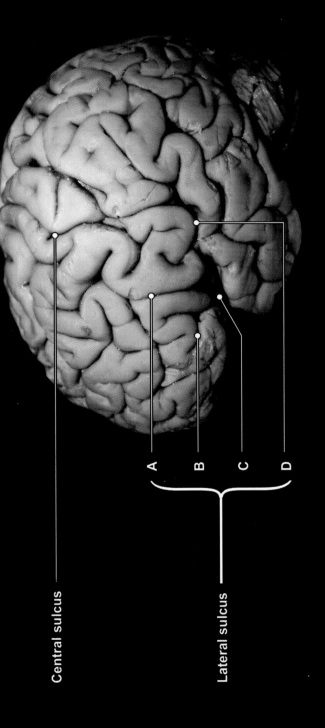

Central sulcus

Lateral sulcus

A

B

C

D

Plate 1: Superolateral surface of the brain
(A- Ascending ramus, B- Anterior ramus, C- Stem, D- Posterior ramus)

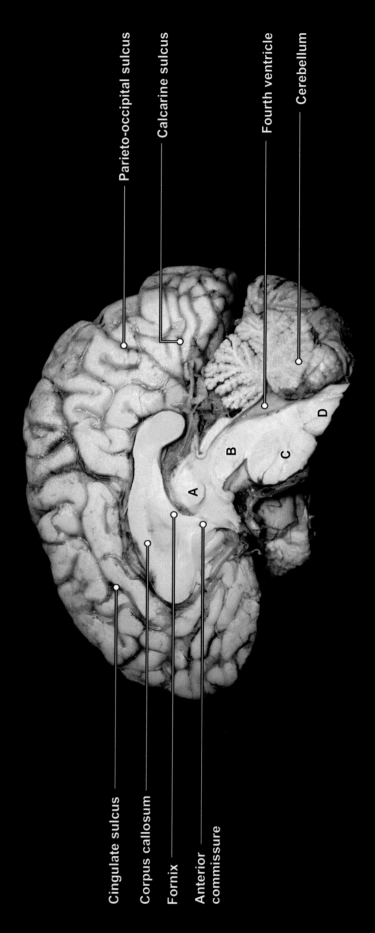

Cingulate sulcus

Corpus callosum

Fornix

Anterior commissure

Parieto-occipital sulcus

Calcarine sulcus

Fourth ventricle

Cerebellum

A

B

C

D

Plate 2: Medial surface of cerebrum
A- Diencephalon B- Midbrain C- Pons D- Medulla oblongata

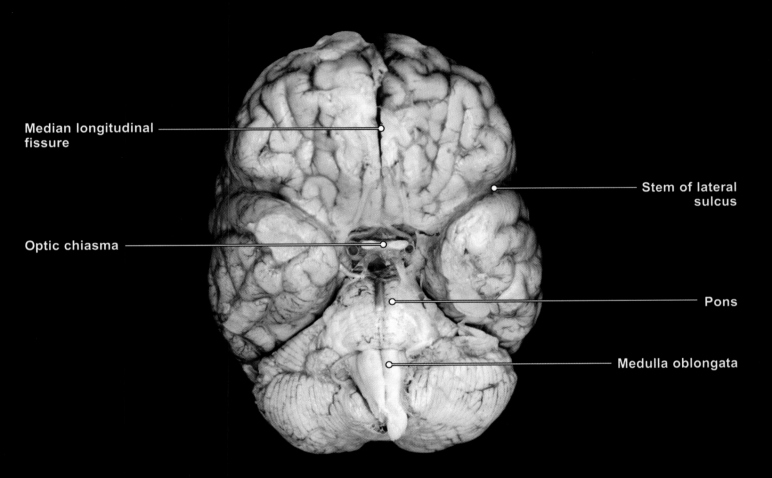

Median longitudinal fissure

Stem of lateral sulcus

Optic chiasma

Pons

Medulla oblongata

Plate 3: Inferior surface of cerebrum

Frontal pole

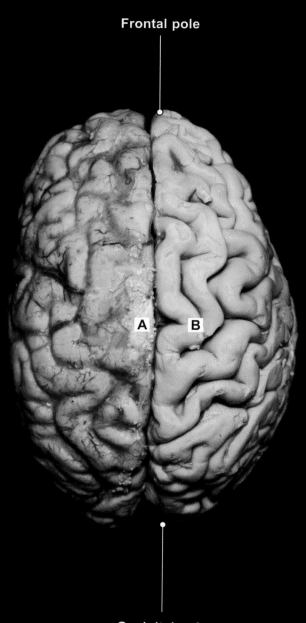

A   B

Occipital pole

Plate 4: Superior view of cerebrum
A- Arachnoid granulations seen on the left side
B- Arachnoid mater removed on the right side

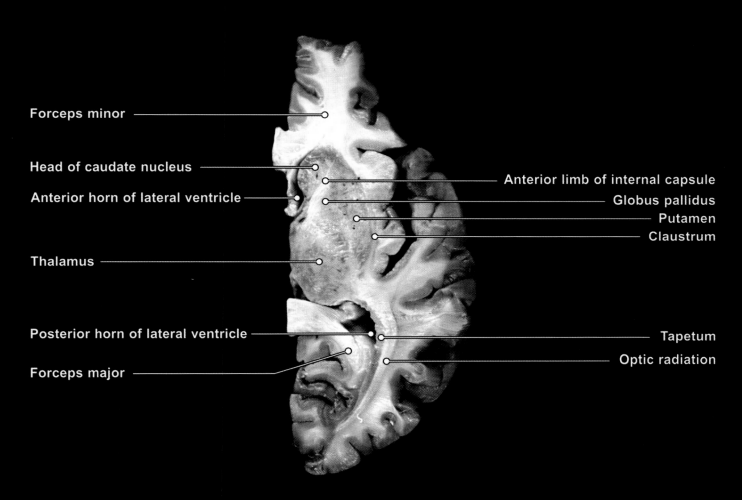

Forceps minor

Head of caudate nucleus

Anterior horn of lateral ventricle

Thalamus

Posterior horn of lateral ventricle

Forceps major

Anterior limb of internal capsule

Globus pallidus

Putamen

Claustrum

Tapetum

Optic radiation

Plate 5: Horizontal section of cerebrum

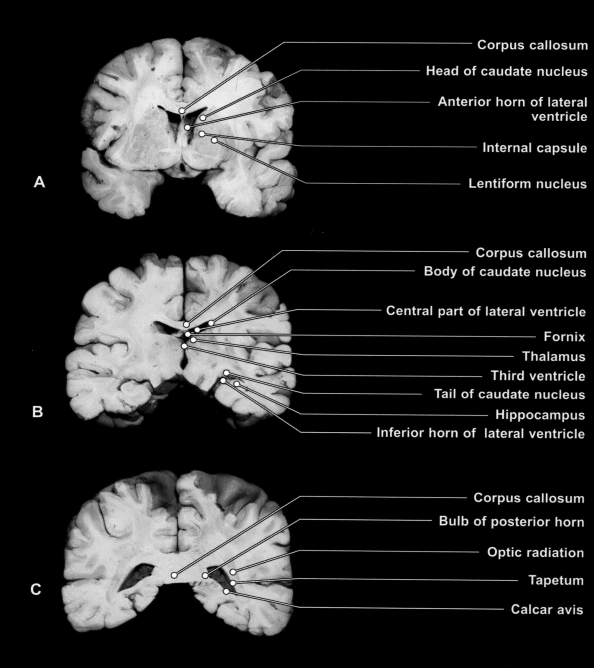

A

Corpus callosum
Head of caudate nucleus
Anterior horn of lateral ventricle
Internal capsule
Lentiform nucleus

B

Corpus callosum
Body of caudate nucleus
Central part of lateral ventricle
Fornix
Thalamus
Third ventricle
Tail of caudate nucleus
Hippocampus
Inferior horn of lateral ventricle

C

Corpus callosum
Bulb of posterior horn
Optic radiation
Tapetum
Calcar avis

Plate 6: Coronal sections of the brain passing through the lateral ventricle
A- Anterior horn B- Central part and inferior horn C- Posterior horn

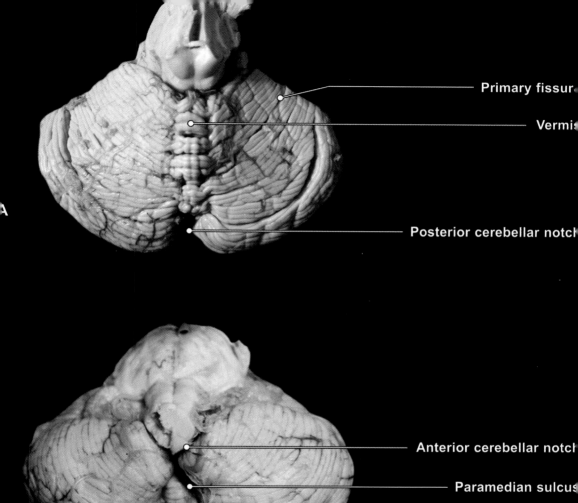

Primary fissure

Vermis

Posterior cerebellar notch

Anterior cerebellar notch

Paramedian sulcus

Vermis

Horizontal fissure

Plate 7: Cerebellum
A. Superior surface B. Inferior surface

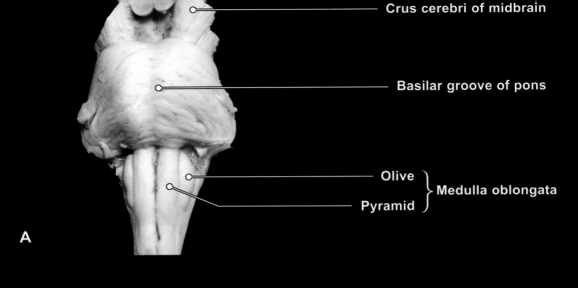

Crus cerebri of midbrain

Basilar groove of pons

Olive ⎫
⎬ Medulla oblongata
Pyramid ⎭

A

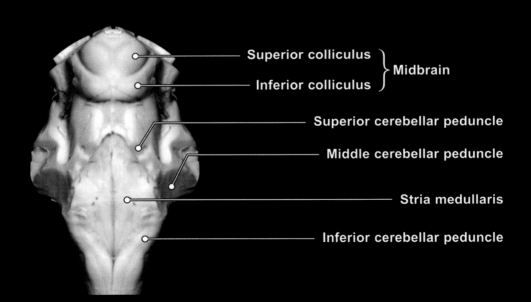

Superior colliculus ⎫
⎬ Midbrain
Inferior colliculus ⎭

Superior cerebellar peduncle

Middle cerebellar peduncle

Stria medullaris

Inferior cerebellar peduncle

B

Plate 8: Brainstem

Chapter 1 | Introduction to Nervous System

INTRODUCTION

The human body consists of numerous tissues and organs, which are diverse in structure and function, yet they function together and in harmony for the well-being of the body as a whole. There has to be some kind of influence that monitors and controls the working of different parts of the body. The overwhelming role in directing the activities of the body rests with the nervous system. Neuroanatomy is the study of the structural aspects of the nervous system. It cannot be emphasized too strongly that the study of structure is meaningless unless correlated with function.

DIVISIONS OF NERVOUS SYSTEM

The nervous system may be divided into the **central nervous system** (CNS), made up of the brain and spinal cord, the **peripheral nervous system** (PNS), consisting of the peripheral nerves and the ganglia associated with them (Figures 1.1 and 1.2, Table 1.1). The brain consists of the **cerebrum, diencephalon**, **midbrain**, **pons**, **cerebellum** and **medulla oblongata**. The midbrain, pons, and medulla oblongata together form the **brainstem**. The medulla oblongata is continuous below with the spinal cord (Figure 1.2).

TISSUES CONSTITUTING NERVOUS SYSTEM

The nervous system is made up, predominantly, of tissue that has the special property of being able to conduct impulses rapidly from one part of the body to another. The specialized cells that constitute the functional units of the nervous system are called **neurons**. Within the brain and spinal cord, neurons are supported by a special kind of connective tissue that is called **neuroglia**.

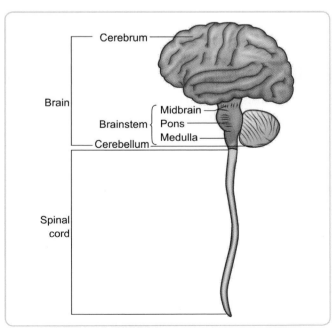

Figure 1.1: Anatomical divisions of the nervous system

TABLE 1.1: Classification of nervous system

Central nervous system			Peripheral nervous system
Brain (encephalon)	Forebrain (prosencephalon)	Telencephalon (cerebrum)	Cranial nerves I and II
		Diencephalon	
	Midbrain (mesencephalon)		Cranial nerves III and IV
	Hindbrain (rhombencephalon)	Metencephalon (pons and cerebellum)	Cranial nerves V to XII
		Myelencephalon (medulla oblongata)	
Spinal cord (myelon)			31 pairs of spinal nerves

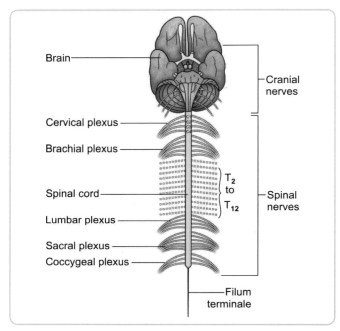

Figure 1.2: Parts of the central and peripheral nervous system

STRUCTURE OF A TYPICAL NEURON

A neuron consists of a **cell body** that gives off a number of **processes** called **neurites** (Figures 1.3A and B).

Cell Body

The cell body is also called the soma or **perikaryon**. The cytoplasm contains a large central nucleus (usually with a prominent nucleolus), numerous mitochondria, lysosomes and Golgi complex (Figure 1.3B). The cytoplasm also shows the presence of a granular material that stains intensely with basic dyes called **Nissl substance** (also called Nissl bodies or granules) (Figure 1.3C). These bodies are rough endoplasmic reticulum (Figure 1.3B).

The **neurofibrils** in the cytoplasm consist of microfilaments and microtubules (Figure 1.3D). The centrioles present in neurons are concerned with the production and maintenance of microtubules. Some neurons contain pigment granules (for example, neuromelanin in neurons of the substantia nigra). Aging neurons contain a pigment, lipofuscin (made up of residual bodies derived from lysosomes).

Neurites

The processes arising from the cell body of a neuron are called **neurites**. These are of two kinds. Most neurons give off a number of short branching processes called **dendrites** and one longer process called an **axon**. The differences between axon and dendrite are summarized in Table 1.2 (Figure 1.3C).

Axoplasmic Flow

The cytoplasm of neurons is in constant motion. Movement of various materials occurs through axons. This **axoplasmic flow** takes place both away from and towards the cell body. Axoplasmic transport of tracer substances introduced experimentally can help trace neuronal connections.

> **Clinical Anatomy**
>
> **Role of Axoplasmic Transport in Spread of Disease**
> Some infections, which affect the nervous system travel along nerves.
> - Rabies virus, from the site of bite, travels along nerves by reverse axoplasmic flow.
> - Polio virus is also transported from the gastrointestinal tract through reverse axoplasmic flow.
> - Tetanus bacteria, in contrast, travels from the site of infection to the brain along the endoneurium of nerve fibres.

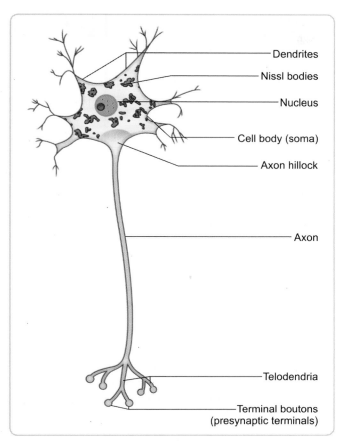

Dendrites

Nissl bodies

Nucleus

Cell body (soma)

Axon hillock

Axon

Telodendria

Terminal boutons
(presynaptic terminals)

Figure 1.3A: Parts of a typical neuron

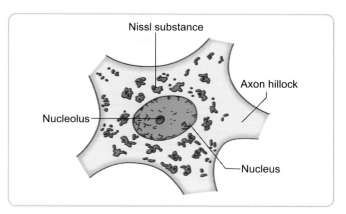

Nissl substance

Axon hillock

Nucleolus

Nucleus

Figure 1.3C: Neuronal cell body showing Nissl substance

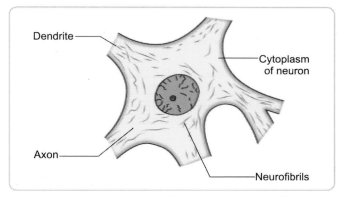

Dendrite

Cytoplasm
of neuron

Axon

Neurofibrils

Figure 1.3D: Neuronal cell body showing neurofibrils

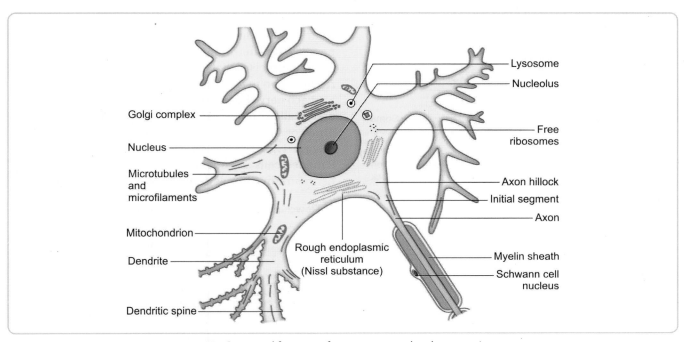

Lysosome

Nucleolus

Golgi complex

Free
ribosomes

Nucleus

Microtubules
and
microfilaments

Axon hillock

Initial segment

Axon

Mitochondrion

Dendrite

Myelin sheath

Schwann cell
nucleus

Rough endoplasmic
reticulum
(Nissl substance)

Dendritic spine

Figure 1.3B: Structural features of neuron as seen by electron microscope

TABLE 1.2: Difference between axons and dendrites

Axons	Dendrites
Axon is a single, long, thin process of a nerve cell, which terminates away from the nerve cell body	Dendrites are multiple, short, thick and tapering processes of the nerve cell which terminate near the nerve cell body
Axon ends by dividing into many fine processes called axon terminals	Dendrites are highly branched to form a dendritic tree
It has uniform diameter and smooth surface	The thickness of dendrite reduces as it divides repeatedly
It is free of Nissl granules	Nissl granules are present in dendrites
The nerve impulses travel away from the cell body	The nerve impulses travel towards the cell body

CLASSIFICATION OF NEURONS

Neurons are classified based on:
- **Variation in the shape of neuronal cell bodies:** Depending on the shapes of their cell bodies, some neurons are referred to as stellate (star-shaped) or pyramidal
- **Polarity:** Unipolar, bipolar, multipolar (Figure 1.4, Flowchart 1.1)
- **Variations in Axons:** Golgi type I and Golgi type II
  Examples of different types of neurons are given in Table 1.3.

NERVE FIBRES

Axons (and some dendrites, which resemble axons in structure) constitute what are commonly called nerve fibres. The bundles of nerve fibres found in CNS are called as **tracts,** while the bundles of nerve fibres found in PNS are called **peripheral nerves.**

Basic Structure of Peripheral Nerve Fibres

Each nerve fibre has a central core formed by the axon. This core is called the **axis cylinder.** The plasma membrane surrounding the axis cylinder is the **axolemma.** The axis cylinder is surrounded by a myelin sheath. This sheath is in the form of short segments that are separated at short intervals called the **nodes of Ranvier.** The part of the nerve fibre between two consecutive nodes is the **internode.** Each segment of the myelin sheath is formed by one Schwann cell.

Outside the myelin sheath, there is a thin layer of Schwann cell cytoplasm and an external lamina (similar to the basal lamina of epithelium). This layer of cytoplasm and external lamina is called the **neurilemma.** Neurilemma is important in the regeneration of peripheral nerves after their injury. Such neurilemma is absent in oligodendrocytes that form myelin sheath in CNS. Hence, regeneration in the CNS is not possible.

Each nerve fibre is surrounded by a layer of connective tissue called **endoneurium** (Figure 1.5). A bundle of nerve fibres or **fasciculus** is surrounded by the **perineurium** (Figure 1.5). The perineurium is made up of layers of flattened cells separated by layers of collagen fibres. The perineurium controls diffusion of substances in and out of

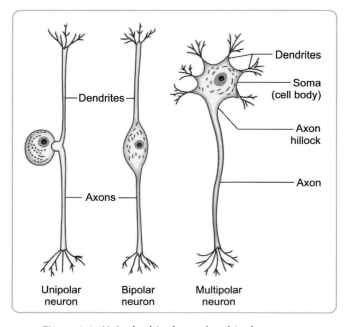

Figure 1.4: Unipolar, bipolar, and multipolar neurons

Flowchart 1.1: Types of neurons—anatomical classification

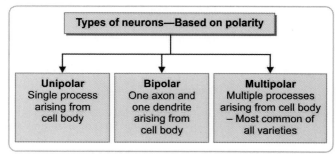

TABLE 1.3: Morphological classification of neurons

Morphology	Location and example
According to polarity • Unipolar • Bipolar • Multipolar	• Posterior root ganglia of spinal nerves, sensory ganglia of cranial nerves • Retina, sensory ganglia of cochlear and vestibular nerves • Motor neurons of anterior grey column of spinal cord, autonomic ganglia
According to size of nerve fibre • Golgi type I (long axons) • Golgi type II (short axons)	• Pyramidal cells of cerebral cortex • Stellate cells of cerebral cortex

axons. The fasciculi are held together by the epineurium (which surrounds the entire nerve).

> **Clinical Anatomy**
>
> • The epineurium contains fat that cushions nerve fibres. Loss of this fat in bedridden patients can lead to pressure on nerve fibres and paralysis.
> • Blood vessels to a nerve travel through the connective tissue that surrounds it. Severe reduction in blood supply can lead to ischaemic neuritis and pain.

Blood–Nerve Barrier

Peripheral nerve fibres are separated from circulating blood by a blood–nerve barrier. Capillaries in nerves are nonfenestrated and their endothelial cells are united by tight junctions. There is a continuous basal lamina around the capillary. The blood-nerve barrier is reinforced by cell layers present in the perineurium.

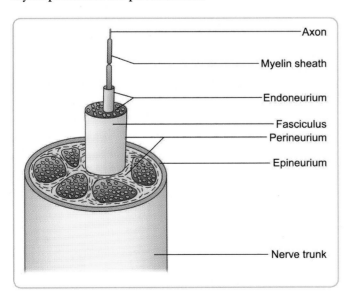

Figure 1.5: Connective tissue supporting nerve fibres of a peripheral nerve

(Labels: Axon, Myelin sheath, Endoneurium, Fasciculus, Perineurium, Epineurium, Nerve trunk)

CLASSIFICATION OF PERIPHERAL NERVE FIBRES

Peripheral nerves are classified in many ways.

According to Function

• Some nerve fibres carry impulses from the spinal cord or brain to peripheral structures like muscle or gland; they are called **efferent** or **motor** fibres.
• Other nerve fibres carry impulses from peripheral organs to the brain or spinal cord. These are called **afferent** fibres.

According to Area of Innervation

• **Somatic afferent fibres:** Carry impulses from skin, bones, muscles, and joints to the CNS
• **Somatic efferent fibres:** Carry impulses from CNS to the skeletal muscles
• **Visceral afferent fibres:** Carry impulses from visceral organs and blood vessels to the CNS
• **Visceral efferent fibres:** Carry impulses from CNS to the cardiac muscle, glands, and smooth muscles

According to Diameter and Velocity of Conduction

• A (subdivided into α, β, γ, δ)
• B
• C (unmyelinated)

Sensory nerve fibres are also classified into I, II, III and IV

Details of diameter and conduction velocity in the peripheral nerves with examples are given in Table 1.4.

Presence of myelin sheath

• Myelinated
• Unmyelinated

MYELIN SHEATH AND PROCESS OF MYELINATION

The nature of myelin sheath is best understood by considering the mode of its formation (Figures 1.6A to E). An axon lying near a Schwann cell invaginates into the cytoplasm of the Schwann cell. In this process, the axon comes to be suspended by a fold of the cell membrane of the Schwann cell. This fold is called the **mesaxon.**

In some situations, the mesaxon becomes greatly elongated and comes to be spirally wound around the axon, which is thus surrounded by several layers of cell membrane. Lipids are deposited between adjacent layers of the membrane. These layers of the mesaxon, along with the lipids, sphingomyelin, form the **myelin sheath**.

Outside the myelin sheath, a thin layer of Schwann cell cytoplasm and an external lamina persists to form an additional sheath, which is called the **neurilemma** (also called the neurilemmal sheath or Schwann cell sheath).

An axon is related to a large number of Schwann cells over its length. Each Schwann cell provides the myelin sheath for a short segment of the axon (Figure 1.7). At the junction of any two such segments, there is a short gap in the myelin sheath. These gaps are called the **nodes of Ranvier**. When an impulse travels down a nerve fibre, it does not proceed uniformly along the length of the axis cylinder, but jumps from one node to the next. This is called **saltatory conduction**. In unmyelinated neurons, the impulse travels along the axolemma. Such conduction is much slower than saltatory conduction.

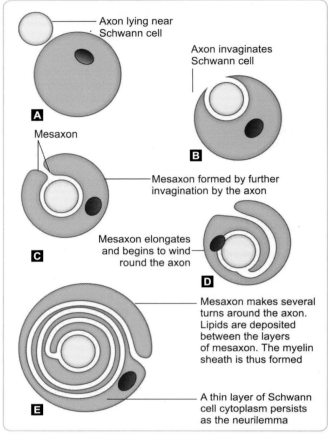

Figures 1.6A to E: (A) Stages in the formation of the myelin sheath by a Schwann cell—the axon, which first lies near the Schwann cell; (B and C) Then it invaginates into its cytoplasm, and comes to be suspended by a mesaxon. (D and E) The mesaxon elongates and comes to be spirally wound around the axon

TABLE 1.4: Classification of fibres in the peripheral nerves

Fibre type	Function	Sensory classification	Diameter (µm)	Velocity (m/s)
A α	Muscle spindle, annulo-spiral ending Golgi tendon organ Somatic motor	Ia Ib –	13–20	70–120
A β	Muscle spindle, flower-spray ending Touch, pressure	II II	6–12	30–70
A γ	Motor to muscle spindles	–	3–6	15–30
A δ	Pricking pain, cold, touch	III	2–5	12–30
B	Preganglionic autonomic	–	1–5	3–15
C	Burning pain, temperature, itch, tickle Postganglionic autonomic	IV –	0.2–1.5	0.5–2

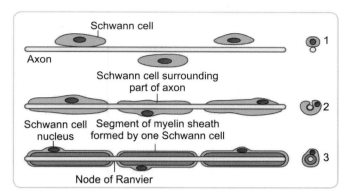

Figure 1.7: Each Schwann cell forms a short segment of the myelin sheath. The figures to the right are transverse sections through the nerve fibre, at the corresponding stages

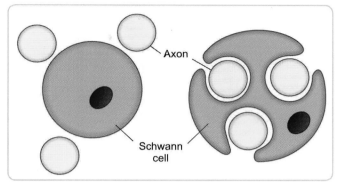

Figure 1.8: Relationship of unmyelinated axons to a Schwann cell

---

Clinical Anatomy

Myelination can be seriously impaired, and there can be abnormal collections of lipids, in disorders of lipid metabolism. Various proteins have been identified in myelin sheaths and abnormality in them can be the basis of some neuropathies.

In multiple sclerosis, myelin formed by oligodendrocytes undergoes degeneration, but that derived from Schwann cells is spared.

Functions of the Myelin Sheath

- The presence of a myelin sheath increases the velocity of conduction (for a nerve fibre of the same diameter).
- It reduces the energy expended in the process of conduction.
- It is responsible for the colour of the white matter of the brain and spinal cord.

Nonmyelinated Fibres

There are some axons, which are devoid of myelin sheaths and examples include postganglionic autonomic fibres and fibres carrying "slow", burning pain. The nonmyelinated fibres are also surrounded by Schwann cells. These **unmyelinated axons** invaginate into the cytoplasm of Schwann cells, but the mesaxon does not spiral around them (Figure 1.8). Another difference is that several such axons may invaginate into the cytoplasm of a single Schwann cell.

Types of Reflexes

A reflex action is defined as an immediate, involuntary motor response of the muscles in response to a specific sensory stimulus. For example, if the skin of the sole of a sleeping person is scratched, the leg is reflexly drawn up.

Monosynaptic: The stimulus applied to a muscle or a tendon is carried by a unipolar neuron which terminates by synapsing with an anterior horn cell supplying the muscle (Figure 1.9). Here, there are only two neurons—one afferent and the other efferent. As only one synapse is involved, the reflex is monosynaptic.

Polysynaptic: Some reflexes are made up of three (or more) neurons as shown in Figure 1.10. The central process of the dorsal nerve root ganglion cell ends by synapsing with a neuron lying in the posterior grey column. This neuron has a short axon that ends by synapsing with an anterior horn cell. Such a reflex is said to be polysynaptic.

Clinical Anatomy

Nerve Injuries
- **Neurapraxia** is a disorder due to pressure on a nerve. There is a temporary loss of function due to damage to the myelin sheath but the axon is intact.
- **Axonotmesis** is an injury usually due to stretch of a nerve. The axons and their myelin sheath are damaged, but Schwann cells and the connective tissue are intact. It leads to Wallerian degeneration but the nerve recovers completely due to intact neurilemma.
- **Neurotmesis** is an injury due to division of a nerve. In this type of injury, both the nerve fibres and the nerve sheath are disrupted. Sometimes surgical approximation of the two cut ends of the nerve is required. Even then, only partial recovery is possible. If the gap between the two cut ends in neurotmesis is more, the growing axonal buds get mixed up with connective tissue to form a mass called a **neuroma.** Sometimes, during regeneration of a mixed nerve, axons may establish contact with the wrong end organs. For example, fibres that should reach a gland may reach the skin. When this happens in the auriculotemporal nerve, it gives rise to Frey's syndrome. Instead of salivation there is increased perspiration, increased blood flow, and pain over skin.

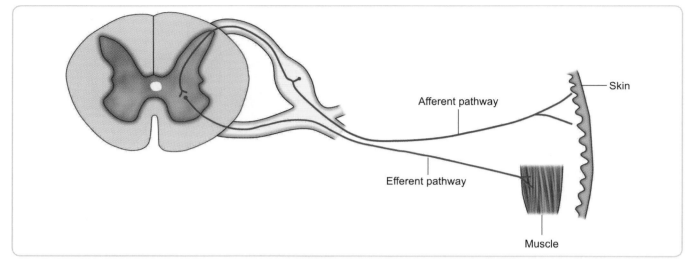

Figure 1.9: A monosynaptic spinal reflex arc composed of two neurons

NEUROGLIA

In addition to neurons, the nervous system contains several types of supporting cells called neuroglia (Flowchart 1.2).

Types of Neuroglia (Flowchart 1.2; Figures 1.11 and 1.12)

- **Astrocytes** act as insulators, nourish the neurons, help form blood-brain barrier.
- **Oligodendrocytes** form myelin sheath in CNS.
- **Microglia** act as phagocytes in CNS.
- **Ependymal cells** line the ventricular system and forms blood CSF barrier.
- **Schwann cells** form myelin sheath in PNS.
- **Capsular cells** (also called satellite cells or capsular gliocytes) support and nourish ganglia.

NEUROBIOTAXIS

(Origin: Greek. Neuro = nerve + bio = life + taxis = arrangement; literally, a law governing the arrangement of neuronal cell bodies and their fibres during life).
- Neuronal cell body **migrates towards the greatest density of stimuli**, e.g. facial nerve nuclei migrate towards trigeminal nucleus to complete the reflex arc.
- Neuronal cell body has a tendency for **centralization and encephalization**, e.g. an evolutionary process by which functions that were governed by lower centres (in lower animals) are progressively being controlled by the higher centres.

- Neuronal processes with **similar function run together,** e.g. in the brainstem descending fibres run in basilar part; ascending fibres in tegmentum.

NEURAL STEM CELLS

Nervous tissue within the central nervous system, till recently, used to be considered as post-mitotic, i.e. neurons are incapable of regeneration. However, recent research has identified cells which are capable of forming new neurons as well as glial cells in the subventricular zone of lateral ventricle and in the hippocampal gyrus. These areas are known as adult neurogenic zone. These cells which are called neural stem cells are capable of self-renewal and show plasticity.

SYNAPSES

A synapse transmits an impulse only in one direction. The two elements taking part in a synapse can, therefore, be spoken of as **presynaptic** and **postsynaptic** (Figure 1.13). In some areas several neurons may take part in forming complex synapses encapsulated by neuroglial cells to form **synaptic glomeruli** (Figure 1.14).

Classification of Synapses

- **Morphological classification:** Figures 1.15A to C show three common types of synapses—(1) axodendritic (2) axosomatic and (3) axoaxonal
- **Functional classification:** From a physiological viewpoint, a synapse may be **excitatory or inhibitory.**

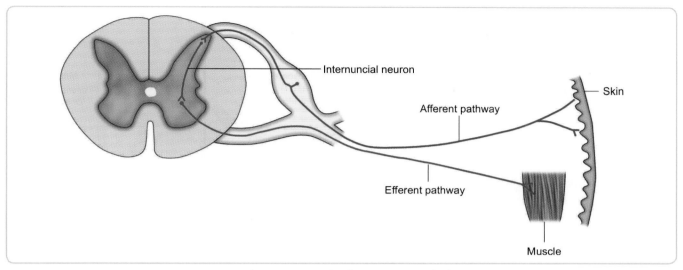

Figure 1.10: A polysynaptic spinal reflex arc composed of three neurons

Flowchart 1.2: Types of neuroglia found in central and peripheral nervous systems

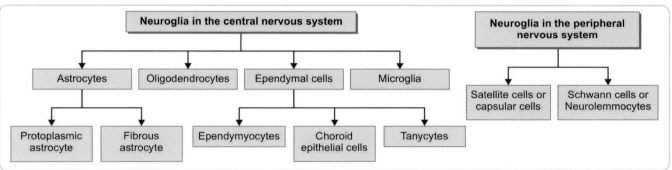

Note: • Astrocytes and oligodendrocytes are together called as macroglia.
 • Macroglia cells are derived from ectoderm of neural tube. Microglia cells are of mesodermal origin.
 • Schwann cells and satellite cells are derived from neural crest.

NEUROTRANSMITTERS

The transmission of impulses through synapses involves the release of chemical substances called **neurotransmitters** into the synaptic cleft. Depending on the neurotransmitter (excitatory of inhibitory), the postsynaptic neuron becomes depolarized or hyperpolarized.

When an action potential reaches the presynaptic terminal, there is an **influx of calcium** ions leading to changes in the synaptic vesicles which pour the neurotransmitter stored in them into the synaptic cleft.

The neurotransmitter released into the synaptic cleft acts only for a **very short duration**. It is either destroyed (by enzymes) or is withdrawn into the terminal bouton.

Important neurotransmitters are acetylcholine, noradrenaline, adrenaline, dopamine, histamine, serotonin, gamma amino butyric acid, glutamate, glycine, and aspartate.

Some chemical substances do not influence synaptic transmission directly, but influence the effects of neurotransmitters. Such chemical substances are referred to as **neuromodulators**, e.g. substance P, vasoactive intestinal polypeptide (VIP), and somatostatin.

NEUROMUSCULAR JUNCTIONS

Each skeletal muscle fibre receives its own direct innervation. The site where the nerve ending comes into intimate contact with the muscle fibre is a neuromuscular junction. In this junction, axon terminals are lodged in grooves in the sarcolemma covering the sole plate (Figure 1.16). Acetylcholine is released when nerve

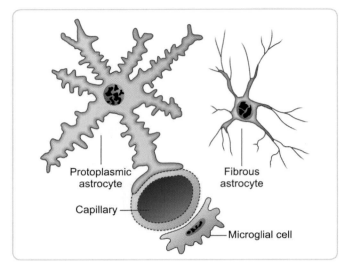

Figure 1.11: Astrocytes form the perivascular feet around a capillary

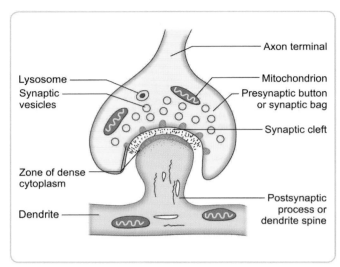

Figure 1.13: Structure of a typical synapse as seen under electron microscope

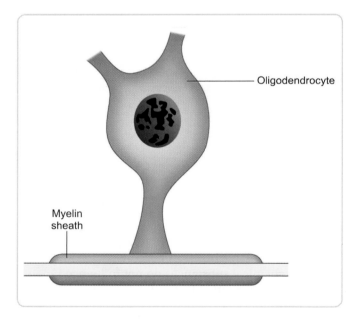

Figure 1.12: Oligodendrocyte and its relationship to a neuron

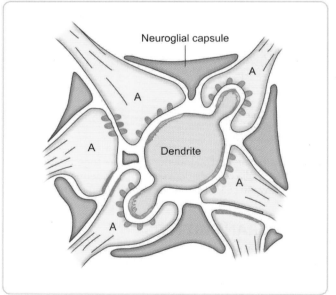

Figure 1.14: Synaptic glomerulus

impulses reach the neuromuscular junction. It initiates a wave of depolarization in the sarcolemma resulting in contraction of the entire muscle fibre.

Some Facts about Muscle Action

- **All or none law:** When a stimulus above the threshold strength is applied, the muscle (and the motor unit, innervated by a single axon) contracts to its full extent.

- **Fatigue:** Depletion of neurotransmitter causes failure of muscle to contract.
- **Muscle tone:** Some fibres, in a resting muscle, are always in a state of contraction.
- **Endurance:** The capacity of a muscle to maintain activity over a period of time.
- **Trophic effect:** Nerve supply maintains the integrity of the muscle.

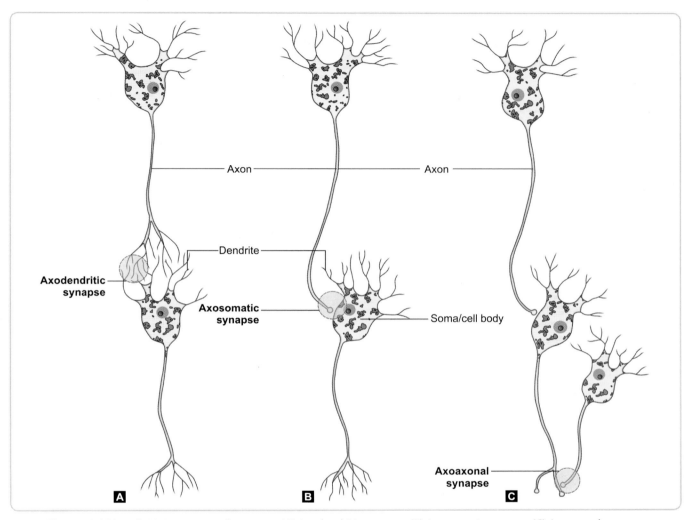

Figures 1.15A to C: Various types of synapses: (A) Axodendritic synapse; (B) Axosomatic synapse; (C) Axoaxonal synapse

Clinical Anatomy

- **Myasthenia gravis**: This is a disease marked by great weakness of skeletal muscle. The body produces antibodies against acetylcholine receptors. As a result many of these are destroyed. Transmission at the myoneural junction is much reduced resulting in weakness of muscles. Some improvement is obtained by administration of anticholine-esterase drugs like neostigmine.
- **Neuromuscular block during administration of general anaesthesia**: Whenever a patient is administered general anaesthesia for surgery, to relax the skeletal muscle, a neuromuscular blocking agent is given. Therefore, the patient cannot breathe on his/her own.

At the end of surgery, the neuromuscular blockade has to be reversed by administering an antidotal drug and the patient resumes breathing on his/her own.

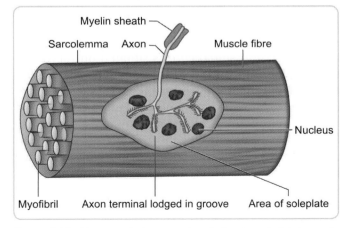

Figure 1.16: Motor end plate seen in relation to a skeletal muscle fibre (surface view)

SENSORY RECEPTORS

The peripheral endings of afferent nerve fibres make contact with receptors that respond to various kinds of sensory stimuli.

Classification of Sensory Receptors

- **Functional classification:** Exteroceptors, proprioceptors and interoceptors
- **Mode of stimulation:** Mechanoreceptors, chemoreceptors, photoreceptors, thermoreceptors, osmoreceptors
- **Structural classification**: Neuronal receptors (most exteroceptors), epithelial receptors (rods and cones), neuroepithelial receptors (olfactory mucosa)

Exteroceptive Receptors (Figure 1.17)

- **Free nerve endings:** Pain
- **Tactile corpuscles of Meissner:** Touch
- **Lamellated corpuscles of Pacini:** Pressure
- **Bulbous corpuscles of Krause:** Cold
- **Merkel cell receptors:** Touch
- **Ruffini endings:** Warmth

Proprioceptive Receptors

- **Golgi tendon organs** (Figure 1.18)
- **Muscle spindles** (Figure 1.19)
  - Annulospiral endings (nuclear bag, nuclear chain)
  - Flower spray endings

FORMATION OF NEURAL TUBE

At the time when the nervous system begins to develop, the embryo is in the form of a three-layered disc, i.e. the gastrula (Figures 1.20 and 1.21).

The part of the ectoderm that is destined to give origin to the brain and spinal cord is situated on the dorsal aspect of the embryonic disc, in the midline and overlies the developing notochord (Figure 1.22A). It soon becomes thickened to form the **neural plate** (Figure 1.22B).

The neural plate becomes depressed along the midline, as a result of which the **neural groove** is formed (Figure 1.22C). This groove becomes progressively deeper. By the end of 3rd week, the two raised edges of the neural plate, which are called **neural folds**, come near each other and eventually fuse, thus converting the neural groove into the **neural tube** (Figure 1.22D). The neural tube is formed from the ectoderm overlying the notochord and, therefore, extends from the prochordal plate to the primitive knot

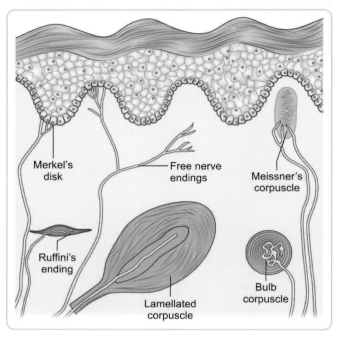

Figure 1.17: Sensory receptors present in relation to skin

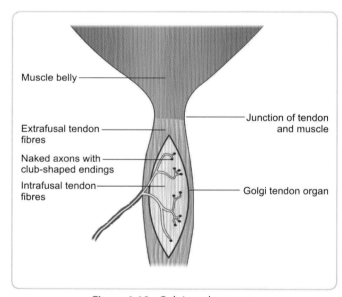

Figure 1.18: Golgi tendon organ

(Figures 1.20 and 1.21). The process of formation of the neural tube is referred to as **neurulation**.

The middle part is the first to become tubular, so that for some time, the neural tube is open cranially and caudally. These openings are called the **anterior** and **posterior neuropores**, respectively. The fusion of the two edges of the neural plate extends cranially (25th day from fertilization) and caudally (27th day from fertilization),

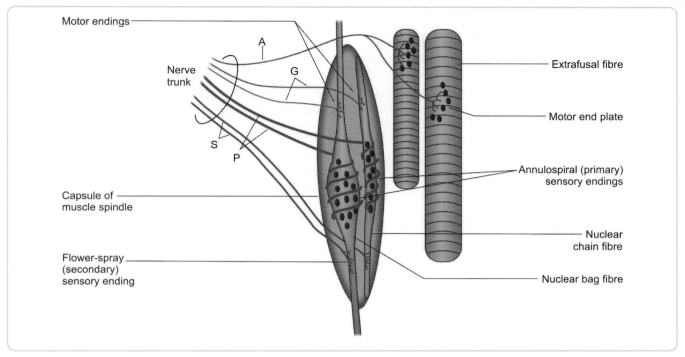

Figure 1.19: Structure of a muscle spindle (A = axon of alpha-neuron supplying extrafusal fibre; G = axons of gamma neurons supplying intrafusal fibres; P and S = afferents from primary and secondary sensory endings, respectively)

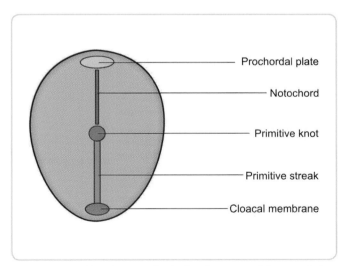

Figure 1.20: Early embryonic disc before formation of the neural plate

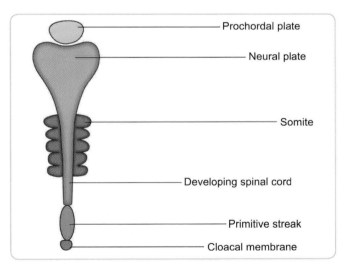

Figure 1.21: Embryonic disc showing the neural plate

and eventually, the neuropores disappear leaving a closed tube.

Even before the neural tube has completely closed, it is divisible into an enlarged cranial part and a caudal tubular part (Figure 1.21). The enlarged cranial part forms the **brain**. The caudal tubular part forms the **spinal cord**. It is at first short but gradually gains in length as the embryo grows.

DEVELOPMENT OF BRAIN

The brain develops from the enlarged cranial part of the neural tube (Figure 1.23A). At about the end of 4th week, the cavity of the developing brain shows three dilatations (Figure 1.23B). Craniocaudally, these are the **prosencephalon (forebrain vesicle)**, **mesencephalon** (**midbrain vesicle**), and **rhombencephalon (hindbrain vesicle)**. The prosencephalon becomes subdivided into the **telencephalon** and the **diencephalon** (Figure 1.23C). The telencephalon consists of right and left **telencephalic vesicles.** The rhombencephalon also becomes subdivided into a cranial part, the **metencephalon**, and a caudal part, the **myelencephalon**. The parts of the brain that are developed from each of these divisions of the neural tube are shown in Figure 1.23D and Flowchart 1.3.

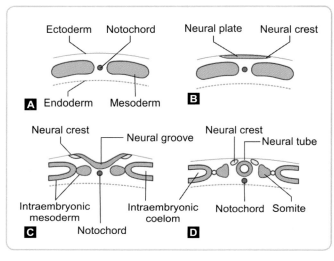

Figure 1.22: Neurulation

Congenital Anomalies of the Brain and the Spinal Cord

Faulty formation of neural tube
The whole length of the neural tube remains unclosed. This results in the condition called **posterior rachischisis**.

Anencephaly
The neural tube remains open in the region of the brain because of nonclosure of the anterior neuropore. This results in **anencephaly**. Brain tissue, which is exposed, degenerates.

Spina bifida: Nonfusion of the neural tube can be associated with nonclosure of the cranium (**cranium bifidum**) or of the vertebral canal (**spina bifida**). As a result of nonfusion of the neural tube or of overlying bones (e.g. spina bifida), neural tissue may lie outside the cranial cavity or vertebral canal. When this happens in the region of the brain the condition is called **encephalocoele or meningoencephalocoele**, and when it occurs in the spinal region it is called myelocoele or **meningomyelocoele** (Figures 1.24A to E).

FLEXURES OF BRAIN

The prosencephalon, mesencephalon, and rhombencephalon are at first arranged craniocaudally (Figure 1.25A). Their relative position is greatly altered by the appearance of a number of flexures. These are:

- The **cervical flexure**, at the junction of the rhombencephalon and the spinal cord (Figure 1.25B)
- The **mesencephalic flexure** (or **cephalic flexure**) in the region of the midbrain (Figure 1.25C)

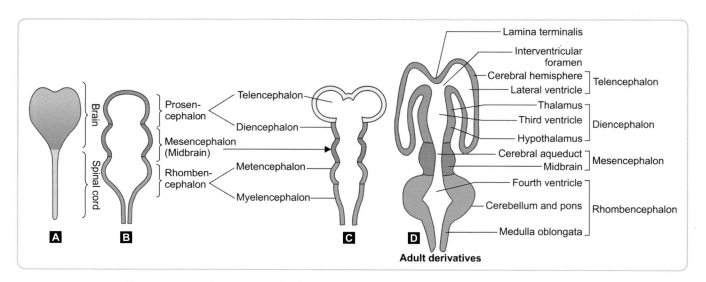

Figures 1.23A to D: Stages in the development of brain vesicles and the ventricular system

Flowchart 1.3: Development of various parts of brain

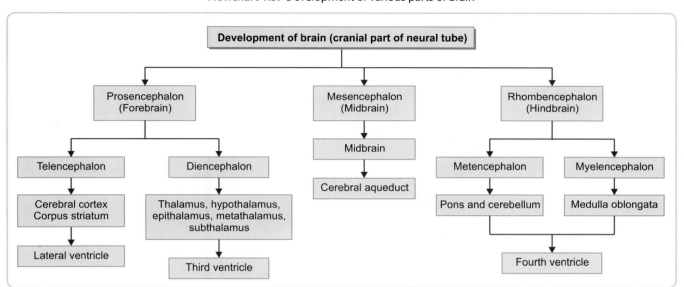

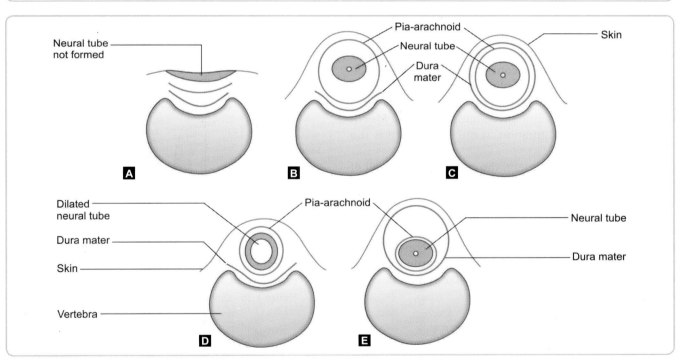

Figures 1.24A to E: Anomalies of the neural tube; (A) Posterior rachischisis; (B to D) Varieties of meningomyelocoele; (E) Meningocoele

- The **pontine flexure**, at the middle of the rhombencephalon, dividing it into the metencephalon and myelencephalon (Figure 1.25D)
- The **telencephalic flexure** that occurs much later between the telencephalon and diencephalon
These flexures lead to the orientation of the various parts of the brain as in the adult.

DEVELOPMENT OF VENTRICULAR SYSTEM

Each of the subdivisions of the developing brain encloses a part of the original cavity of the neural tube (Figure 1.26).
- The cavity of each telencephalic vesicle becomes the **lateral ventricle.**

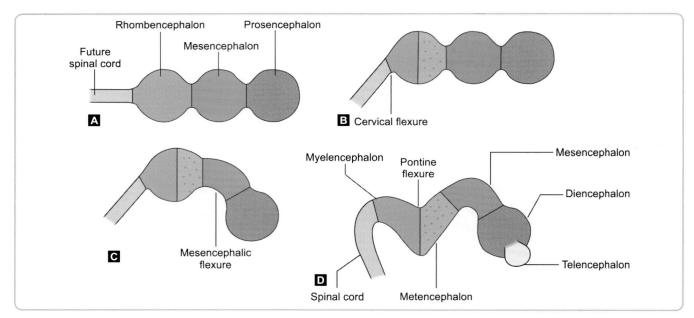

Figures 1.25A to D: (A) Neural tube before formation of flexures; (B) Cervical flexure; (C) Mesencephalic flexure; (D) Pontine flexure

- The cavity of diencephalon (along with the central part of the telencephalon) becomes the **third ventricle**.
- The cavity of the mesencephalon remains narrow, and forms the **cerebral aqueduct** (aqueduct of Sylvius).
- The cavity of the rhombencephalon forms the **fourth ventricle**. Its continuation in the spinal cord is the **central canal.**

With further development, the cells lining the wall of the neural tube proliferate to form thickenings. Ventrally, the thickenings are called basal laminae, and dorsally, they form alar laminae. The line separating the thickened ventral part from the dorsal part is called the **sulcus limitans** (Figure 1.27). This division is of considerable functional importance. The cells of basal lamina develop into motor neurons and the cells of alar lamina develop into sensory neurons and interneurons.

FORMATION OF NEURAL CREST

At the time when the neural plate is being formed, some cells at the junction between the neural plate and the rest of the ectoderm become specialized (on either side) to form the primordia of the **neural crest** (Figures 1.22B and C). With the separation of the neural tube from the surface ectoderm, the cells of the neural crest appear as groups of cells lying along the dorsolateral sides of the neural tube (Figure 1.22D). The neural crest cells soon become free (by losing the property of cell-to-cell adhesiveness). They migrate to distant places throughout the body. In

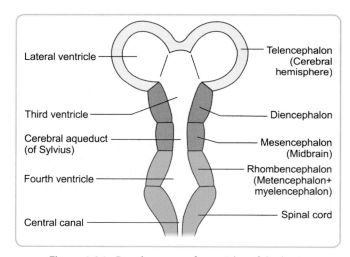

Figure 1.26: Development of ventricles of the brain

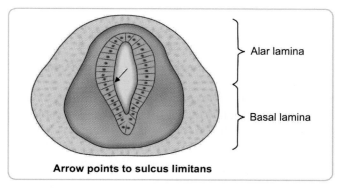

Arrow points to sulcus limitans

Figure 1.27: Sulcus limitans

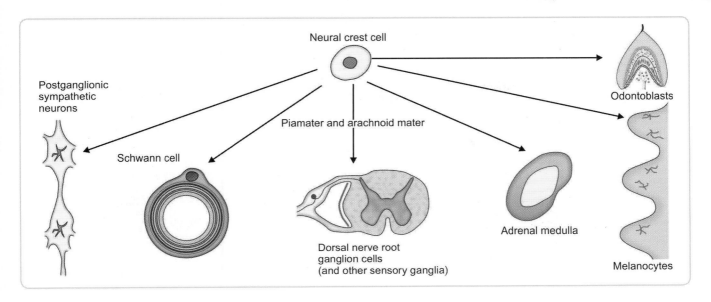

Figure 1.28: Derivatives of neural crest cells

subsequent development, several important structures are derived from the neural crest. These include some neurons of sensory and autonomic ganglia, Schwann cells, and the pia mater and the arachnoid mater. Many other derivatives of the neural crest are recognized in widespread tissues (Figure 1.28).

Clinical Anatomy

Several diseases and syndromes are associated with the disturbances of the neural crest, i.e. Hirschsprung's disease (aganglionic megacolon), aorticopulmonary septal defects of heart, cleft lip, cleft palate, frontonasal dysplasia, neurofibromatosis, tumour of adrenal medulla, and albinism, etc.

PRINCIPLES OF NEUROIMAGING TECHNIQUES

Diagnosing a neurological disease involves a thorough history-taking and physical examination aided by an array of basic to sophisticated investigations so as to anatomically localize the lesion and also to know its pathology. The investigative techniques used in the diagnosis of neurological disorders vary from plain radiography of skull and vertebral column to complex MR tractography. The neuroimaging modalities are classified based on the technique used as given Flowchart 1.4.

Plain Skiagraphy/Radiography

The basic principle in plain radiography is that the X-rays incident on bone, soft tissue or fluid/air get absorbed to a different extent and the emergent beam after such absorption reacts differently with the chemical on the X-ray plate. So, bone produces a dense white shadow, air produces a black shadow and the soft tissue produces varying shades of grey.

Myelography

In this investigation, a radio-opaque dye is injected into the spinal subarachnoid space after lumbar puncture.

Angiography

A radio-opaque dye is injected into the blood vessels supplying the brain, namely the internal carotid artery and the vertebral artery. This is followed by taking serial radiographs of skull to show the arterial, the capillary and the venous phases of flow of the dye which helps to visualize the normal anatomy of the arterial system (Figures 1.29 and 1.30).

Computed Tomography Scan (CT Scan)

This technique uses a collimated beam of X-rays which is passed circumferentially around a transverse slice of

Flowchart 1.4: Neuroimaging modalities based on techniques used

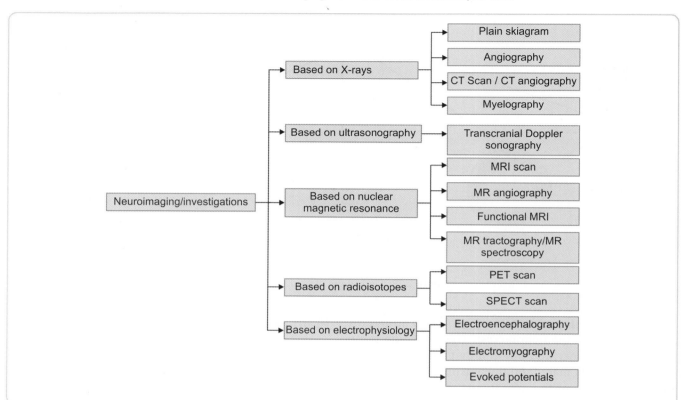

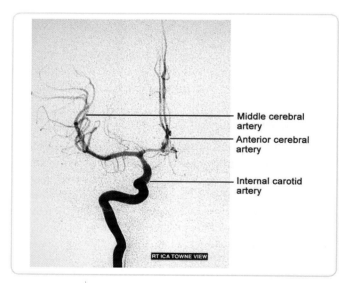

Figure 1.29: Internal carotid angiogram-Digital Subtraction Angiogram (DSA) (*Courtesy:* Dr HD Deshmukh, Professor & Head, Department of Radiology, Seth GS Medical College & KEM Hospital, Mumbai.)

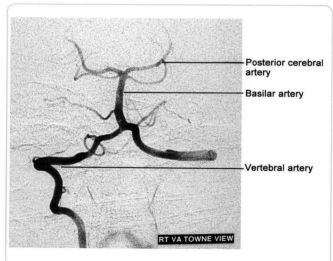

Figure 1.30: Vertebral angiogram. (*Courtesy:* Dr HD Deshmukh, Professor & Head, Department of Radiology, Seth GS Medical College & KEM Hospital, Mumbai.)

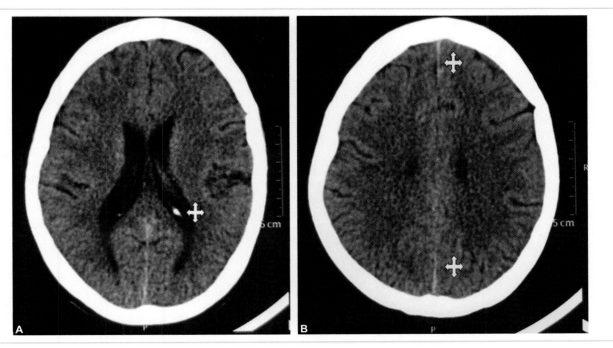

Figures 1.31A and B: (A) CT scan image showing CSF as black shadow within lateral ventricle–quad arrow shows a white spec within the ventricle–choroid plexus in the collateral trigone; (B) CT scan image showing falx cerebri as a thin white line in the midline-quad arrow–Sulci and gyri can be appreciated in the periphery. (*Courtesy:* Dr HD Deshmukh, Professor & Head, Department of Radiology, Seth GS Medical College & KEM Hospital, Mumbai.)

head and multiple detectors around the slice capture the emerging X-rays to produce multiple images. These are then put together with the help of a computer to get an axial tomogram (Figures 1.31A and B).

Magnetic Resonance Imaging (MRI)

This investigation uses the principle of nuclear magnetic resonance which states that the atoms of a tissue/substance oscillate and release energy when subjected to a strong magnetic field. This energy is captured in the form of an image (T1 weighted image). Later when the oscillating atoms are subjected to radiofrequency waves, the direction of oscillation changes and releases energy in another direction and a diametrically opposite image is produced (T2 weighted image).

Transcranial Doppler Ultrasonography

This is based on Doppler effect in which the frequency of the ultrasound waves gets changed when they strike a moving object such as the blood flowing in a vessel.

Positron Emission Tomographic Scan (PET Scan)

Positron emitting radioisotopes such as ^{15}O and ^{18}F are used in this study. When brain tissue is scanned after administration of these isotope containing substances, high metabolic areas with more blood flow or neurons with higher glucose intake will show up as hot spots. The advantage over CT is PET gives information about function because of neuronal activity or blood flow.

MR Tractography

This imaging technique is based on the principle of diffusion weighted imaging (DWI). Water molecules in live tissues are in constant motion due to the thermal energy carried by them, and this is called as Brownian motion. In white matter of the brain, this motion is along the longitudinal axis of the white fibres because the axolemma limits their perpendicular motion. MR signals catch these motions and different computer algorithms are used to reconstruct the fibre tracts called as diffusion tensor imaging (DTI) or MR tractography (Figure 1.32).

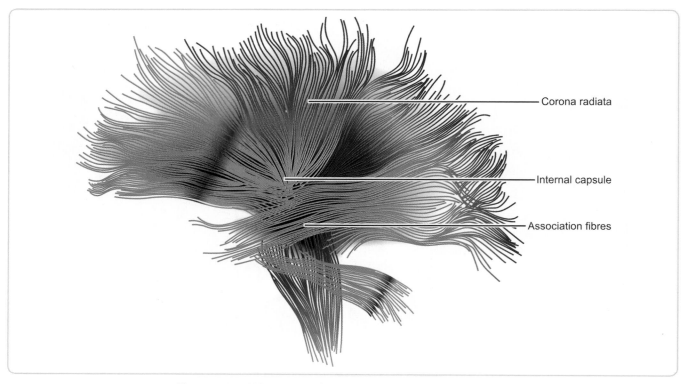

Figures 1.32: MR tractography showing white matter of cerebrum

MULTIPLE CHOICE QUESTIONS

Q1. The "Nissl substance" represents which organelle of neuron?
A. Golgi complex
B. Nucleolus
C. Rough endoplasmic reticulum
D. Mitochondria

Q2. Which of the following provides myelin sheath to the axons of the CNS?
A. Astrocytes
B. Oligodendrocytes
C. Microglia
D. Ependymocytes

Q3. The perivascular foot of the "blood–brain barrier" is an extension from the:
A. Oligodendrocyte
B. Ependymocyte
C. Astrocyte
D. Microglia

Q4. Sensation of pain is detected by:
A. Mechanoreceptor
B. Chemoreceptor
C. Nociceptor
D. Thermoreceptor

Q5. The cerebral aqueduct is developed from the cavity of:
A. Rhombencephalon
B. Mesencephalon
C. Telencephalon
D. Diencephalon

Q6. The failure of closure of the cranial end of neural tube gives rise to:
A. Anencephaly
B. Hydrocephalus
C. Microcephaly
D. Meningomyelocoele

Q7. By which week of intrauterine life does the neural tube close?
- A. Fourth
- B. Fifth
- C. Sixth
- D. Seventh

Q8. The cervical flexure of the neural tube occurs:
- A. Between the forebrain and midbrain
- B. In the midbrain
- C. Between hindbrain and spinal cord
- D. In the hindbrain

ANSWERS

1. C   2. B   3. C   4. C   5. B   6. A   7. A   8. C

SHORT NOTES

1. Describe myelination
2. Classify neurons with examples
3. Differentiate an axon from a dendrite
4. Classify peripheral nerve fibres with examples
5. Classify receptors
6. Specify the different parts of neural tube and enumerate their derivatives
7. Enumerate the derivatives of neural crest cells
8. Define neurobiotaxis with an example

Clinical Cases

1.1: During surgery on parotid salivary gland in a patient, the auriculotemporal nerve got damaged. When recovery occurred, the secretomotor fibres of auriculotemporal nerve got exchanged with the sympathetic fibres supplying the sweat glands of the skin over the parotid gland.
- A. What is the type of nerve injury to auriculotemporal nerve in this patient?
- B. In what type of nerve injury will the auriculotemporal nerve recover completely?

Chapter 2 Spinal Cord—External Features

Specific Learning Objectives

At the end of learning, the student shall be able to:
➤ Describe the external features of the spinal cord
➤ Define a spinal segment and correlate the spinal segmental level with the vertebral level
➤ Specify the segmental innervations of skin and spinal segments responsible for important movements
➤ Describe spinal reflexes and specify spinal segments responsible for important reflexes
➤ Describe the meninges covering the spinal cord and their specializations
➤ Specify the anatomical basis of lumbar puncture and epidural anaesthesia
➤ Specify the blood supply of various parts of spinal cord

INTRODUCTION

The spinal cord or the spinal medulla (medulla spinalis L.) is the most important content of the vertebral canal. In adults, it occupies only the upper two-thirds of the vertebral canal.

It begins as a downward extension of medulla oblongata at the level of the upper border of the first cervical vertebra (C1) and extends down to the level of the lower border of the first lumbar vertebra (L1) (Figure 2.1). The level varies with flexion or extension of the spine.

The lowest part of the spinal cord is conical and is called the **conus medullaris**. The conus is continuous, below, with a fibrous cord called the **filum terminale**, which is a prolongation of pia mater and is attached to the posterior surface of the first piece of coccyx.

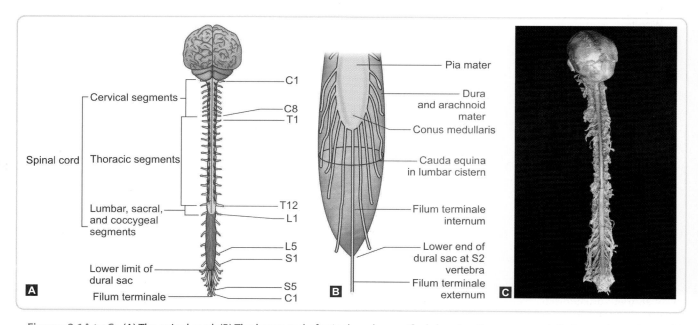

Figures 2.1A to C: (A) The spinal cord; (B) The lower end of spinal cord magnified showing the conus medullaris, cauda equina and filum terminale; (C) Specimen of brain and spinal cord—posterior view

DIMENSIONS OF THE CORD

The length of the cord is about 45 cm. The spinal cord is not of uniform thickness. It resembles a flattened cylinder. The transverse diameter shows two enlargements at the cervical level and lumbar level. The spinal segments that contribute to the nerves of the upper limbs (from third cervical to second thoracic segments) are enlarged to form the **cervical enlargement** of the cord. Similarly, the segments innervating the lower limbs (first lumbar to third sacral segments) form the **lumbar enlargement** (Figure 2.2).

AGE-WISE CHANGES IN THE CORD

In early fetal life (3rd month), the spinal cord is as long as the vertebral canal and each spinal nerve arises from the cord at the level of the corresponding intervertebral foramen. In subsequent development, the spinal cord does not grow as much as the vertebral column, and its lower end, therefore, gradually ascends to reach the level of the third lumbar vertebra at the time of birth and to the lower border of the first lumbar vertebra in the adult (Figure 2.3).

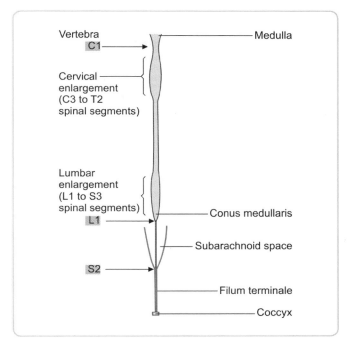

Figure 2.2: Important vertebral levels in relation to the spinal cord

---

> ### Clinical Anatomy
>
> **Lumbar puncture**
> Lumbar puncture is performed to obtain samples of cerebrospinal fluid (CSF) for various diagnostic and therapeutic purposes. In this procedure, a needle is introduced into the subarachnoid space through the interval between the third and fourth lumbar vertebrae (Figure 2.4A).
>
> With the patient lying on his or her side, with the vertebral column well-flexed, the space between adjoining laminae in the lumbar region is increased to a maximum. Taking full aseptic precautions, the lumbar puncture needle is inserted into the vertebral canal above or below the third lumbar spine. An imaginary line joining the highest points on the iliac crests passes over the fourth lumbar spine and this is taken as a landmark to insert the spinal needle.
> Structures through which the needle passes during a lumbar puncture are (Figure 2.4B):
> * Skin
> * Superficial fascia
> * Supraspinous ligament
> * Interspinous ligament
> * Ligamentum flavum
> * Areolar tissue containing the internal vertebral venous plexus
> * Dura mater
> * Arachnoid mater
>
> **Purpose of lumbar puncture**
> * The pressure of CSF can be estimated roughly by counting the rate at which drops of CSF flow out of the needle or more accurately, by connecting the needle to a manometer.
> * Samples of CSF can be collected for examination. The important points to note about CSF are its colour, its cellular content and its chemical composition (specially the protein and sugar content).
> * Lumbar puncture may be used for introducing air or radiopaque dyes into the subarachnoid space for certain investigative procedures, e.g. myelography. Drugs may also be injected for treatment.
> * Anaesthetic drugs injected into the subarachnoid space act on the lower spinal nerve roots and render the lower part of the body insensitive to pain. This procedure, called spinal anaesthesia, is frequently used for operations on the lower abdomen or on the lower extremities.

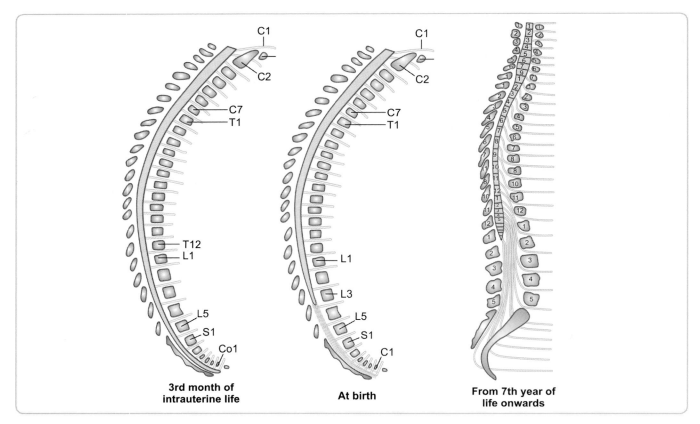

3rd month of
intrauterine life

At birth

From 7th year of
life onwards

Figure 2.3: Scheme to show the effect of recession of the spinal cord (during development) on the course of the roots of spinal nerves

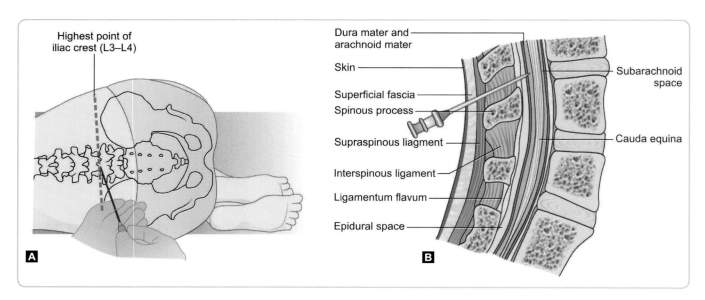

Highest point of
iliac crest (L3–L4)

A

Dura mater and
arachnoid mater

Skin

Superficial fascia

Spinous process

Supraspinous liagment

Interspinous ligament

Ligamentum flavum

Epidural space

Subarachnoid
space

Cauda equina

B

Figures 2.4A and B: (A) The site of lumbar puncture; (B) Anatomical layers pierced to reach the subarachnoid space

As a result of this upward migration of the cord, the roots of spinal nerves have to follow an oblique downward course to reach the appropriate intervertebral foramen (Figure 2.3). This also makes the spinal nerve roots longer. The obliquity and length of the roots are most marked in the lower nerves and many of these roots occupy the vertebral canal below the level of the spinal cord. These roots constitute the **cauda equina** (Figures 2.1 and 2.3).

FUNCTIONS OF SPINAL CORD

The spinal cord has three major functions:
1. It acts as a pathway for motor information, which travels down the spinal cord.
2. It serves as a passage for sensory information in the reverse direction.
3. It is a centre for coordinating simple reflexes.

EXTERNAL FEATURES OF SPINAL CORD

The anterior surface of the spinal cord is marked by a deep **anterior median fissure**, which contains anterior spinal artery (Figure 2.5A). The posterior surface is marked by a shallow **posterior median sulcus** (Figure 2.5B). The anterior median fissure and posterior median sulcus divide the surface of the cord into two symmetrical halves.

Each half of the cord is further subdivided into posterior, lateral and anterior regions by **anterolateral and posterolateral sulci** (Figures 2.5A and B). The **rootlets of the dorsal or sensory roots** of spinal nerves enter the cord at the posterolateral sulcus on either side. The **rootlets of the ventral or motor roots** of spinal nerves emerge through the anterolateral sulcus on either side.

SPINAL NERVES

The spinal cord gives attachment on either side to 31 pairs of spinal nerves: 8 cervical, 12 thoracic, 5 lumbar, 5 sacral and 1 coccygeal.

Each spinal nerve arises by two roots: (1) anterior motor root and (2) posterior sensory root (Flowchart 2.1 and Figure 2.6). Just proximal to the junction of the two roots, the dorsal root is marked by a swelling called the **dorsal nerve root ganglion or spinal ganglion** (Figure 2.6).

Both the roots of spinal nerve receive a tubular prolongation from the **spinal meninges** and enter the corresponding **intervertebral foramen**. In the intervertebral foramen, anterior and posterior spinal nerve roots unite to form the **mixed spinal nerve trunk**. Thus, a spinal nerve is made-up of a mixture of motor and sensory fibres.

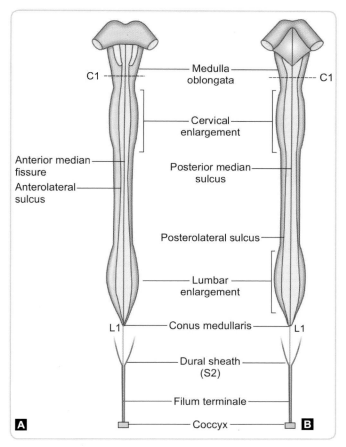

Figures 2.5A and B: External features of the spinal cord: (A) anterior aspect; (B) posterior aspect

Flowchart 2.1: Formation of a spinal nerve

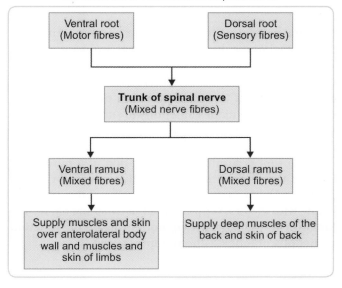

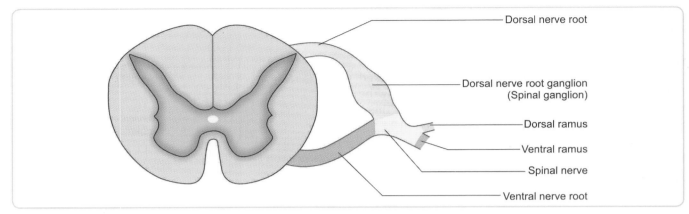

Figure 2.6: Relationship of a spinal nerve to the spinal cord

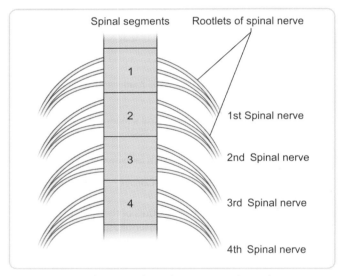

Figure 2.7: Scheme to show the concept of spinal segments

SPINAL SEGMENTS

The part of the spinal cord giving origin to the rootlets for one pair of spinal nerves constitutes one **spinal segment** (Figure 2.7). So, the spinal cord is made-up of 31 such segments—8 cervical, 12 thoracic, 5 lumbar, 5 sacral and 1 coccygeal.

Vertebral Levels of Spinal Segments

Since, the length of spinal cord (45 cm) is smaller than that of vertebral column (65 cm), the spinal segments are thinner and crowded, more so in the lower part of the cord. Thus, the spinal and vertebral segments (vertebral bodies) do not lie at the same level. **The spinal segments as a rule always lie above their numerically corresponding vertebral bodies.** As a rough guide, it may be stated that in the cervical region, there is a difference of one segment (for example, the fifth cervical spine overlies the sixth cervical segment); in the thoracic region, there is a difference of two to three segments (for example, the fourth thoracic spine overlies the sixth thoracic segment; the ninth thoracic spine lies opposite the twelfth thoracic segment). Approximate spinal segments and the corresponding vertebral level are shown in Table 2.1.

After emerging from the intervertebral foramen, each spinal nerve divides into **dorsal and ventral rami** (Flowchart 2.1 and Figure 2.6). The dorsal ramus passes posteriorly around the vertebral column to supply the **deep muscles of the back and skin of the back**. The ventral ramus continues anteriorly to supply the **muscles and skin over the anterolateral body wall and all the muscles and skin of the limbs**.

Each root is formed by aggregation of a number of rootlets that arise from the cord over a certain length (Figure 2.7). The last rootlet of hypoglossal nerves arises in line with the first ventral rootlet of C1 spinal nerve. The **junction between these two rootlets marks the junction of medulla oblongata and the spinal cord**.

Clinical Anatomy

Transection of spinal cord at different vertebral segments
- **Hangman's fracture:** When a person is hanged, the second cervical vertebra is fractured. From Table 2.1, we can see that the spinal segment damaged is C2. This disconnects the respiratory centres of medulla oblongata from C3, C4 and C5 segments of phrenic nerves. This causes respiratory arrest and death.
- **Quadriplegia**: Damage to spinal segment C5 (due to disease **between vertebrae C4 and C5**), results in paralysis of both upper limbs and both lower limbs which is called quadriplegia.
- **Burst fracture of T3 vertebrae**: From Table 2.1, we find that this damages the spinal segment T5.
- **Deep traumatic injury at T6 spinous process**: The palpable tips of spinous processes of middle four thoracic vertebrae (T5 to T8) reach the vertebral body, which is numerically two below, due to their long and down sloping spinous processes. The T6 spinous process lies opposite T8 vertebral body. From Table 2.1, the spinal segment that will be damaged is T11.
- **Spondylolisthesis (slipping of upper vertebral body over the lower one)**: This is more common between L4 and L5. This will not damage any spinal segment as the spinal cord in adults ends at L1, but may compress the cauda equina.

TABLE 2.1: Relation between vertebral levels and spinal segments

Vertebral level	Formula—(to get the number of spinal segment underlying, add the numeral to the number of vertebra)	Example
Upper cervical C1–C4	Add 0 to the number of vertebra to get the underlying spinal segment	Third cervical vertebra overlies the third cervical segment
Lower cervical C5–C7	Add 1 to the number of vertebra to get the underlying spinal segment	Fifth cervical vertebra overlies the sixth cervical segment
Upper thoracic T1–T6	Add 2 to the number of vertebra to get the underlying spinal segment	Fourth thoracic vertebra overlies the sixth thoracic segment
Lower thoracic T7–T9	Add 3 to the number of vertebra to get the underlying spinal segment	Ninth thoracic vertebra overlies the 12th thoracic segment
T10	—	L1–L2 segments
T11	—	L3–L4 segments
T12	—	L5–S1 segments
L1	—	S2–Co segments

Exit of Spinal Nerves

Each spinal nerve emerges through the intervertebral foramen. The cervical nerves leave the vertebral canal above the corresponding vertebrae with the exception of eighth, which emerges between seventh cervical and first thoracic vertebrae. The remaining spinal nerves emerge below the pedicles of the corresponding vertebrae.

As the spinal cord ends at the level of L1 vertebra, the lower spinal nerves below L1 level descend down with the filum terminale as a leash, which resembles a horse's tail and hence called as cauda equina.

Clinical Anatomy

- **Cervical spondylosis:** Osteophytes growing from the facet joints between C4 and C5 compress C5 spinal nerve resulting in paralysis of deltoid (see myotomes below).
- **Prolapsed intervertebral disc between L5 and S1**: Spares the spinal nerve L5, since it is deeply snug in the groove below the pedicle of L5, significantly above the disc below the body of L5.

SEGMENTAL INNERVATION

Any condition that leads to pressure on the spinal cord, or on spinal nerve roots, can give rise to symptoms in the region supplied by nerves. In such cases, it is important to be able to localize the particular spinal segments or roots involved. For this purpose, it is necessary to know which areas of skin and which muscles are innervated by each segment. Spinal segments responsible for muscle stretch reflexes also give an indication about the level of spinal cord involvement.

Dermatomes

Areas of skin supplied by individual spinal nerves are called **dermatomes**. To understand the arrangement of dermatomes, it is necessary to know some facts about the development of the limbs.

The upper and lower limbs are derived from limb buds. These are paddle-shaped outgrowths that arise from the side-wall of the embryo. They are at first directed forward and laterally from the body of the embryo

(Figure 2.8). Each bud has a **preaxial (or cranial) border** and a **postaxial border** (Figure 2.9). The thumb and great toe are formed on the preaxial border.

The forelimb bud is derived from the part of the body wall belonging to segments C4, C5, C6, C7, C8, T1 and T2. It is, therefore, innervated by the corresponding spinal nerves. The hindlimb bud is formed opposite the segments L1, L2, L3, L4, L5, S1, S2 and S3. As the limbs grow, skin supplied by these nerves gets "pulled away" into the limbs. This has a great effect on the arrangement of dermatomes (Figures 2.10 and 2.11).

The dermatomes of the body are shown in Figure 2.12. The following **dermatomes** are of clinical significance:

- Spinal nerve **C1** does not supply any area of skin (**C1 has no dermatome**).
- Spinal nerve **C4** supplies the tip of shoulder.
- Spinal nerves **C6, C7, C8** supplies the skin of the hand.
- Spinal nerve **T4** supplies the skin over the nipple.
- Spinal nerve **T10** supplies the skin over the umbilicus.
- Spinal nerves **L5, S1** supplies the skin of the sole.

> ### Clinical Anatomy
>
> **Referred pain**: The pain of an internal organ or structure is projected (referred) to that part of the body wall that is innervated by the same spinal segment (dermatome).
>
> Examples are:
> - **Heart**: T1 to T5 (referred over **precordium and inner border of upper limb**)
> - **Diaphragm**: C3, C4, C5 (referred to tip of **shoulder**)
> - **Appendix**: T10 (referred to **umbilicus**)

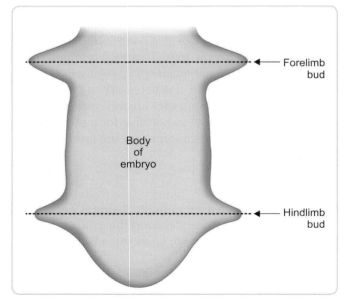

Figure 2.8: Scheme to show that the longitudinal axis of the limb buds is transverse to the long axis of the embryonic body

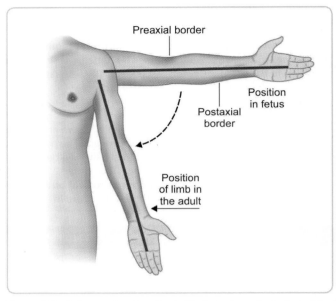

Figure 2.9: Scheme showing that with the external rotation of the embryonic limb, the preaxial border becomes the lateral border

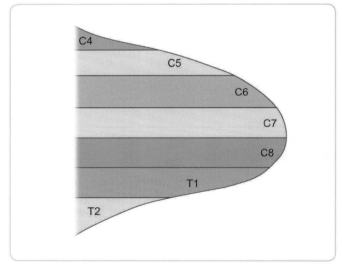

Figure 2.10: Dermatomes of the upper limb in an embryo

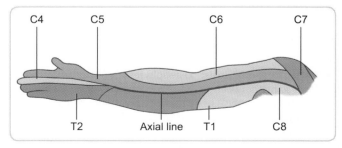

Figure 2.11: Dermatomes of the upper limb in an adult—anterior view

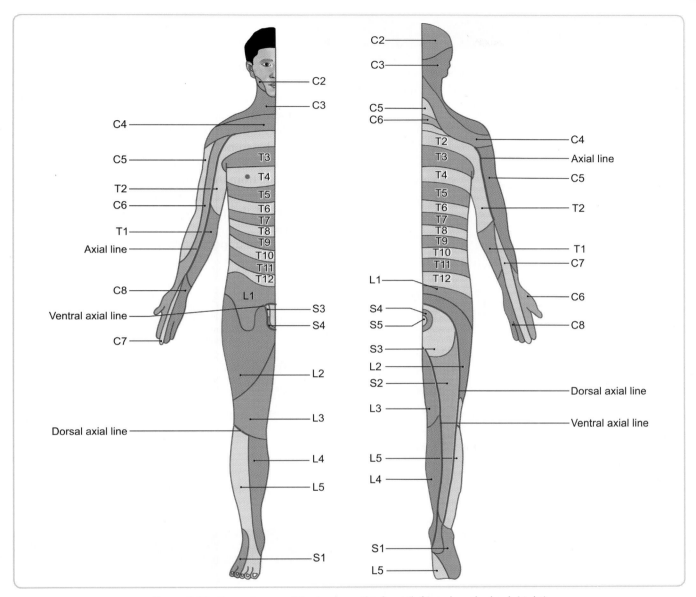

Figure 2.12: Dermatomes of the body on the front (left) and on the back (right)

Myotomes

Group of muscles supplied by a single spinal nerve is called **myotomes**. Some significant features of myotomes are as follows:

- It is rare for a muscle to be supplied only by one segment. Some exceptions are shoulder abductor (deltoid), C5; intrinsic muscles of the hand, T1; invertor of foot, L4.

- The segment supplying muscles acting on a joint, supply the joint itself and also the skin over the joint (Hilton's law).
- Muscles having a common action are usually supplied by the same spinal segments.

The segmental innervation of certain muscles producing the movements is enumerated in Table 2.2.

TABLE 2.2: Segmental innervation of muscles producing various movements

Movements		Spinal segments (segments in brackets signify minor contribution)
Movements of the head		C1 to C4
Movements of the diaphragm		(C3) C4 (C5)
Movements of the upper limb		*C5 to T1*
Abduction of shoulder		C5
Adduction of shoulder		C6, C7, C8
Flexion of elbow		C5, C6
Extension of elbow		C7, C8
Supination of forearm		C6 (C7)
Pronation of forearm		(C6) C7
Flexion of wrist		(C6) C7
Extension of wrist		C6 (C7)
Movements of fingers		C8, T1
Movements of lower limb		*L2 to S3*
Flexion of hip		L2, L3
Extension of hip		L4, L5
Extension of knee		L3, L4
Flexion of knee		L5, S1
Dorsiflexion of ankle		L4, L5
Plantar flexion of ankle		S1, S2
Inversion of foot		L4
Eversion of foot		(L5) S1
Movements of toes		S2, S3
Evacuation of bladder and bowel		S2 to S4

Clinical Anatomy

- Injury of spinal cord above C3 causes paralysis of all respiratory muscles and death due to paralysis of diaphragm.
- Injury of spinal cord at C4–C5 level paralyses all four limbs—**quadriplegia**.
- Injury to spinal nerves C5 and C6 (**Erb's paralysis**) causes loss of abduction of shoulder, loss of flexion of elbow, loss of supination and loss of extension of wrist. Unopposed action of antagonists produces policeman's tip deformity.
- Injury to spinal nerves C8 and T1 (**Klumpke's paralysis**) causes paralysis of intrinsic muscles of the hand causing claw hand.
- Injury of spinal cord between T2 and L1 paralyses both the lower limbs—**paraplegia**.

SPINAL REFLEXES

The integrity of spinal segments can also be tested by examining reflexes mediated by the segment.

Myotatic or Muscle Stretch Reflexes or Deep Reflex

Sudden stretching of a muscle (by tapping its tendon) produces reflex contraction of the muscle. The pathway for this reflex involves two neurons only (monosynaptic). Stretching of the muscle stimulates proprioceptive nerve endings located in muscle spindles. These impulses are carried to the spinal cord by neurons that synapse with motor neurons in the ventral grey columns (Figure 2.13). Fibres arising from these motor neurons reach the muscle and produce contraction. Stretch reflexes are abolished, if any part of the pathway for it (i.e. the reflex arc) is interrupted.

Some of the important deep reflexes are described in Table 2.3.

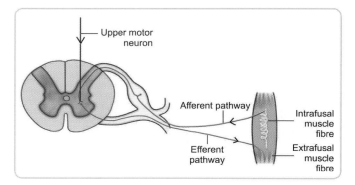

Figure 2.13: A spinal reflex arc showing pathway for muscle stretch reflex or myotatic reflex

TABLE 2.3: Spinal segments responsible for deep or stretch reflex

Reflex	Description	Spinal segments
Knee jerk or patellar tendon reflex	Extension of the leg by contraction of the quadriceps when the ligamentum patellae are tapped	L3, L4
Ankle jerk or Achilles tendon reflex	Plantar flexion of the foot on tapping the tendo calcaneus	S1, S2
Biceps tendon reflex	Flexion of the forearm on tapping the biceps tendon	C5, C6
Triceps tendon reflex	Extension of the forearm on tapping the triceps tendon	C7, C8
Supinator jerk	Flexion of the forearm when the distal end of the radius is tapped (brachioradialis)	C6, C7

Superficial Reflexes

Superficial reflexes are polysynaptic (Figure 2.14). One of the superficial reflexes is the plantar reflex. The normal **plantar reflex** consists of plantar flexion and adduction of the toes on stroking the skin of the sole (L5, S1). When there is an injury to the corticospinal system, an abnormal response is obtained. There is extension (dorsiflexion) of the great toe and fanning out of other toes. This response is referred to as **Babinski sign**. Some of the important superficial reflexes are described in Table 2.4.

> **Clinical Anatomy**
>
> - Stretch reflexes are exaggerated in upper motor neuron (corticospinal tract) lesion.
> - Superficial reflexes are abolished in corticospinal tract lesions.
> - Both reflexes are lost in lower motor neuron lesion.

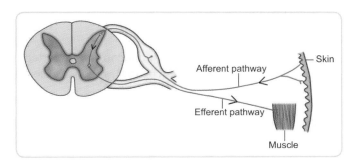

Figure 2.14: A spinal reflex arc showing pathway for superficial reflex

TABLE 2.4: Spinal segments responsible for superficial reflexes

Reflex	Description	Spinal segments
Abdominal reflexes: • Upper • Middle • Lower	Contraction of underlying muscles on stroking the skin of the abdomen in its upper, middle and lower parts	T7, T8 T9, T10 T11, T12
Cremasteric reflex	Elevation of the scrotum on stroking the skin of the medial side of the thigh	L2
Gluteal reflex	Contraction of the glutei on stroking the overlying skin	L4 to S1
Plantar reflex	Plantar flexion and adduction of the toes on stroking the skin of the sole	L5, S1
Anal reflex	Contraction of the external anal sphincter on stroking the perianal region	S4, S5, Co

SPINAL MENINGES (FIGURE 2.15)

Dura Mater

The spinal dura mater forms a loose tubular covering for the spinal cord. The spinal dura mater **does not fuse with the endosteum** of the vertebral canal. Hence, there is a well-developed **epidural space** surrounding the spinal cord. The spinal epidural space is filled with the internal vertebral venous plexus (Batson's plexus) and fat.

> **Clinical Anatomy**
>
> **Epidural anaesthesia**: As the spinal nerves pass through the spinal epidural space, they may be anaesthetized by injecting a local anaesthetic drug into the spinal epidural space. This type of epidural anaesthesia is used in obstetric procedures during childbirth. One has to be careful about the venous plexus while introducing the needle for anaesthesia as it may injure the veins and cause an epidural haematoma.

The dorsal and ventral roots of spinal nerves pass through the spinal dura mater separately. The dura-arachnoid partially enclose the dorsal nerve root ganglion. The dura and arachnoid (along with the subarachnoid space containing CSF) extend up to the level of second sacral vertebra. Beyond that level, the dura covers the filum terminale and distally gets attached to the dorsal surface of the first coccygeal vertebra.

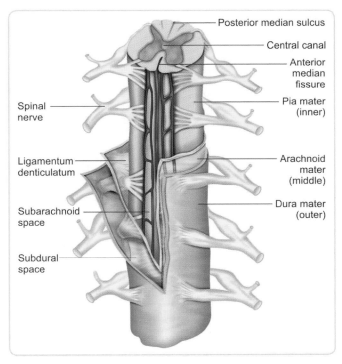

Figure 2.15: Spinal meninges

Arachnoid Mater

The spinal arachnoid mater is present deep to the dura and extends up to the level of second sacral vertebra. The subarachnoid space extends up to this level (**lumbar cistern**). The lumbar cistern is broadest between L2 and L4 level. Lumbar puncture is therefore done at L3-L4 space or L2-L3 space.

Pia Mater

The spinal pia mater is a thin membrane closely applied to the spinal cord and specialized in some areas and continues above with the cranial pia mater. The modifications of pia mater are as follows:

- **Linea splendens**: Along the anteromedian fissure, the pia mater is thickened to form a glistening band called as linea splendens (Figure 2.16). The branches from the anterior spinal artery pierce this to enter the spinal cord.

- **Ligamenta denticulata**: Along the lateral aspect of spinal cord, between the dorsal and the ventral roots, the pia forms triangular thickenings, which pierce the arachnoid and are attached to the dura. These tooth-like thickenings are called as ligamenta denticulata (Figures 2.15 and 2.17). There are 21 pairs of ligamenta denticulata.

- **Filum terminale**: At the lower end of the spinal cord, the pia mater extends as a thin filament called filum terminale surrounded by the leash of nerves, i.e. cauda equina (Figures 2.1 and 2.3). This filum terminale passes through the sacral hiatus and gets attached to the dorsal surface of the first coccygeal vertebra.

BLOOD SUPPLY OF SPINAL CORD

Arterial Supply

The arterial supply of the cord is derived from following arteries (Figure 2.18):
- Anterior spinal artery
- Two posterior spinal arteries
- The radicular arteries

The pia mater covering the spinal cord has an arterial plexus (called the **arterial vasocorona**), which also sends branches into the substance of the cord.

Anterior Spinal Artery

The anterior spinal artery is formed in the posterior cranial fossa by the union of the right and left anterior spinal arteries (which are the branches of the fourth part of the vertebral artery). The anterior spinal artery descends through the foramen magnum and runs down in the anterior median fissure of the spinal cord.

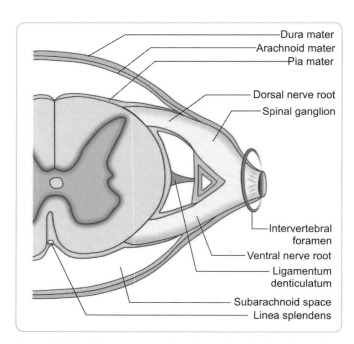

Figure 2.16: Transverse section through spinal cord to show the formation of meningeal sheaths over the roots of a spinal nerve

Labels: Dura mater, Arachnoid mater, Pia mater, Dorsal nerve root, Spinal ganglion, Intervertebral foramen, Ventral nerve root, Ligamentum denticulatum, Subarachnoid space, Linea splendens

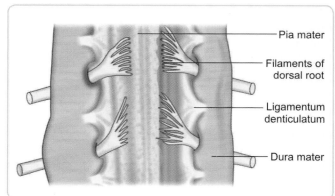

Figure 2.17: Spinal pia mater seen from posterior aspect. Note the extension of pia mater as ligamenta denticulata attached to the dura mater

Labels: Pia mater, Filaments of dorsal root, Ligamentum denticulatum, Dura mater

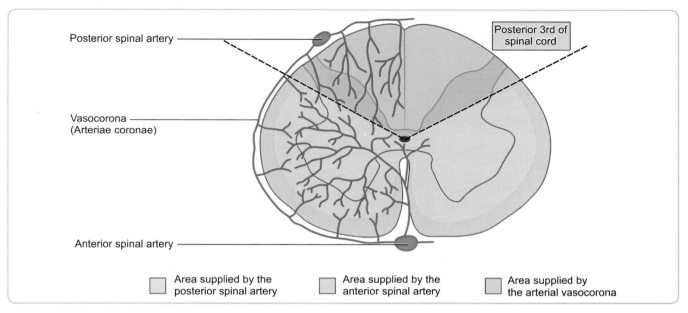

Figure 2.18: Intrinsic arterial supply of the spinal cord

Posterior Spinal Arteries

The right and left posterior spinal arteries are the branches of the fourth part of the vertebral arteries. Each posterior spinal artery descends through the foramen magnum as two branches, which pass one in front and the other behind the dorsal roots of the spinal nerves.

Radicular Arteries

The main source of blood to the spinal arteries is from the vertebral arteries (from which the anterior and posterior spinal arteries take origin). However, the blood from the vertebral arteries reaches only up to the cervical segments of the cord. Lower down, the spinal arteries receive blood through radicular arteries that reach the cord along the roots of spinal nerves. These radicular arteries arise from spinal branches of the vertebral, intercostal, lumbar and sacral arteries (Figure 2.19).

Arteria Radicularis Magna

Many of these radicular arteries are small and end by supplying the nerve roots. A few of them, which are larger, join the spinal arteries and contribute blood to them. One of the radicular branches, usually from the right or left 11th intercostal artery is very large and is called the **arteria**

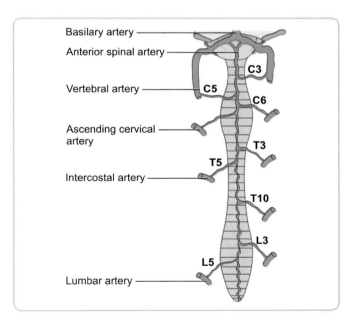

Figure 2.19: Radicular arteries that contribute blood to the spinal arteries

radicularis magna (artery of Adamkiewicz). Its position is variable. This artery may be responsible for supplying blood to as much as the lower two-thirds of the spinal cord especially the lumbar enlargement.

Intrinsic Blood Supply

The greater part of the cross-sectional area of the spinal cord, roughly the anterior two-thirds, is supplied by branches of the anterior spinal artery (Figure 2.18). These branches enter the anterior median fissure (or sulcus) and are, therefore, called **sulcal branches.** Alternate sulcal branches pass to the right and left sides. They supply the anterior and lateral grey columns and the central grey matter. They also supply the anterior and lateral funiculi. The rest (posterior one-third) of the spinal cord is supplied by the posterior spinal arteries (Figure 2.18). As already mentioned, branches from the arteria vasocorona also supply the cord.

Venous Drainage

The veins draining the spinal cord are arranged in the form of six longitudinal channels (Figure 2.20). These are:

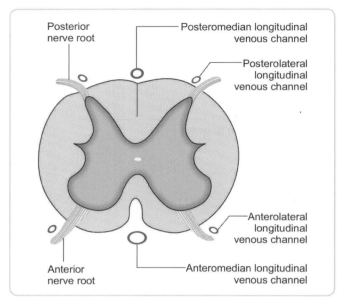

Figure 2.20: Venous drainage of the spinal cord

- **Two median longitudinal channels**, one in the anterior median fissure called the anteromedian channel, and the other in the posteromedian sulcus called the posteromedian channel
- **The paired anterolateral channels**, one on either side, posterior to the anterior nerve roots
- **The paired posterolateral channels**, one on either side posterior to the posterior nerve roots

These channels are interconnected by a plexus of veins that form a **venous vasocorona**. The blood from these veins is drained into radicular veins that open into a venous plexus lying between the dura mater and the bony vertebral canal (**internal vertebral venous plexus**) and through it, into various segmental veins.

<hr />

MULTIPLE CHOICE QUESTIONS

Q1. At birth, the lower end of spinal cord lies at the level of which vertebra?
  A. L1
  B. L3
  C. S2
  D. S4

Q2. In adults, the length of the spinal cord in centimeter is:
  A. 25
  B. 35
  C. 45
  D. 55

Q3. Inferior continuation of the pia mater of spinal cord is called as:
  A. Conus medullaris
  B. Cauda equina
  C. Filum terminale
  D. Ganglion impar

Q4. Ligamentum denticulatum is an extension from the:
A. Posterior longitudinal ligament
B. Pia mater
C. Ligamentum flavum
D. Dura mater

Q5. The surface landmark used for inserting the needle while doing lumbar puncture is:
A. Highest point of iliac crest
B. Posterosuperior iliac spine
C. Tubercle of iliac crest
D. Anterosuperior iliac spine

Q6. Total number of spinal segments is:
A. 30
B. 31
C. 32
D. 33

Q7. Ninth thoracic spine corresponds to which spinal segment?
A. T9
B. T10
C. T11
D. T12

Q8. Cervical enlargement of the spinal cord extends between which of the following spinal segments?
A. C1 and C8
B. C1 and T2

C. C3 and C8
D. C3 and T2

Q9. Spinal segments responsible for biceps tendon reflex are:
A. C5, C6
B. C6, C7
C. C7, C8
D. C8, T1

Q10. Spinal segments responsible for plantar reflex are:
A. L3, L4
B. L5, S1
C. S2, S3, S4
D. S3, S4

Q11. Which artery gives rise to arteria radicularis magna (artery of Adamkiewicz)?
A. Vertebral
B. Fifth intercostal
C. 11th intercostal
D. First lumbar

Q12. Anterior spinal artery is a branch of which of the following arteries?
A. Internal carotid
B. Vertebral
C. Subclavian
D. Posteroinferior cerebellar

ANSWERS

1. B   2. C   3. C   4. B   5. A   6. B   7. D   8. D   9. A   10. B
11. C   12. B

SHORT NOTES

1. Specializations of pia mater of spinal cord
2. Spinal segments
3. Arterial supply of spinal cord
4. Lumbar puncture

Clinical Cases

2.1: In a case of vehicular accident, a radiogram showed crush fracture of the body of the seventh thoracic vertebra.
A. Which spinal segment is affected in this person?
B. Below which part of the trunk would this person have loss of sensation?

2.2: In a person with anterior spinal artery syndrome at spinal segment C8, what would be the effect on?
A. Biceps jerk; Knee jerk
B. Plantar reflex; Cremasteric reflex

2.3: During lumbar epidural anaesthesia, the patient was asked to flex the vertebral column.
A. What are the structures pierced by the needle (in sequence) in lumbar epidural anaesthesia?
B. Why was the patient asked to flex the vertebral column?

Chapter 3

Spinal Cord—Internal Features

Specific Learning Objectives

At the end of learning, the student shall be able to:
- Describe the various nuclei in the anterior, posterior and lateral grey columns of the spinal cord
- Describe the various tracts in the anterior, lateral and posterior funiculi of the spinal cord
- Draw and label a transverse section of the spinal cord depicting important nuclear groups in the grey columns and important ascending and descending tracts in the white columns
- Explain the anatomical basis of clinical conditions affecting the grey and white matter of the spinal cord

INTRODUCTION

A transverse section of the spinal cord shows grey matter surrounded by white matter. The grey matter is formed by neurons (dendrites, cell bodies and unmyelinated axons) and glial cells. The white matter is composed of myelinated axons.

The grey matter forms an H-shaped or a butterfly-shaped mass (Figure 3.1). In a cross-section, the grey matter is called as **ventral horn, dorsal horn** and central grey. Three-dimensionally it forms **anterior (ventral) grey column and posterior (dorsal) grey column** and the **grey commissure** (Figure 3.2). In the thoracic and the

sacral parts of the spinal cord, a small lateral projection of grey matter is seen between the ventral and dorsal grey columns. This is the **lateral grey column**.

The white matter of the spinal cord is divided into right and left halves, in front by the **anterior median fissure** and behind by the **posterior median septum**. In each half of the cord the white matter between the dorsal grey column and the posteromedian septum forms the **posterior funiculus** (posterior white column). The white matter between the anterior grey column and the anteromedian fissure forms the **anterior funiculus** (anterior white column), while the white matter lateral to the anterior and posterior grey columns between the anterolateral sulcus

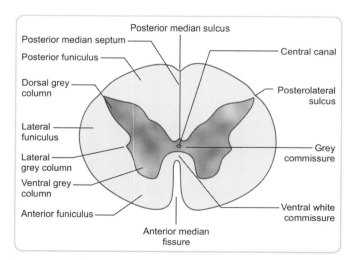

Figure 3.1: Transverse section through the spinal cord showing grey and white matter

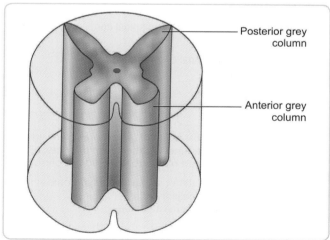

Figure 3.2: Three-dimensional view of grey matter of the spinal cord

and the posterolateral sulcus forms the **lateral funiculus** (lateral white column). (The anterior and lateral funiculi are sometimes collectively referred to as the **anterolateral funiculus**) (Figure 3.1). The white matter of the right and left halves of the spinal cord is continuous across the midline as the **anterior white commissure**, which lies anterior to the grey commissure.

Variation in the Internal Structure of Spinal Cord at Different Levels

- The shape of the transverse section of the spinal cord varies at different levels. It is transversely oval in the cervical region, round in thoracic region, round to oval in lumbar region and round in sacral region.
- The relative amount of grey and white matter and the shape and size of the grey columns vary at different levels of the spinal cord (Figure 3.3).
- The amount of grey matter to be seen at a particular level can be correlated with the mass of tissue to be supplied. It is, therefore, greatest in the region of the cervical and lumbar enlargements, which supply the limbs.
- The amount of white matter undergoes progressive increase from the lower part of the spinal cord to the upper part. This is because:
  - Progressively more and more ascending fibres are added as the upper levels of the cord are reached.
  - The number of descending fibres decrease as lower levels of the cord are reached as some of them terminate in each segment.

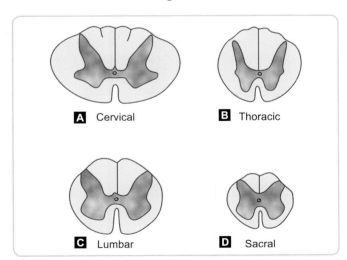

Figures 3.3A to D: Differences in appearance of transverse sections through various levels of the spinal cord

NUCLEI IN GREY MATTER

Discrete collections of neurons (or nuclei) occur in various regions of the spinal grey matter. The cell groups correspond with one or more of ten cell layers, known as Rexed laminae.
- Lamina I to IV lie at the dorsal part of dorsal horn.
- Lamina V and VI lie at the base of dorsal horn.
- Lamina VII lies in the intermediate (lateral) grey column.
- Lamina VIII and IX lie in the ventral horn.
- Lamina X corresponds to the central grey.

The correlation of the nuclei with the Rexed laminae is illustrated in Figure 3.4 and Table 3.1.

Nuclei in the Posterior Grey Column (Dorsal Horn)

This group consists of sensory and integrative nerve cells (Figure 3.5). The type of cells and their connections are given in Table 3.2.

> **Clinical Anatomy**
>
> **The "gate control" theory of pain inhibition:**
> Large-diameter afferents are excitatory to the neurons of lamina IV and to interneurons in the substantia gelatinosa.
> In contrast, fine nonmyelinated pain afferents are excitatory to the neurons of lamina IV but inhibitory to substantia gelatinosa.
> The axons of substantia gelatinosa inhibit presynaptically the terminals of all afferents that synapse with lamina IV (Figure 3.6).
> Therefore, impulses in the large-diameter afferents would close the gate to lamina IV in the interneurons by presynaptic inhibition and thus pain inhibition.

Nuclei in the Lateral Grey Column

This group consists of proprioceptive and visceral nerve cells (Figure 3.5). The type of cells and their connections are given in Table 3.3.

Nuclei in the Anterior Grey Column (Ventral Horn)

This group consists of proprioceptive and somatic efferent neurons and their interneurons (Figure 3.7A). Motor neurons can be subdivided into:
- **Medial group:**
  - Ventromedial nucleus (entire spinal cord)
  - Dorsomedial nucleus (entire spinal cord)

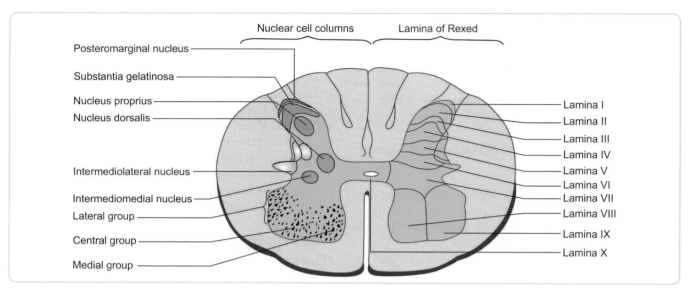

Figure 3.4: Nuclei and laminae of Rexed

TABLE 3.1: Nerve cell groups in the spinal grey columns

Rexed lamina	Nuclei in grey column	Extent in the spinal cord	Functions
I	Posteromarginal nucleus	Entire cord	Relay station for "fast" pain
II	Substantia gelatinosa	Entire cord	Interneurons for modification of pain and other sensory input
III and IV	Nucleus proprius	Entire cord	Gives origin to ventral and lateral spinothalamic tracts
V	Diffuse spinal reticular nucleus	Entire cord	Integration of exteroceptive, nociceptive, proprioceptive and visceral senses
VI	Interneurons for spinal reflexes	Prominent in limb enlargements	Propriospinal polysynaptic reflexes like flexion or withdrawal reflex
VII	Central cervical nucleus	C1–C4	Tonic neck reflexes
	Posterior thoracic (Clarke's column)	C8–L3	Unconscious proprioception from lower limb; gives origin to posterior spinocerebellar tract
	Intermediomedial nucleus	T1–L2 and S2–S4	Visceral afferents
	Intermediolateral nucleus	T1–L2 and S2–S4	Visceromotor
VIII	Spinal border nucleus	Lateral border of L1–L5	Unconscious proprioception from lower limb
	Interneurons for motor neurons	Entire cord	Influence motor neurons
IX	Motor neurons (α and γ)	Entire cord	Innervates the striated muscles
X	Central grey	Entire cord	Diffuse and nondiscriminatory

- **Central group**:
  - Spinal accessory (C1–C5)
  - Phrenic nucleus (C3–C5)
  - Nucleus of Onuf (S2–S4)

- **Lateral group**:
  - Ventrolateral (C5–C8 and L2–S2)
  - Dorsolateral (C5–C8 and L2–S2)
  - Retrodorsolateral (C8, T1 and S2, S3)

  The cells of anterior grey column and their connections are given in Table 3.4.

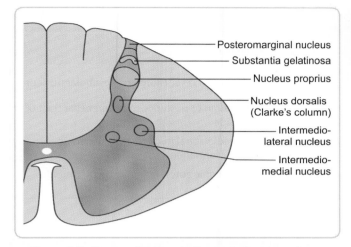

Figure 3.5: Nerve cell groups in the posterior grey column

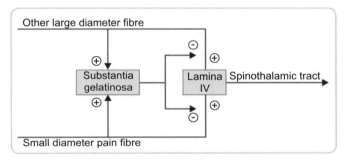

Figure 3.6: The sensory "gate" mechanism in the spinal cord showing presynaptic inhibition by substantia gelatinosa

TABLE 3.2: Nerve cell groups and their connections (Posterior grey column)

Rexed lamina	Nuclei in grey column	Afferent connections	Efferent connections
I	Posteromarginal nucleus	"Fast" pin-pricking type of pain from dorsolateral tract of Lissauer	Gives origin to lateral spinothalamic tract of the opposite side
II	Substantia gelatinosa	Stimulation from large diameter sensory fibres; inhibitory from pain fibres	Presynaptic inhibition to nucleus proprius (See Figure 3.6)
III and IV	Nucleus proprius	Fibres carrying sensation of crude touch, pressure, thermal and "slow" burning pain	Gives origin to anterolateral spinothalamic tracts of the opposite side
V	Diffuse spinal reticular nucleus	Exteroceptive, nociceptive, proprioceptive and visceral senses; corticospinal tract and subcortical inputs	Gives origin to spinoreticular, spinotectal and spino-olivary tracts
VI	Interneurons for spinal reflexes	Exteroceptive, nociceptive, proprioceptive senses; corticospinal tract	Motor neurons for superficial spinal reflexes

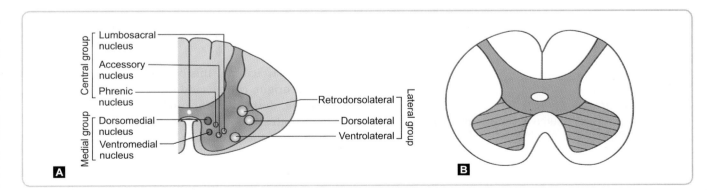

Figures 3.7A and B: (A) Nerve cell groups in the anterior grey column; (B) *Poliomyelitis* affecting the nerve cell groups in the anterior grey column

TABLE 3.3: Nerve cell groups and their connections (Lateral grey column)

Rexed lamina	Nuclei in grey column	Afferent connections	Efferent connections
VII	Central cervical nucleus	Proprioception from neck, semicircular canals	Contralateral cerebellum and vestibular nucleus
	Posterior thoracic (Clarke's column)	Proprioception from lower limbs	Gives origin to posterior spinocerebellar tract of same side
	Intermediomedial nucleus	Interoception from viscera	Intermediolateral nucleus, hypothalamus, reticular formation
	Intermediolateral nucleus	Hypothalamus, reticular formation, intermediomedial nucleus	Preganglionic autonomics to smooth muscles and glands

TABLE 3.4: Nerve cell groups and their connections (Anterior grey column)

Rexed lamina	Nuclei in grey column	Afferent connections	Efferent connections
VIII	Spinal border nucleus	Proprioception from lower limbs	Gives origin to anterior spinocerebellar tract of opposite side
	Interneurons for motor neurons	Corticospinal and extrapyramidal tracts, other spinal neurons	Motor neurons
IX	Ventromedial nucleus	Corticospinal, spinal interneurons, muscle spindle	Dorsal muscles of trunk
	Dorsomedial nucleus	Corticospinal, spinal interneurons and muscle spindle	Ventral muscles of trunk
	Spinal accessory	Corticospinal, spinal interneurons, muscle spindle	Sternocleidomastoid and trapezius
	Phrenic nucleus	Corticospinal, spinal interneurons, medullary respiratory centre	Diaphragm
	Nucleus of Onuf	Spinal interneurons and visceral afferents	Pelvic diaphragm, voluntary sphincters of urethra and anal canal
	Ventrolateral	Corticospinal, spinal interneurons and muscle spindle	Dorsal muscles of limbs
	Dorsolateral	Corticospinal, spinal interneurons and muscle spindle	Ventral muscles of limbs
	Retrodorsolateral	Corticospinal, spinal interneurons and muscle spindle	Muscles of hand and foot

Clinical Anatomy

Poliomyelitis (Figure 3.7B):
Lesion of ventral grey column neurons as in poliomyelitis or as in progressive muscular atrophy results in lower motor neuron (LMN) paralysis of the affected segments. It would be flaccid paralysis, with absent superficial and deep reflexes. If the virus affects the grey matter of the medulla (bulbar polio), it can result in respiratory arrest.

TRACTS IN WHITE MATTER

A collection of nerve fibres within the central nervous system, that connects two masses of grey matter, is called a tract (or fasciculus). This collection of nerve fibres has a similar origin, course, and termination. Tracts may be ascending, descending or intersegmental (which could include both ascending and descending). They are usually named after the masses of grey matter connected by them. Thus, a tract beginning in the cerebral cortex and descending to the spinal cord is called the **corticospinal tract**, while a tract ascending from the spinal cord to the thalamus is called the **spinothalamic tract**. Tracts are sometimes referred to as lemnisci (ribbons). The major tracts passing through the spinal cord are shown schematically in Figure 3.8 and in Table 3.5. The position of the tracts in a transverse section of the spinal cord is shown in Figure 3.9.

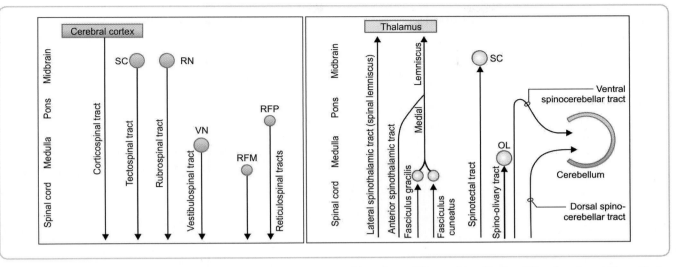

Figure 3.8: Major tracts of spinal cord passing through the brainstem (*Abbreviation*: SC, superior colliculus; RN, red nucleus; VN, vestibular nuclei; RFP, reticular formation of pons; RFM, reticular formation of medulla; OL, inferior olivary nucleus)

TABLE 3.5: Important ascending and descending tracts in various funiculi		
Funiculus	*Ascending tracts*	*Descending tracts*
Posterior	• Fasciculus gracilis • Fasciculus cuneatus	• Septomarginal tract • Fasciculus interfascicularis (Semilunar tract/ Comma tract of Schultze)
Lateral	• Posterior spinocerebellar • Anterior spinocerebellar • Lateral spinothalamic • Spinotectal • Spino-olivary • Dorsolateral (Lissauer's tract)	• Lateral corticospinal • Rubrospinal • Lateral reticulospinal • Olivospinal • Hypothalamospinal • Raphespinal
Anterior	• Anterior spinothalamic • Spinoreticular	• Anterior corticospinal • (Lateral) vestibulospinal • Medial vestibulospinal (Medial longitudinal fasciculus) • Tectospinal • Medial reticulospinal

Clinical Anatomy

Cordotomy

Sometimes, a patient may be in severe pain that cannot be controlled by drugs. As an extreme measure pain may be relieved by cutting the lateral spinothalamic tracts (which carries pain sensation). The operation is called cordotomy. The ligamentum denticulatum serves as a guide to the surgeon. For relief of pain the incision is placed anterior to this ligament (anterolateral cordotomy), so as not to involve lateral corticospinal tract (which lie behind ligamentum denticulatum), responsible for skillful voluntary movement.

Pain can also be relieved by cutting the posterior nerve roots in the region. This operation is called posterior rhizotomy.

ASCENDING TRACTS

Sensory modalities are either special senses or general senses. The general senses are classified as follows:

- **Exteroception**: Sensations perceived by the body, arising from external world and include touch, pressure, vibration, pain, thermal sensation, itch, tickle, etc.
- **Proprioception**: Sensations perceived by the body, generated by the own tissues and include perception of posture, joint position and movement, muscle contraction and stretch.
- **Interoception**: Sensations perceived by the body, arising from internal world and include sensations

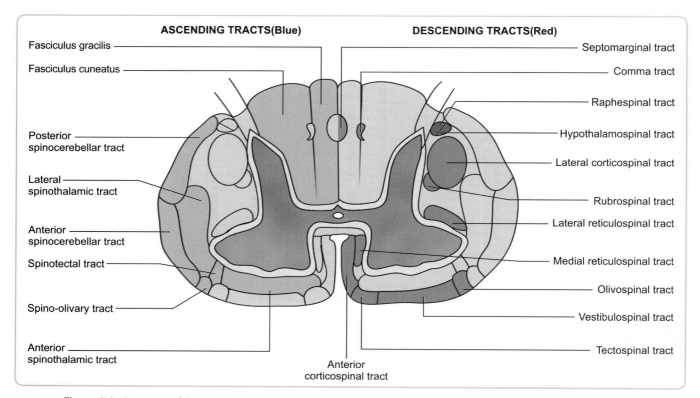

ASCENDING TRACTS(Blue)   **DESCENDING TRACTS(Red)**

Fasciculus gracilis

Fasciculus cuneatus

Posterior spinocerebellar tract

Lateral spinothalamic tract

Anterior spinocerebellar tract

Spinotectal tract

Spino-olivary tract

Anterior spinothalamic tract

Septomarginal tract

Comma tract

Raphespinal tract

Hypothalamospinal tract

Lateral corticospinal tract

Rubrospinal tract

Lateral reticulospinal tract

Medial reticulospinal tract

Olivospinal tract

Vestibulospinal tract

Tectospinal tract

Anterior corticospinal tract

Figure 3.9: Positions of the main ascending and descending tracts present in a transverse section of the spinal cord

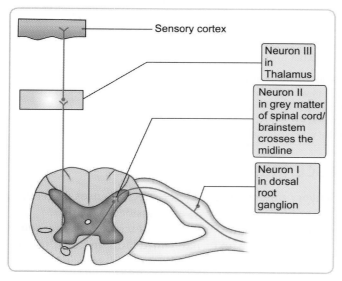

Sensory cortex

Neuron III in Thalamus

Neuron II in grey matter of spinal cord/ brainstem crosses the midline

Neuron I in dorsal root ganglion

Figure 3.10: Levels of neurons in ascending or sensory tract

from viscera like hunger, thirst, bladder fullness, urge to defecate, etc.

Ascending tracts related to the conscious general senses consist of a sequence of three neurons that extends from

peripheral receptor to the cerebral cortex. These are often referred to as primary, secondary and tertiary neurons or first-order neurons, second-order neurons and third-order neurons (Figure 3.10). Unconscious proprioception and some exteroception going to cerebellum consist of only two neurons, as also those terminating in brainstem.

Ascending Tracts Projecting to the Cerebral Cortex

The **first-order neurons** of these pathways are located in spinal (dorsal nerve root) ganglia (Figure 3.11). The neurons in these ganglia are unipolar. Each neuron gives off a peripheral process and a central process. The peripheral processes of the neurons end in relation to sensory end organs (receptors) situated in various tissues. The central processes of these neurons enter the spinal cord through the dorsal nerve roots. The **second-order neurons** (located in the spinal cord or medulla oblongata) cross the midline and end by synapsing with neurons in the thalamus. **Third-order neurons** are located in the thalamus and carry the sensations to the cerebral cortex.

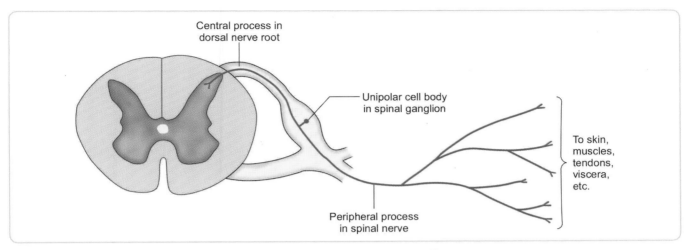

Figure 3.11: Typical arrangement of a primary afferent neuron

Posterior Columns

The **fasciculus gracilis** (Tract of Goll) **and cuneatus** (Tract of Burdach) are central processes of first-order neurons synapsing with nucleus gracilis and cuneatus in the medulla oblongata (which are the second-order neurons) (Figure 3.12A). The sensory modalities that they carry are:

- Fine touch (tactile localization, two-point discrimination)
- Vibration
- Joint position
- Muscle proprioception

> **Clinical Anatomy**
>
> **Sensory neuron disease** (Figure 3.12B): Involvement of posterior columns, as in hereditary sensory neuropathy or tertiary syphilis causes bilateral loss of fine touch, two-point discrimination, joint position and vibration sense. However, crude sensations carried by spinothalamic tracts remain intact.

Anterolateral Spinothalamic Tract

The other sensations are carried by **anterolateral spinothalamic tract** (Figure 3.13A). The first-order neurons ascend two or three segments in the **dorsolateral tract of Lissauer** before they terminate in **posteromarginal** nucleus (for "pin-pricking" pain) and **nucleus proprius** (for crude touch, pressure, "burning" pain and thermal sensation). These nuclei are the second-order neurons. The fibres of pain and thermal sensation cross the midline in the anterior white commissure and ascend up as lateral part of anterolateral spinothalamic tract. The crude touch

and pressure sensation (after crossing) ascend up as anterior part of anterolateral spinothalamic tract.

> **Clinical Anatomy**
>
> **Syringomyelia (Figure 3.13B):** A destructive process around the central canal of the spinal cord results in increase in the size of the cavity and affects the crossing spinothalamic fibres in the anterior white commissure. So, there will be bilateral loss of pain and temperature sensations but the posterior column sensations are preserved as they do not get affected initially. This produces "dissociated sensory loss".

Different modalities of sensations are carried by different portions of anterolateral spinothalamic tract. The spinothalamic tract carries sensations from the opposite side of the body.

> **Clinical Anatomy**
>
> **Tract of Lissauer:** A unilateral lesion of the spinothalamic tract will result in loss of crude touch, pressure, pain and thermal sensation. The sensation will be lost on the opposite side below the level of lesion. The contralateral loss of pain and temperature sensations, however, occur **2–3 segments below the level of the lesion** because pain and thermal sense rise 2–3 levels up in the tract of Lissauer before they terminate.

Ascending Tracts Projecting to the Cerebellum (Figure 3.14)

Posterior Spinocerebellar Tract

This tract carries unconscious proprioception from **individual muscles** of the **lower limb**. The dorsal nerve

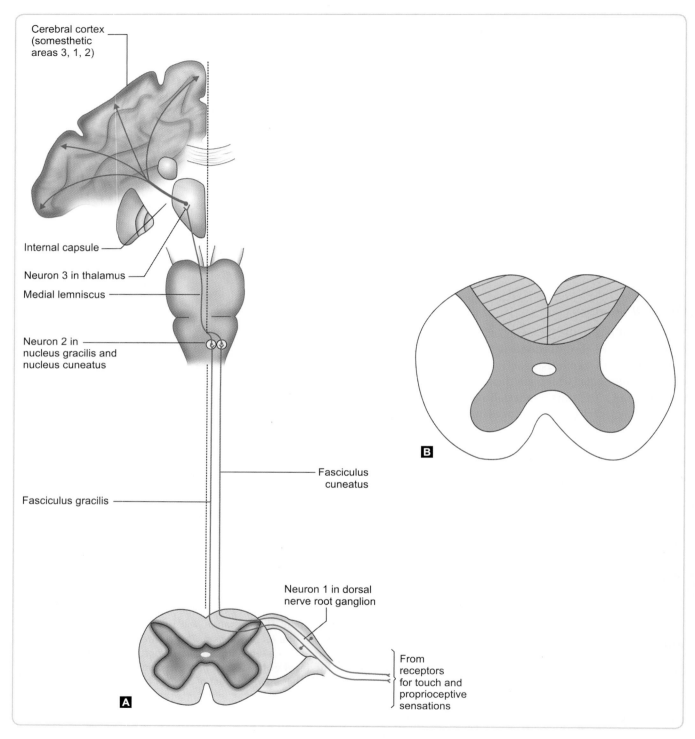

Figures 3.12A and B: (A) Main features of the posterior column medial lemniscus pathway; (B) Tabes dorsalis affecting the posterior column pathway

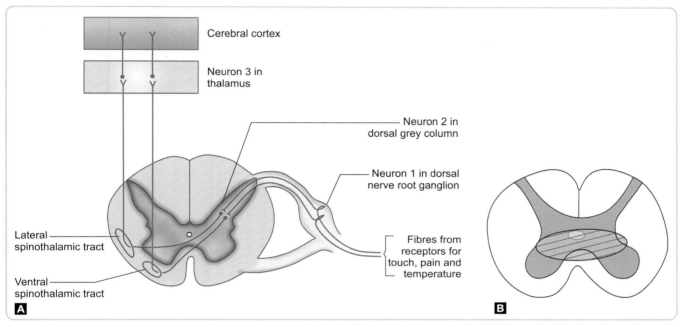

Figures 3.13A and B: (A) Main features of the spinothalamic pathways (Red: pain; Blue: crude touch);
(B) Syringomyelia (destructive lesions of central canal)

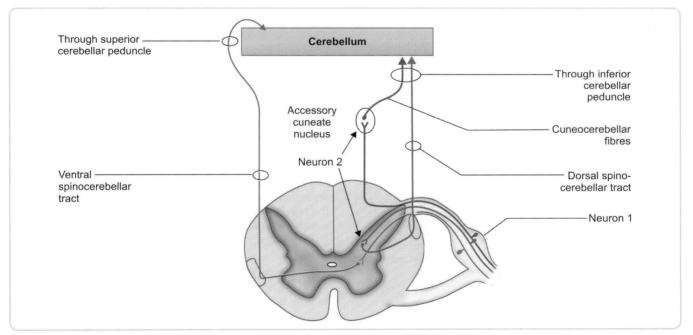

Figure 3.14: Main features of the spinocerebellar pathways

root ganglion is the first-order neuron. The central process of the neuron synapses with posterior thoracic nucleus (Clarke's column). Axons from Clarke's column **do not cross** the midline and enter the cerebellum through the inferior cerebellar peduncle.

Anterior Spinocerebellar Tract

This tract carries unconscious proprioception from **lower limb as a whole**. The dorsal nerve root ganglion is the first-order neuron. The central process of the neuron synapses with spinal border cells. Axons from spinal border cells **cross the midline** and enter the cerebellum through the superior cerebellar peduncle and most of the fibres **recross** in the cerebellum.

Clinical Anatomy

A unilateral lesion of spinal cord will show **bilateral ataxia of lower limbs**, if the ventral spinocerebellar tract (carrying contralateral proprioceptive impulses) and dorsal spinocerebellar tract (carrying ipsilateral proprioceptive impulses) are affected.

The upper limb equivalent of posterior spinocerebellar tract is **cuneocerebellar tract** (which lies in the medulla oblongata).

The upper limb equivalent of ventral spinocerebellar tract is **rostral spinocerebellar tract** arising from diffuse neurons in the base of the posterior horn of cervical part of spinal cord. The existence of this pathway is doubtful in humans.

Clinical Anatomy

Disorders of equilibrium: Inability to maintain the equilibrium of the body, while standing or while walking, is referred to as **ataxia**. This may occur as a result of interruption of afferent proprioceptive pathways, i.e. tracts in the posterior column and the spinocerebellar pathways (sensory ataxia).

Lack of proprioceptive information can be compensated to a considerable extent by information received through the eyes. The defects are, therefore, much more pronounced with the eyes closed (**Romberg's sign positive**).

Ascending Tracts Projecting to the Brainstem

The spinotectal, spino-olivary and spinoreticular fibres start from lamina V of spinal cord and terminate in the respective nuclei of the brainstem.

A summary of the ascending tracts is seen in Table 3.6.

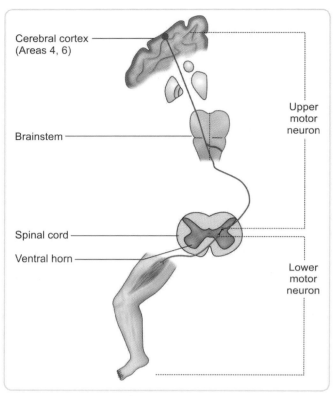

Figure 3.15: Position of upper motor neuron and lower motor neuron in brain and spinal cord

---

Clinical Anatomy

The second-order neurons of both the tracts of dorsal funiculus (carrying fine sensations) and spinothalamic tracts (carrying pain sensation) decussate. The level of decussation is different.

Fasciculi gracilis and cuneatus decussate at medulla; spinothalamic tract decussates at spinal cord.

Hence, spinal cord lesions cause ipsilateral loss of fine senses and contralateral loss of pain. A lesion anywhere in the brainstem or higher will cause contralateral loss of both senses—a **great localizing** sign.

DESCENDING TRACTS

The grey matter of lamina IX of Rexed (alpha and gamma motor neurons) sends axons that innervate skeletal muscles through the anterior root of spinal cord. This pathway is called as final common pathway or Lower Motor Neuron (LMN) pathway. The LMN (Figure 3.15) can be activated by:

- Pyramidal tract or corticospinal tract or upper motor neuron (UMN) starting from cerebral cortex for voluntary movements

TABLE 3.6: Ascending tracts of spinal cord

Tract	Function	First-order neuron			Second-order neuron			Third-order neuron	
		Peripheral process	Cell body	Central process	Cell body	Crossing	Ascent	Cell body	Axons
Fasciculus gracilis	Fine touch, proprioception, vibration, joint position sense from below T6	Skin, joint, tendon	Dorsal nerve root ganglia	Fasciculus gracilis in the posterior funiculus	Nucleus gracilis in medulla oblongata	Internal arcuate fibres	Medial lemniscus	Ventral postero-lateral nucleus of thalamus	Superior thalamic radiation to postcentral gyrus
Fasciculus cuneatus	Fine touch, proprioception, vibration, joint position sense from above T6	Skin, joint, tendon	Dorsal nerve root ganglia	Fasciculus cuneatus in the posterior funiculus	Nucleus cuneatus in medulla oblongata	Internal arcuate fibres	Medial lemniscus	Ventral postero-lateral nucleus of thalamus	Superior thalamic radiation to postcentral gyrus
Anterior spino-thalamic tract	Crude touch, pressure	Skin	Dorsal nerve root ganglia	Synapses with nucleus proprius of spinal cord	Nucleus proprius in spinal cord	Anterior white commissure of spinal cord	Joins medial lemniscus in medulla oblongata	Ventral postero-lateral nucleus of thalamus	Superior thalamic radiation to postcentral gyrus
Lateral spino-thalamic tract	Pain and thermal sensation	Skin	Dorsal nerve root ganglia	Ascends few segments up in dorso-lateral tract of Lissauer	Nucleus postero-marginal and nucleus proprius	Anterior white commissure of spinal cord	Continues as spinal lemniscus in brainstem	Ventral postero-lateral nucleus of thalamus	Superior thalamic radiation to postcentral gyrus
Posterior spinocerebellar	Unconscious proprioception from lower limb	Muscles and joints of lower limb	Dorsal nerve root ganglia	Ascends in fasciculus till Clarke's column	Posterior thoracic nucleus	—	Terminates in anterior lobe of cerebellum	—	—
Anterior spinocerebellar	Unconscious proprioception from lower limb	Muscles and joints of lower limb	Dorsal nerve root ganglia	Synapses with spinal border cells	Spinal border cells	Anterior white commissure of spinal cord	Terminates in anterior lobe of cerebellum	—	—
Spino-reticular tract	Deep pain	Deep tissues	Dorsal nerve root ganglia	Synapses with cells in lamina V	Lamina V of Rexed	Anterior white commissure of spinal cord; some fibres do not cross	Reticular formation of brainstem	—	—
Spino-olivary tract	Feedback about performance	Muscles and joints	Dorsal nerve root ganglia	Synapses with cells in lamina V	Lamina V of Rexed	Anterior white commissure of spinal cord	Inferior olivary nucleus of medulla oblongata	—	—
Spinotectal tract	Reflex movements of the head and eyes	Skin, joint, muscles	Dorsal nerve root ganglia	Synapses with cells in lamina V	Lamina V of Rexed	Anterior white commissure of spinal cord	Superior colliculus of midbrain	—	—

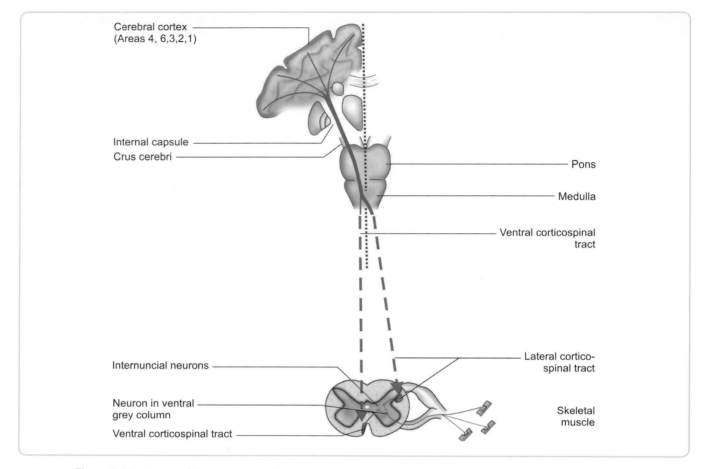

Figure 3.16: Course of the corticospinal tracts (Note the position of the tracts at various levels of the brainstem)

- Extrapyramidal tracts starting from brainstem for postural control of proximal muscles and controlling the output of autonomic nervous system
- Spinal reflexes (monosynaptic stretch reflex or polysynaptic reflexes) through intersegmental tracts

Corticospinal Tract (or Pyramidal Tract)

About 30% of fibres of this tract arise from the neurons lying in the motor area of the cerebral cortex (area 4), 30% arise from the premotor area (area 6) and 40% from the somatosensory area (areas 3, 1, 2). The fibres starting from sensory cortex influence sensory input to the central nervous system. A few fibres also arise from association areas of parietal, temporal and occipital lobes.

After passing through the internal capsule, the fibres enter the crus cerebri (of the midbrain) and then descend through the ventral part of the pons to enter the pyramids in the upper part of the medulla. Near the lower end of the medulla about 80% of the fibres cross to the opposite side and enter the lateral funiculus of the spinal cord and descend as the **lateral corticospinal** tract (Figure 3.16). The fibres of this tract terminate in grey matter of the spinal cord.

The corticospinal fibres that do not cross in the pyramidal decussation enter the anterior funiculus of the spinal cord to form the **anterior corticospinal** tract. On reaching the appropriate level of the spinal cord, many of the fibres of this tract cross the midline (through the anterior white commissure) to reach grey matter on the opposite side of the cord. A few terminate on the same side and are responsible of bilateral activities of the trunk.

The corticospinal tract constitutes the upper motor neuron (UMN). Majority of the fibres of UMN terminate in an interneuron, although a few may terminate directly on the lower motor neuron (LMN).

TABLE 3.7: Differences between upper motor neuron lesion and lower motor neuron lesion

Feature	Upper motor neuron lesion	Lower motor neuron lesion
Paralysis	Groups of muscles of one or more limbs paralyzed	Individual muscles paralyzed
Muscle tone	Spasticity/rigidity (spastic paralysis)	Flaccid (flaccid paralysis)
Deep tendon reflexes	Exaggerated	Absent
Superficial reflexes like abdominal and cremasteric reflexes	Absent	Absent
Plantar response	Extensor (Babinski sign positive)	No response
Muscle atrophy	May not be marked (may occur late and will be due to disuse)	Will be early and severe and due to denervation
Fasciculations and fibrillations	Do not occur	Are common

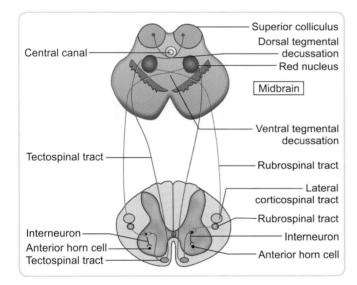

Figure 3.17: Main features of tectospinal and rubrospinal tracts. Note that the fibres of both the tracts cross to the opposite side in midbrain (in dorsal and ventral tegmental decussations)

Clinical Anatomy

The cerebral cortex controls voluntary movement through the corticospinal tract. Inability to move a part of the body is referred to as paralysis. This can be produced by interruption of motor pathways anywhere between the motor area of the cerebral cortex and the muscles themselves (UMN or LMN). From a clinical point of view, Table 3.7 will help to differentiate the two.

Extrapyramidal Tracts

Descending tracts arising from subcortical centres are called extrapyramidal tracts.

Rubrospinal Tract

This tract is made up of axons of neurons lying in the red nucleus (which lies in the upper part of the midbrain). The fibres of the tract cross to the opposite side of the midbrain and pass through the pons and medulla to enter the lateral funiculus of the spinal cord (Figure 3.17). The tract terminates in the cervical segments of spinal cord and is facilitatory to flexors of upper limb.

Tectospinal Tract

The fibres of this tract arise from neurons in the superior colliculus (midbrain). The fibres cross to the opposite side in the midbrain and descend through the pons and medulla into the anterior funiculus of the spinal cord (Figure 3.17). The tract terminates in the upper cervical segments of the spinal cord. This tract is responsible for reflex postural movements of neck in response to visual stimuli.

Medial Reticulospinal Tract

Fibres arise from the medial part of the reticular formation of pons. The fibres are largely uncrossed and descend in the anterior funiculus. The tract is facilitatory to the extensor muscles of the trunk and limbs. The tract is concerned with postural adjustments of the head, trunk and limbs (Figure 3.18). Control of bladder and bowel is also done through this tract.

Lateral Reticulospinal Tract

This tract is constituted by fibres arising in the reticular formation of the medulla oblongata. The fibres are crossed and uncrossed. They descend in the lateral funiculus

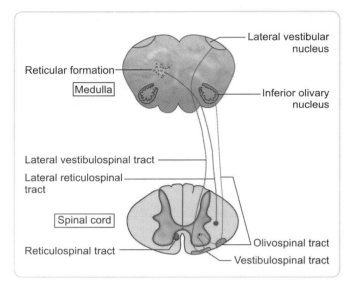

Figure 3.18: Main features of vestibulospinal, olivospinal and reticulospinal tracts

(Figure 3.18). The tract is facilitatory to the flexor muscles of the trunk and limbs. Automatic breathing is also controlled by lateral reticulospinal tract. It also influences transmission of pain through the ascending tracts.

Lateral Vestibulospinal Tract

The neurons of origin of the lateral vestibulospinal tract lie in the lateral vestibular nucleus located at pontomedullary junction. This tract is uncrossed and lies in the anterior funiculus of the spinal cord (Figure 3.18). This tract is an important efferent path for equilibrium.

The lateral vestibulospinal tract is facilitatory to motor neurons supplying extensor muscles.

Medial Vestibulospinal Tract or Medial Longitudinal Fasciculus (MLF)

The medial vestibulospinal tract arises mainly from the medial vestibular nucleus located at the pontomedullary

TABLE 3.8: Descending tracts of spinal cord

Tract	Origin	Crossing	Termination	Funiculus of cord	Function
Lateral corticospinal	Cerebral cortex area 4, area 6, and areas 3, 1, 2	Lower medulla	Interneuron and alpha motor neuron	Lateral	Fine motor function of distal muscles of limb and modulation of senses
Anterior corticospinal	Cerebral cortex area 4, area 6, and areas 3, 1, 2	Just before termination in the spinal cord	Interneuron and alpha motor neuron	Anterior	Gross motor function of axial musculature
Rubrospinal	Red nucleus	Upper midbrain	Gamma motor neuron	Lateral	Facilitates flexors of upper limb
Tectospinal tract	Superior colliculus	Upper midbrain	Interneurons	Anterior	Reflex postural movements of neck
Medial reticulospinal tract	Pontine reticular formation	—	Gamma motor neuron	Anterior	Facilitates extensors and bladder, bowel control
Lateral reticulospinal tract	Medullary reticular formation	Various levels	Gamma motor neuron	Lateral	Facilitates flexors, automatic breathing, modulation of pain
Lateral vestibulospinal tract	Lateral vestibular nucleus	—	Alpha motor neuron	Anterior	Facilitates extensors
Medial vestibulospinal tract (MLF)	Medial vestibular nucleus	Upper midbrain	Alpha motor neuron	Anterior	Turning of head
Olivospinal	Inferior olivary nucleus	Upper medulla	Interneurons	Lateral	Feedback to spino-olivary tract
Descending autonomic	Limbic lobe, hypothalamus	—	Preganglionic autonomic neurons	Lateral	Control autonomic output
Raphespinal	Raphe magnus nucleus	—	Dorsal horn	Lateral	Pain inhibition by release of serotonin

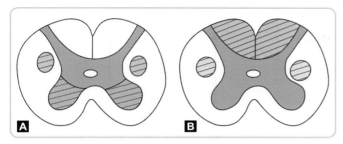

Figures 3.19A and B: (A) Lesion in amyotrophic lateral sclerosis; (B) Lesion in subacute combined degeneration

junction (with some fibres from the inferior and superior nuclei). The tract descends through the anterior funiculus. This tract is a downward continuation of medial longitudinal fasciculus and terminates in the upper cervical spinal cord. The tract is responsible for the neck righting reflex in response to stimulus received from vestibular apparatus.

Olivospinal Tract

This tract arises from the inferior olivary nucleus (medulla). It provides a feedback to spino-olivocerebellar pathway.

Descending Autonomic Fibres

Hypothalamospinal fibres descend uncrossed in the lateral funiculus and control the output of preganglionic autonomic neurons of thoracolumbar and sacral segments of spinal cord.

Raphespinal Tract

Raphespinal fibres descend uncrossed in the lateral funiculus and terminate in the dorsal horn. These are serotoninergic fibres involved in the inhibition of pain.

Clinical Anatomy

Spinothalamic tract gives off numerous collaterals to reticular formation of brainstem. These collaterals also stimulate the ascending reticular-activating system. A person can be easily awoken from a sleeping state by these pathways.

These collaterals are also responsible for pain inhibition via descending fibres from periaqueductal grey matter. Some fibres descend from the periaqueductal grey matter to nucleus raphe magnus of medulla, while others pass directly to the spinal cord.

Descending **raphespinal** tract from medulla pass to the substantia gelatinosa. Neurons in these sites secrete serotonin, GABA, substance P, enkephalin and endorphin. All of these are intimately concerned with the control of pain inputs.

A summary of the descending tracts is seen in Table 3.8.

Clinical Anatomy

Amyotrophic lateral sclerosis (Figure 3.19A): A combination of lesions of pyramidal tracts and anterior horn cells results in both UMN and LMN signs as in motor neuron disease (MND) or amyotrophic lateral sclerosis (ALS). This is a progressive degenerative disorder.

In the earlier stages, depending of the site of involvement, there will be LMN signs at the level of lesion and UMN signs below the level of lesion. Plantar reflex will show Babinski sign positive. As the disease progresses, death occurs due to paralysis of respiratory muscles. Death occurs much earlier in bulbar ALS.

Subacute combined degeneration (Figure 3.19B): Involvement of both posterior columns and pyramidal tracts is seen in subacute combined degeneration due to vitamin B12 deficiency.

This causes bilateral loss of fine touch, two-point discrimination, joint position and vibration sense and bilateral spastic paralysis and Babinski sign positive.

SOMATOTOPIC LAMINATION

The **orderly arrangement** of different levels of the body in a tract is somatotopic lamination of a tract.

In the posterior funiculus, since it is an uncrossed tract first-order neuron, sacral fibres which are added first, are pushed most medially, followed by lumbar, thoracic and cervical. Cervical, thoracic, lumbar and sacral fibres are arranged from medial to lateral in spinothalamic and corticospinal tracts (Figures 3.20 and 3.21).

Clinical Anatomy

A tumour in relation to the spinal cord can either grow from outside (meningioma) or from within (neuroglioma).

If the meningioma is pressing the cervical part of spinal cord from the lateral aspect, it initially involves:
• The sacral and lumbar fibres of lateral corticospinal tract causing ipsilateral monoplegia of lower limb
• The sacral and lumbar fibres of lateral spinothalamic tract causing contralateral loss of pain from lower limb and perianal region

If the neuroglioma is growing in the cervical part spinal cord laterally, it initially involves:
• The cervical and thoracic fibres of lateral corticospinal tract causing ipsilateral monoplegia of upper limb
• The cervical and thoracic fibres of lateral spinothalamic tract causing contralateral loss of pain from upper limb and trunk. Lower limb and perianal region are last to be involved

Some of the clinical conditions produced due to lesions of various funiculi of spinal cord are shown in Figure 3.22 and Table 3.9.

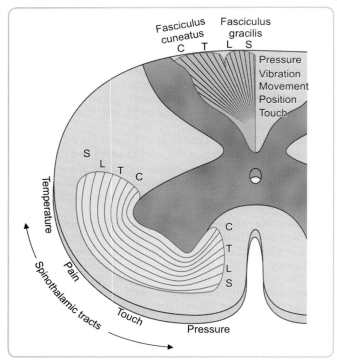

Figure 3.20: Pattern of lamination of the spinothalamic and posterior column tracts (*Abbreviation:* SLTC, sacral, lumbar, thoracic, cervical)

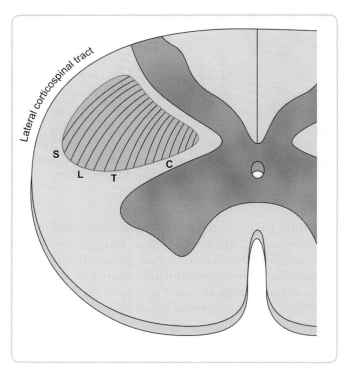

Figure 3.21: Somatotopic lamination of corticospinal tract (*Abbreviation:* SLTC, sacral, lumbar, thoracic, cervical)

TABLE 3.9: The clinical conditions produced due to lesions of various funiculi of spinal cord		
Site of lesion in the spinal cord	*Name of the clinical condition*	*Tracts or neurons affected*
One-half of spinal cord	Brown-Séquard syndrome	All the ascending and the descending tracts of one-half
Anterior two-thirds of spinal cord	Anterior spinal artery occlusion	Tracts in anterior and lateral funiculi of both sides
Anterior grey columns	Poliomyelitis	Anterior grey columns
Anterior grey columns and lateral funiculi	Amyotrophic lateral sclerosis or motor neuron disease	Anterior grey columns and corticospinal tracts of both sides
Around the central canal	Syringomyelia	Crossing fibres of spinothalamic tracts
Posterior columns	Hereditary sensory neuropathy	Fasciculus gracilis and fasciculus cuneatus of both sides
Lateral and posterior columns	Subacute combined degeneration due to vitamin B12 deficiency	Fasciculus gracilis and fasciculus cuneatus and corticospinal tracts of both sides

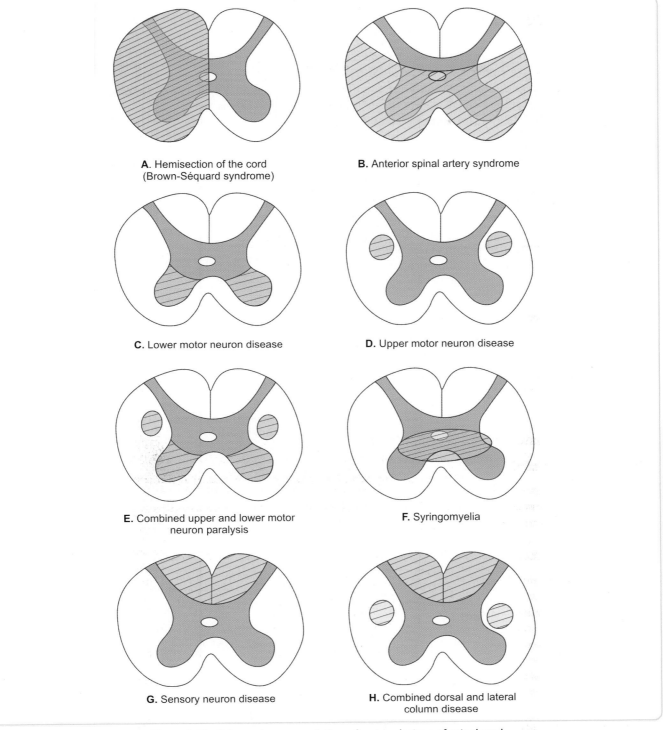

A. Hemisection of the cord
(Brown-Séquard syndrome)

B. Anterior spinal artery syndrome

C. Lower motor neuron disease

D. Upper motor neuron disease

E. Combined upper and lower motor
neuron paralysis

F. Syringomyelia

G. Sensory neuron disease

H. Combined dorsal and lateral
column disease

Figure 3.22: Schematic representation of various lesions of spinal cord

INTERSEGMENTAL TRACT OR PROPRIOSPINAL TRACT

Tracts originating and terminating in spinal cord (**spinospinal tracts**) are called as propriospinal tracts. More than half of all ascending and descending tracts in the spinal cord are propriospinal! These are short ascending or descending tracts. They exist in the anterior, lateral and posterior funiculi. Fasciculus septomarginalis and fasciculus interfascicularis are examples of descending tracts in the posterior funiculus. Posterolateral tract of Lissauer is another example. Propriospinal tracts connect the neurons of different spinal segments and are important in intersegmental spinal reflexes. Some examples include:

- Flexor withdrawal reflex on nociceptive stimulus
- Crossed extensor reflex on flexion of one limb
- Reciprocal inhibition on stimulation of agonist
- Postural adjustments on local stretching
- Evacuation reflexes on a full bladder or colon
- Paralytic ileus on peritoneal irritation

Clinical Anatomy

Transection of Spinal Cord: Paraplegia in Flexion or Paraplegia in Extension

In a transection of the thoracic part of spinal cord, both lower limbs get paralyzed (paraplegia).

In an incomplete transection, fibres in the lateral funiculus get affected, i.e. lateral reticulospinal tract and rubrospinal tract (both facilitatory to flexors). Vestibulospinal tract and medial reticulospinal tract lying in anterior funiculus (both facilitatory to extensors) are spared. This results in paraplegia in extension.

In a complete transection, all descending fibres are involved. Lower limbs go into flexor withdrawal reflex (spinal reflex). Hence, there is paraplegia in flexion.

MULTIPLE CHOICE QUESTIONS

Q1. The somatic efferent cells of the ventral grey column of spinal cord are known as:
  A. Alpha motor neurons
  B. Ganglion cells
  C. Gamma motor neurons
  D. Renshaw cells

Q2. The fibres of posterior spinocerebellar tract arise from:
  A. Visceral afferent nucleus
  B. Substantia gelatinosa
  C. Nucleus dorsalis
  D. Nucleus proprius

Q3. The LMNs are located in the:
  A. Dorsal root ganglion
  B. Pontine nuclei
  C. Sympathetic chain
  D. Anterior grey column of the spinal cord

Q4. Which of the following is the most posterior in the dorsal grey column of the spinal cord?
  A. Substantia gelatinosa (of Rolando)
  B. Nucleus dorsalis (Clarke's column)

  C. Nucleus proprius
  D. Visceral afferent nucleus

Q5. Which of the following tracts is concerned with reflex head and neck movements in response to the stimulation of body parts?
  A. Spino-olivary
  B. Spinoreticular
  C. Spinotectal
  D. Spinovestibular

Q6. Which of the following funiculi of the spinal cord contains the fasciculus cuneatus?
  A. Anterior
  B. Lateral, anterior half
  C. Lateral, posterior half
  D. Posterior

Q7. The fibres of the medial reticulospinal tract begins from:
  A. Medulla oblongata
  B. Pons
  C. Midbrain
  D. Diencephalon

ANSWERS

1. A   2. C   3. D   4. A   5. C   6. D   7. B

SHORT NOTES

1. Draw and label a transverse section of the cervical part of spinal cord to depict various ascending and descending tracts
2. Describe the various nuclei in the anterior, posterior and lateral grey columns of the spinal cord
3. Describe the various tracts in the anterior funiculus of the spinal cord
4. Describe the various tracts in the lateral funiculus of the spinal cord
5. Describe the various tracts in the posterior funiculus of the spinal cord

---

Clinical Cases

3.1: Brown-Séquard Syndrome

A person had a stab injury in the back of his neck between C7 and T1 vertebra. Magnetic resonance imaging (MRI) scan showed that the left half of the spinal cord was damaged at the T1 spinal segment. Left-sided motor paralysis and left-sided fine touch sensations were lost from T1 segment downwards. Pain sensation was lost on the right side from T4 segment.

A. Why was the pain sensation lost contralaterally from T4 segment?
B. Which group of muscles will show LMN type of paralysis?

3.2: Poliomyelitis

A 4-year-old child suffered from fever and gastroenteritis. This was followed by acute flaccid paralysis with fasciculation of the quadriceps muscle and absence of knee jerk. Atrophy of the muscle soon ensued.

A. Specify the type of neurological lesion.
B. Which segment of the spinal cord is involved in this child?

3.3: Amyotrophic Lateral Sclerosis

A 60-year-old person showed progressive wasting, fasciculation and weakness of upper limbs starting with the intrinsic muscles of the hand. Lower limbs showed spastic weakness with exaggerated stretch reflex. There was no sensory involvement.

A. Specify the spinal segment initially involved.
B. Specify the somatotopic lamination (arrangement of fibres) in the lateral corticospinal tract

3.4: Subacute combined degeneration

A 25-year-old person suffering from pernicious anemia showed loss of kinesthesia and discriminative touch. There was also paraplegia and loss of joint position sense. Superficial reflexes were lost and plantar response was extensor.

A. Which tracts are involved in this condition?
B. What type of motor lesion is seen in the lower limb?

INTRODUCTION

The brainstem consists of the midbrain, pons and medulla oblongata (or, just medulla) from above downwards (Figure 4.1). Superiorly, the brainstem (midbrain) is continuous with the structures forming the forebrain: thalamus, hypothalamus and cerebral hemispheres (Figure 4.2). Inferiorly, it is continuous with the spinal cord (Figure 4.1).

Posteriorly, the pons and medulla are separated from the cerebellum by the fourth ventricle (Figure 4.2). The ventricle is continuous below with the central canal, which traverses the lower part of the medulla and becomes continuous with the central canal of the spinal cord. Cranially, the fourth ventricle is continuous with the aqueduct, which passes through the midbrain (Figure 4.2).

The midbrain, pons and medulla are connected to the cerebellum posteriorly by the superior, middle and inferior cerebellar peduncles, respectively (Figure 4.3).

Ten pairs of cranial nerves are attached to the brainstem. The third and fourth nerves emerge from the

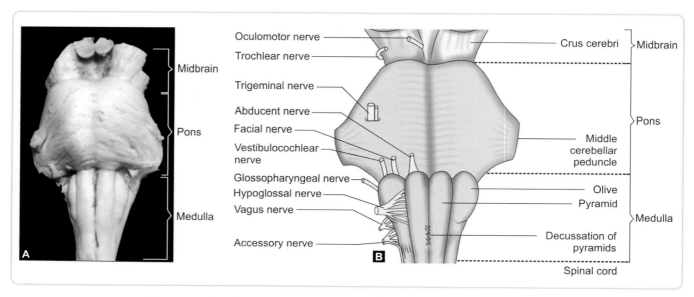

Figures 4.1A and B: Ventral aspect of the brainstem: (A) Specimen; (B) line diagram

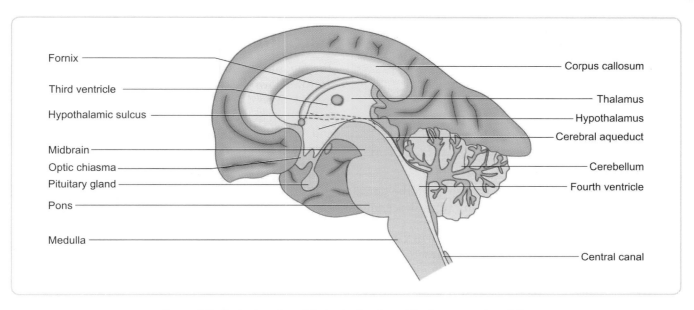

Figure 4.2: Sagittal section of the brain showing midbrain, pons and medulla.
Note that pons and medulla are separated from the cerebellum by the fourth ventricle

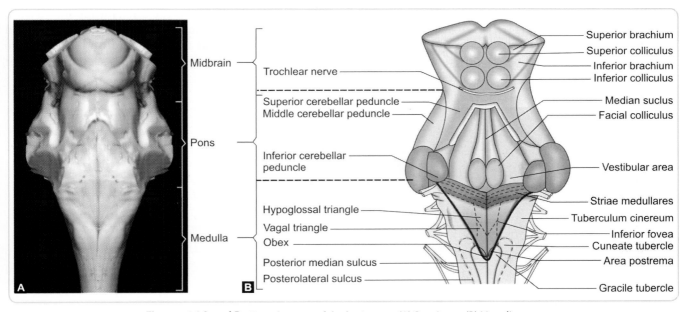

Figures 4.3A and B: Dorsal aspect of the brainstem: (A) Specimen; (B) Line diagram

surface of the midbrain and the fifth from the pons. The sixth, seventh and eighth nerves emerge at the junction of the pons and medulla. The ninth, tenth, cranial part of eleventh and twelfth cranial nerves emerge from the surface of the medulla (Figure 4.1 and Table 4.1).

FUNCTIONS

The functions of the brainstem are:

- Serves as a passage for the ascending tracts and descending tracts connecting the spinal cord to the different parts of the higher centres in the forebrain

TABLE 4.1: Attachment of cranial nerves

Site of attachment	Cranial nerves
Forebrain	I and II
Midbrain	III and IV
Hindbrain:	
Pons	V
Junction of pons and medulla	VI–VIII
Medulla	IX–XII

Ascending tracts, in general, pass through the dorsal part of the brainstem (tegmentum); while descending tracts through the ventral part (basilar part).

- Contains the cranial nerve nuclei from III to XII. Spinal part of accessory extends up to C5 segment of spinal cord.
- Contains important reflex centres associated with the control of respiration and cardiovascular system. Pons contains the pneumotaxic and apneustic centre. This influences the dorsal and ventral respiratory groups of medulla. Cardiovascular centre lies in the medulla.
- Controls consciousness (ascending reticular-activating system), regulates muscle tone (medial and lateral reticulospinal tracts), controls other vegetative functions (autonomic nervous system), inhibits pain (periaqueductal and raphespinal tracts) through reticular formation of brainstem.

EXTERNAL FEATURES OF MEDULLA OBLONGATA

The medulla is broad above where it joins the pons and narrows down below where it becomes continuous with the spinal cord. Its length is about 3 cm, and its width is about 2 cm at its upper end. The junction of the medulla and the spinal cord lies at the level of the upper border of the atlas vertebra. A deep groove demarcates the medulla from the bulging ventral part of pons.

The medulla is divided into a lower closed part, which surrounds the central canal and an upper open part, which is related to the lower part of the fourth ventricle (Figure 4.4). The surface of the medulla is marked by a series of fissures or sulci that divide it into a number of regions.

Anterior (Ventral) Aspect of Medulla

The **anterior median fissure** is the upward continuation of the corresponding feature seen in the spinal cord. Where the anterior median fissure meets the pontomedullary junction, there is a depression called as foramen caecum.

Immediately lateral to the anterior median fissure lies the elevation called **pyramid**. This is produced by the corticospinal tract (pyramidal tract). The decussation of the pyramidal tracts is seen in the lower part of medulla.

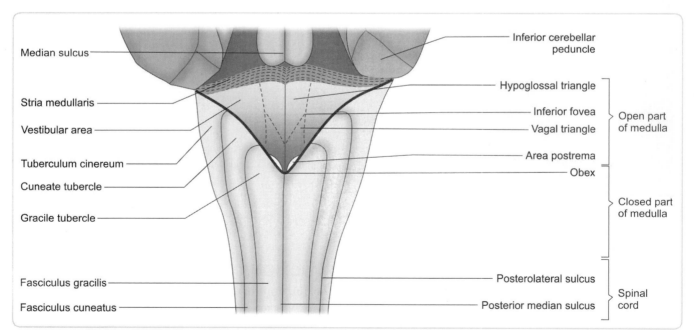

Figure 4.4: Diagram to show the open and closed parts of medulla

The **anterolateral sulci**, which are continuations of the corresponding sulci of the spinal cord, lie lateral to the pyramids. The anterolateral sulcus lies in line with the ventral roots of spinal nerves. The rootlets of the **hypoglossal nerve** emerge from this sulcus. The **ventral rootlet of first cervical nerve** is continuous with the rootlets of hypoglossal nerve. The junction of the last rootlet of hypoglossal nerve and the first ventral rootlet of C1 nerve marks the demarcation between medulla oblongata and spinal cord.

Lateral to the sulcus lies an elevation called **olive**. This is produced by the inferior olivary nuclear complex. This complex sends fibres to the opposite cerebellum and is a part of corticorubro-olivocerebellar pathway (denoting the intention of movement) and

spino-olivocerebellar pathway (feedback about the performance of movement).

The rootlets of **glossopharyngeal, vagus** and **cranial part of accessory** nerves arise from the groove lateral to the olive. The rootlets of **spinal part of accessory nerve** also arise, in line with this groove, from C1 to C5 segments of the spinal cord.

Lateral to the olive, the elevation is produced by the inferior cerebellar peduncles of the left and right side attaching the medulla with the cerebellum. They also form the inferolateral boundaries of the lower half of fourth ventricle.

Posterior (Dorsal) Aspect of Medulla

The posterior surface of the lower part (closed part) of medulla (Figure 4.4), shows the **posterior median sulcus** in the midline. This is the upward continuation of the corresponding feature seen in the spinal cord.

Lateral to the sulcus are two elevations which contain tracts that enter from the posterior funiculus of the spinal cord. These are the fasciculus gracilis, next to the midline and the fasciculus cuneatus placed laterally. These fasciculi end in rounded elevations called **the gracile and cuneate tubercles**. These tubercles are produced by masses of grey matter called the nucleus gracilis and

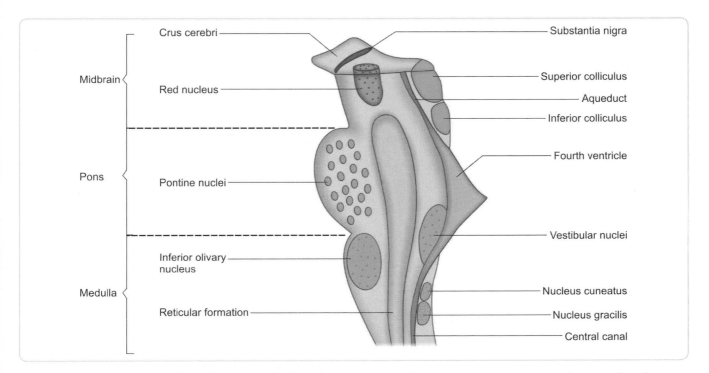

Figure 4.5: Median section through the brainstem. Some important masses of grey matter are shown projected on to median plane

the nucleus cuneatus, respectively (Figure 4.5). The groove in between these two tubercles is called **posterior intermediate sulcus**.

Lateral to the cuneate tubercle and the fasciculus cuneatus lie the **posterolateral sulcus**. This sulcus is in line with the corresponding sulcus of the spinal cord. The **dorsal rootlets of cervical nerves** arise from this sulcus at the level of the spinal cord.

The lower part of the medulla, immediately lateral to the posterolateral sulcus, is marked by another longitudinal elevation called the **tuberculum cinereum**. This elevation is produced by an underlying collection of grey matter of the **spinal nucleus of the trigeminal nerve**. The grey matter of this nucleus is covered by a layer of nerve fibres that form the spinal tract of the trigeminal nerve. The spinal nucleus of the trigeminal nerve is continuous with the **substantia gelatinosa** of spinal cord.

The posterior surface of the upper medulla (open part) forms the lower part of the floor of the fourth ventricle. This fossa is bounded on either side by the inferior cerebellar peduncles. The midline shows the **posterior median sulcus**. Lateral to that is **posterior medial eminence** formed by the nuclei of **hypoglossal and vagus** nerves. The lower part of medial eminence shows **chemoreceptor trigger zone (CTZ) or area postrema**. Limiting this eminence laterally is **sulcus limitans**. The **vestibular area** (marked by the underlying vestibular nuclei) is the elevation a lateral to sulcus limitans. The superior limit of medulla oblongata shows **striae medullares**. The features of this part of medulla are described in further details in Chapter 15.

> ⌐ **Clinical Anatomy** ¬
>
> **Vomiting reflex**: The CTZ is the strongest stimulator of vomiting centre. This area is devoid of blood-brain barrier. Most antiemetic drugs, hence, act at this zone. However, cortical causes of vomiting and motion sickness act directly on vomiting centre. Therefore, they require different drugs to control.

BLOOD SUPPLY OF MEDULLA OBLONGATA

The medulla is supplied by various branches of the vertebral arteries. These are the **anterior and posterior spinal arteries, the posterior inferior cerebellar artery and small direct branches** (Figure 4.6). The anterior spinal artery supplies a triangular area next to the midline. This area includes the pyramid, the medial lemniscus

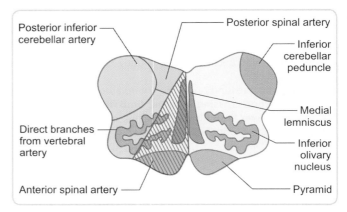

Figure 4.6: Cross-section through the medulla to show the regions supplied by different arteries

and the hypoglossal nucleus. The posterior spinal artery supplies a small area including the gracile and cuneate nuclei. The posterior inferior cerebellar artery supplies the retro-olivary region, i.e. the dorsolateral part of medulla oblongata. This region contains several important structures including the spinothalamic tracts, the vestibular nucleus, the nucleus ambiguus, the dorsal vagal nucleus and descending autonomic fibres. The posterior inferior cerebellar artery also supplies part of the inferior cerebellar peduncle. The rest of the medulla is supplied by direct bulbar branches of the vertebral arteries.

EXTERNAL FEATURES OF PONS

Pons is a part of the brainstem, situated between the medulla below and midbrain above (Figures 4.1 to 4.3). It lies in the posterior cranial fossa on the clivus, anterior to the cerebellum.

Pons, in a literal sense, means "**the bridge**". It is so named because it acts as a conduit for the passage of fibres from one side of the cerebellum to the other by its transverse fibres constituting the middle cerebellar peduncle. Nuclei of the cranial nerves, V (trigeminal), VI (abducent), VII (facial), and VIII (vestibulocochlear) lie in the pons.

Anterior Aspect of Pons

Pons shows a convex anterior surface, marked by prominent transversely running fibres. Laterally, these fibres collect to form a bundle, the **middle cerebellar peduncle**. These fibres intermingle with **corticospinal** and **corticonuclear fibres,** which are responsible for voluntary movements of the body.

The **trigeminal nerve** emerges from the anterior surface and the point of its emergence is taken as a landmark to define the plane of junction between the pons and the middle cerebellar peduncle.

The anterior surface of the pons is marked, in the midline, by a shallow groove, the **sulcus basilaris**, which lodges the basilar artery.

The line of junction between the pons and the medulla is marked by a groove through which a number of cranial nerves emerge. The abducent nerve emerges from just above the pyramid and runs upward in close relation to the anterior surface of the pons. The facial and vestibulocochlear nerves emerge from the interval between the olive and the pons.

Posterior Aspect of Pons

The posterior aspect of the pons forms the upper part of the floor of the fourth ventricle. Above the stria medullaris, in the medial eminence, lies the facial colliculus. Herein, the facial nerve axons wind around the nucleus of abducent nerve. Hence, the facial colliculus is also called as eminentia abducens.

On either side of the lower part of the pons, there is a region called the **cerebellopontine angle**. This region lies near the lateral aperture of the fourth ventricle. The facial nerve, vestibulocochlear nerve, nervus intermedius and the labyrinthine arteries lie in this region.

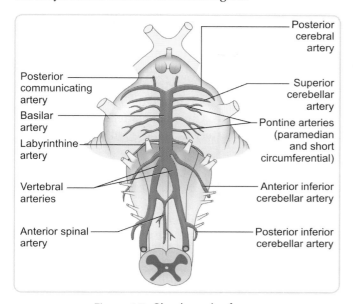

Figure 4.7: Blood supply of pons

BLOOD SUPPLY OF PONS

The pons is supplied by branches from the **basilar artery** (Figure 4.7). The **medial** portion of the ventral part of the pons is supplied by **paramedian branches**. The anterolateral part is supplied by **short-circumferential branches**. The posterolateral part is supplied by **long-circumferential branches**. The posterior part also receives branches from the **anterior inferior cerebellar** and **superior cerebellar arteries**. The paramedian branches of the basilar artery may extend into this region from the ventral part of the pons.

> **Clinical Anatomy**
>
> **Locked-in syndrome**
> This is due to thrombosis of short-circumferential branches of basilar artery. It results in infarction of the basal part of pons. The corticospinal and the corticonuclear fibres (which are responsible for voluntary movements of the body) of both sides are affected.
>
> The patient will present with complete paralysis due to involvement of corticospinal tracts and aphonia due to involvement of corticobulbar fibres.
>
> The person is conscious because of noninvolvement of reticular formation (which is periventricular). Since, the ascending fibres are unaffected, all general and special sensory inputs are normal.
>
> The only way the patient can communicate is by blinking and by vertical gaze (III and IV nerves arising from midbrain are intact).

EXTERNAL FEATURES OF MIDBRAIN

The midbrain is the uppermost part of the brainstem, connecting the hindbrain with the forebrain. It is about 2 cm in length. Its cavity, the cerebral aqueduct, connects the third ventricle to the fourth ventricle (Figure 4.2).

The midbrain contains nuclei of origin for cranial nerves III (**oculomotor**) and IV (**trochlear**). Apart from the cranial nerve nuclei, the midbrain also has nuclei that coordinate the movement of the eyeball in response to visual stimuli, which are located at the level of **superior colliculi**. Nuclei, which coordinate movements of head and trunk in response to auditory stimuli are located at the level of **inferior colliculi** (Figure 4.3).

Anterior Aspect of Midbrain

When the midbrain is viewed from the **anterior aspect**, two large bundles of fibres are seen, one on each side of the midline. These are the **cerebral peduncles**. They are separated by a deep fissure. Near the pons, the fissure is narrow, but broadens as the peduncles diverge to enter the corresponding cerebral hemispheres. The parts of the peduncles, just below the cerebrum, form the posterior boundary of a space called the **interpeduncular fossa**. The oculomotor nerve emerges from the medial aspect of the peduncle of the same side.

Posterior Aspect of Midbrain

The posterior aspect of the midbrain is marked by four rounded swellings (Figure 4.3). These are the **colliculi**, a pair of **superior colliculi** and a pair of **inferior colliculi** on each side. These are also known as **corpora quadrigemina**. Each colliculus is related laterally to a ridge called the **brachium**. The **superior brachium** (also called the superior quadrigeminal brachium or brachium of superior colliculus) connects the superior colliculus to the lateral geniculate body. Similarly, the **inferior brachium** (also called the inferior quadrigeminal brachium or brachium of inferior colliculus) connects the inferior colliculus to the medial geniculate body. Just below the colliculi, there is the uppermost part of a membrane, the

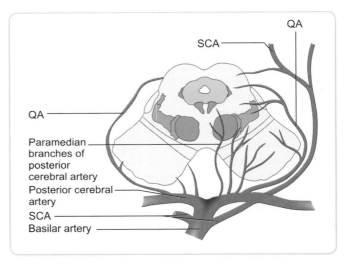

Figure 4.8: Blood supply of midbrain (*Abbreviations*: SCA, Superior Cerebellar Artery; QA, Quadrigeminal Artery

superior medullary velum, which stretches between the two superior cerebellar peduncles and helps to form the roof of the fourth ventricle. The trochlear nerve emerges from the velum and then winds round the side of the midbrain to reach its ventral aspect.

BLOOD SUPPLY OF MIDBRAIN

The midbrain is supplied mainly by branches of the basilar artery (Figure 4.8). These are the **posterior cerebral** and **superior cerebellar arteries** and direct branches from the **basilar artery**. Branches are also received from the **posterior communicating and anterior choroidal arteries**. Branches arising from these vessels may either be paramedian, which supply parts near the midline or circumferential which wind round the midbrain to supply lateral and dorsal parts. One of the latter arteries is called the **quadrigeminal** artery. It is the main source of blood to the colliculi.

MULTIPLE CHOICE QUESTIONS

Q1. The cranial nerve that emerges from the medulla oblongata between the pyramid and the olive is:
A. Glossopharyngeal
B. Vagus
C. Cranial accessory
D. Hypoglossal

Q2. The cranial nerve that emerges lateral to the olive is:
A. Abducent
B. Spinal accessory
C. Glossopharyngeal
D. Hypoglossal

Q3. The structure that lies deep to tuberculum cinereum is:
   A. Nucleus gracilis
   B. Spinal nucleus of trigeminal
   C. Nucleus coeruleus
   D. Hypoglossal nucleus

Q4. One of the cranial nerves that lies at the cerebellopontine angle is:
   A. Vestibulocochlear
   B. Trochlear
   C. Trigeminal
   D. Accessory

Q5. To which structure does the superior brachium connect the superior colliculus?
   A. Medial geniculate body
   B. Cerebellum
   C. Lateral geniculate body
   D. Pulvinar

Q6. The dorsolateral part of medulla oblongata is supplied by which of the following arteries?
   A. Posterior spinal
   B. Basilar
   C. Superior cerebellar
   D. posterior inferior cerebellar

ANSWERS

1. D   2. C   3. B   4. A   5. C   6. D

SHORT NOTES

1. Draw and label the anterior aspect of the brainstem showing the attachments of the cranial nerves
2. Anatomical basis of clinical features of cerebellopontine angle tumour
3. Blood supply of the brainstem

Clinical Cases

4.1: A 50-year-old male developed complete paralysis of all extremities and bilateral facial weakness. His swallowing was impaired, and the patient could not protrude his tongue. Eyes could not move horizontally; only vertical eye movements were maintained. The patient was conscious. Higher mental status was normal. He was able to communicate using eye blinks and vertical eye movements. Sensations tested by simple yes-no questions were intact.
   A. Name the neurological condition.
   B. Specify the blood vessel involved.

4.2: If a patient has paralysis of his right upper limb and left lower limb:
   A. What is this condition called?
   B. Where is the site of lesion?

Chapter 5 — Brainstem: Internal Features

Specific Learning Objectives

At the end of learning, the student shall be able to:

➤ Describe the internal features of medulla oblongata
➤ Draw and label transverse sections (TS) of medulla oblongata at pyramidal decussation, at sensory decussation and at mid-olivary levels
➤ Describe the anatomical basis of clinical syndromes affecting medulla oblongata
➤ Describe the internal features of pons
➤ Draw and label TS of lower pons at the level of facial colliculus and TS upper pons at the level of trigeminal nucleus
➤ Describe the anatomical basis of clinical syndromes affecting pons
➤ Describe the internal features of midbrain
➤ Draw and label TS of midbrain at the level of superior colliculi and at the level of inferior colliculi
➤ Describe the anatomical basis of clinical syndromes affecting midbrain

MEDULLA OBLONGATA

The arrangement of grey and white matter in the lowermost part of medulla is similar to that of spinal cord. However, above this, its internal structure changes gradually. The change in the arrangement of grey and white matter in the upper part of the medulla is mainly due to the presence of the fourth ventricle.

The internal structure of medulla is generally studied at the following levels (Levels A to C in Figure 5.1):
• At the level of the pyramidal decussation
• At the level of the sensory decussation
• At the level of the olivary nucleus

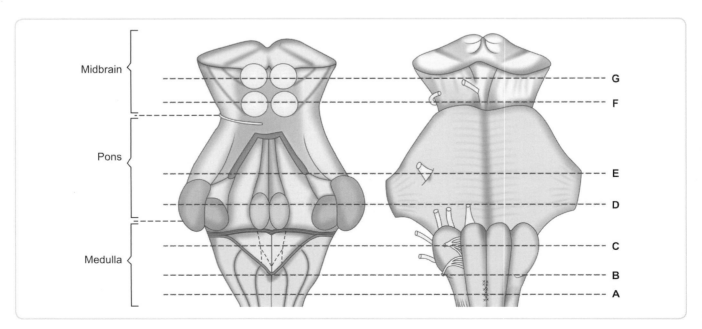

Figure 5.1: Posterior and anterior aspects of brainstem to show the levels of transverse sections (A to G) taken to study its internal features

Clinical Anatomy

Injury to Medulla:
- Injury to the medulla is usually fatal because vital centres controlling the heart and respiration are located here.
- Paralysis due to a lesion in the medulla is called **bulbar palsy**. In this condition, the ninth, tenth, eleventh, and twelfth cranial nerves are affected.
- The tracts are closely packed as they pass through the brainstem. This may result in paralysis of the muscles on the opposite side (due to damage to the corticospinal tract) and loss of sensation of the opposite side (due to damage to ascending sensory tracts).

SECTION THROUGH MEDULLA OBLONGATA AT THE LEVEL OF PYRAMIDAL DECUSSATION (LEVEL A IN FIGURE 5.1)

A section at the level of the pyramidal decussation shows some similarity to sections through the spinal cord.

The **central canal** is surrounded by **central grey matter.** The **ventral grey columns** are present but are separated from the central grey matter by the **decussating pyramidal fibres.**

The area between the ventral grey column and the spinal nucleus of the trigeminal nerve is occupied by a network of fibres and scattered nerve cells called **reticular formation.**

The main structures seen at this level are given in Table 5.1.

The **spinal nucleus of the trigeminal nerve,** when traced inferiorly, reaches the second cervical segment of the spinal cord, where it becomes continuous with the substantia gelatinosa. Above, the nucleus extends as far as the upper part of the pons.

The main descending fibres seen at this level are the **corticospinal fibres,** on their way from the cerebral cortex to the spinal cord. At this level in the medulla, many of these fibres run backward and medially to cross in the midline. These crossing fibres constitute the **decussation**

TABLE 5.1: Section through medulla oblongata at the level of pyramidal decussation (Figure 5.2)

Nuclei	Ascending tracts	Descending tracts
Nucleus gracilis with its tract	Anterior spinothalamic	Corticospinal
Nucleus cuneatus with its tract	Lateral spinothalamic	Medial longitudinal fasciculus
Spinal nucleus of trigeminal with its tract	Anterior spinocerebellar	Tectospinal
Accessory	Posterior spinocerebellar	Vestibulospinal
	Spino-olivary	Olivospinal
	Spinotectal	Rubrospinal

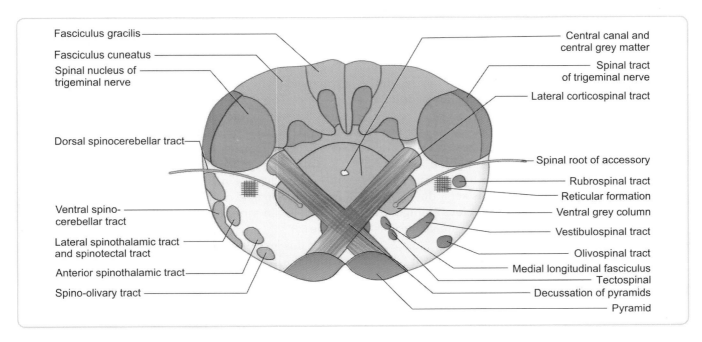

Figure 5.2: Transverse section through the medulla at the level of the pyramidal decussation

of the pyramids. After crossing the midline, these fibres turn downward in the region lateral to the central grey matter to form the **lateral corticospinal tract.** Those fibres of the pyramids that do not cross, descend into the ventral funiculus of the spinal cord to form the **ventral corticospinal tract.**

SECTION THROUGH MEDULLA OBLONGATA AT THE LEVEL OF SENSORY DECUSSATION (LEMNISCAL DECUSSATION) (LEVEL B IN FIGURE 5.1)

The central canal is surrounded by the central grey matter. The nucleus gracilis, the nucleus cuneatus, the spinal nucleus of the trigeminal nerve, and the pyramids occupy the same positions as at lower levels.

The nucleus gracilis and the nucleus cuneatus are, however, much larger and are no longer continuous with the central grey matter. **Internal arcuate fibres** arising in these nuclei arch ventrally and medially around the central grey matter to cross the midline. These crossing fibres constitute the **lemniscal (or sensory) decussation.** After crossing the midline, these fibres turn cranially to constitute the **medial lemniscus.** As the fibres from the nucleus gracilis and the nucleus cuneatus pass ventrally, they cross each other so that the fibres from the nucleus gracilis come to lie ventral to those from the nucleus cuneatus. The most medial fibres (from the legs) lie most anteriorly in the medial lemniscus. These are followed by fibres from the trunk and upper limb in that order.

The **accessory cuneate nucleus** is placed dorsolateral to the cuneate nucleus. It receives proprioceptive impulses from the upper limb through **fasciculus cuneatus.** Efferents of the accessory cuneate nucleus constitute the **posterior external arcuate fibres.** They reach the cerebellum through the **inferior cerebellar peduncle** of the same side.

A number of cranial nerve nuclei can be identified at this level. The **hypoglossal** nucleus is located ventral to the central canal just lateral to the midline. The **dorsal vagal** nucleus lies dorsolateral to the hypoglossal nucleus. The **nucleus of the solitary tract** is seen dorsal to the central canal near the midline. The **nucleus ambiguus** lies in the reticular formation medial to the spinal nucleus of the trigeminal nerve.

The main structures seen at this level are given in Table 5.2.

TABLE 5.2: Section through medulla oblongata at the level of sensory decussation (Figure 5.3)

Nuclei	Ascending tracts	Descending tracts
Gracilis with its tract	Anterior spinothalamic	Corticospinal
Cuneatus (and accessory) with its tract	Lateral spinothalamic	Medial longitudinal fasciculus
Spinal of trigeminal with its tract	Anterior spinocerebellar	Tectospinal
Hypoglossal, dorsal vagal, solitary tract, ambiguus	Posterior spinocerebellar	Vestibulospinal
Inferior olivary and medial accessory	Spino-olivary	Olivospinal
Arcuate	Spinotectal	Rubrospinal

SECTION THROUGH MEDULLA OBLONGATA AT THE LEVEL OF OLIVE (MID-OLIVARY LEVEL) (LEVEL C IN FIGURE 5.1)

The medial lemniscus is, however, much more prominent and is somewhat expanded anteriorly.

Lateral to the spinal nucleus (and tract) of the trigeminal nerve, a large compact bundle of fibres is seen. This is the **inferior cerebellar peduncle,** which connects the medulla to the cerebellum. Posteriorly, the medulla forms the floor of the fourth ventricle.

Several cranial nerve nuclei can be recognized in relation to the floor of the fourth ventricle. From medial to lateral side, these are the **hypoglossal** nucleus, the **dorsal vagal** nucleus, and the **vestibular** nuclei. The **solitary tract** and its nucleus lie ventrolateral to the dorsal vagal nucleus. The nucleus **ambiguus** is located much more ventrally within the reticular formation. The **dorsal and ventral cochlear** nuclei are seen in relation to the inferior cerebellar peduncle.

Other masses of grey matter present are the inferior olivary nuclei, the medial and dorsal accessory olivary nuclei, the arcuate nuclei, and the pontobulbar body.

The main structures seen at this level are given in Table 5.3.

At this level, the **posterior spinocerebellar tract** lies within the inferior cerebellar peduncle.

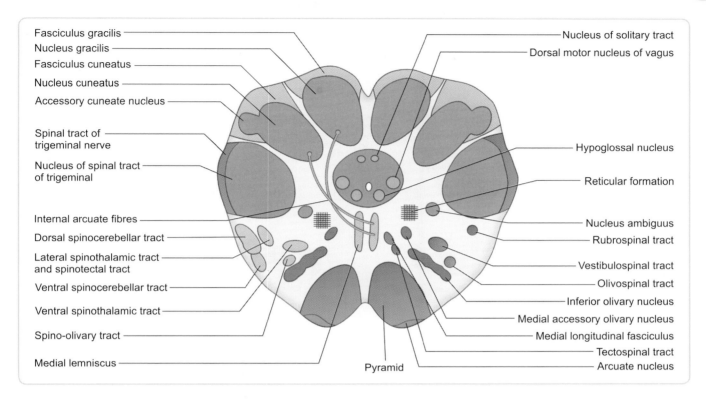

Figure 5.3: Transverse section through the medulla at the level of sensory decussation

Nuclei	Ascending tracts	Descending tracts
Spinal of trigeminal with its tract	Medial lemniscus	Corticospinal
Hypoglossal, dorsal vagal, ambiguus	Anterior spinothalamic	Medial longitudinal fasciculus
Solitary tract, vestibular, cochlear	Lateral spinothalamic	Tectospinal
Arcuate, pontobulbar body	Anterior spinocerebellar	Vestibulospinal
Inferior olivary, medial and dorsal accessory olivary	Spinotectal	Rubrospinal

TABLE 5.3: Section through medulla oblongata at the mid-olivary level (Figure 5.4)

Connections of the Inferior Olivary Complex

Afferent Fibres

The main afferents of the inferior olivary nucleus are from the cerebral cortex and the spinal cord (Figure 5.5).

Efferent Fibres

The main efferents are to the cerebellar cortex through olivocerebellar tract. Other connections of the nucleus are shown in Figure 5.5. The **accessory olivary nuclei** are connected to the cerebellum by **parolivo-cerebellar tract.**

Connections of Arcuate Nuclei and Pontobulbar Body

The **arcuate nuclei** and the **pontobulbar body** are generally regarded as displaced pontine nuclei. So the connections are cortico-arcuato-cerebellar and cortico-pontobulbo-cerebellar.

The arcuate nuclei relay to the cerebellum by fibres which follow two separate pathways. Some of them wind round the anterior and lateral aspect of the medulla as **anterior external arcuate fibres.** Other fibres pass dorsally as fibres of the **striae medullares.** Both reach the inferior cerebellar peduncle of the opposite side.

Fibres arising from pontobulbar body form the **circumolivary bundle.** These fibres join the arcuate nuclei.

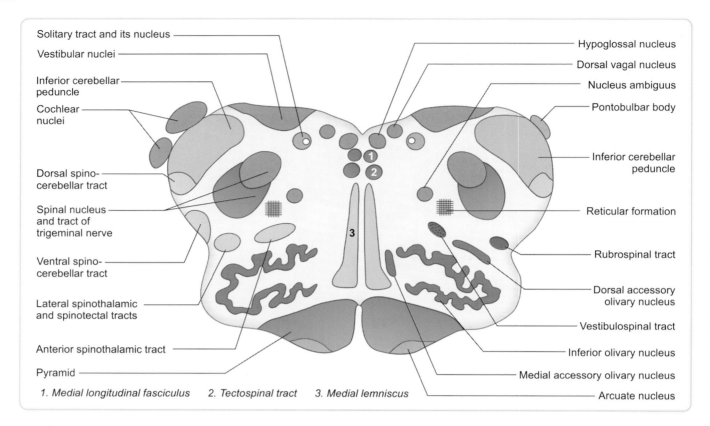

Figure 5.4: Transverse section through the medulla at the level of the olive

Solitary tract and its nucleus

Vestibular nuclei

Inferior cerebellar peduncle

Cochlear nuclei

Dorsal spino-cerebellar tract

Spinal nucleus and tract of trigeminal nerve

Ventral spino-cerebellar tract

Lateral spinothalamic and spinotectal tracts

Anterior spinothalamic tract

Pyramid

Hypoglossal nucleus

Dorsal vagal nucleus

Nucleus ambiguus

Pontobulbar body

Inferior cerebellar peduncle

Reticular formation

Rubrospinal tract

Dorsal accessory olivary nucleus

Vestibulospinal tract

Inferior olivary nucleus

Medial accessory olivary nucleus

Arcuate nucleus

1. Medial longitudinal fasciculus   2. Tectospinal tract   3. Medial lemniscus

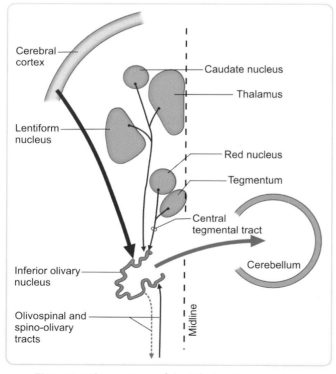

Figure 5.5: Connections of the inferior olivary nucleus

Cerebral cortex

Caudate nucleus

Thalamus

Lentiform nucleus

Red nucleus

Tegmentum

Central tegmental tract

Cerebellum

Inferior olivary nucleus

Olivospinal and spino-olivary tracts

Midline

Clinical Anatomy

Two characteristic syndromes are the **medial medullary syndrome** produced by thrombosis in the anterior spinal artery, and the **lateral medullary syndrome** or **Wallenberg syndrome** produced by thrombosis of the posterior inferior cerebellar artery (Figures 5.6 and 5.7, and Table 5.4).

PONS

The pons is divisible into a **ventral part** (basilar) and a **dorsal part** (tegmentum) (Figure 5.8). The two are separated by **trapezoid body.**

Structure of the Basilar Part of Pons

The ventral (or basilar) part contains numerous transverse and vertical fibres. Amongst the fibres are the groups of cells that constitute the **pontine nuclei** (Figure 5.8).

The Pontine Nuclei

The pontine nuclei are small masses of grey matter scattered between longitudinal and transversely arranged fibres. They form a relay station in the cortico-pontocerebellar

TABLE 5.4: Anatomical basis of clinical syndromes affecting medulla oblongata

Name of the syndrome	Structure affected	Clinical effect produced
Medial medullary syndrome (Dejerine's anterior bulbar syndrome) (Figure 5.6)	Corticospinal fibres (pyramids)	Contralateral hemiplegia
	Hypoglossal nucleus and nerve fibres	Ipsilateral (lower motor neuron type) paralysis of muscles of tongue (on protrusion, tongue deviates to the side of lesion)
	Medial lemniscus	Contralateral loss of sensation of fine touch, sense of movement and sense of position
Lateral medullary syndrome (Wallenberg syndrome or posterior inferior cerebellar artery syndrome (PICA) syndrome) (Figure 5.7)	Inferior cerebellar peduncle	Loss of equilibrium (ataxia) and giddiness
	Lateral spinothalamic tract	Loss of sensation of pain and temperature over the contralateral half of the body
	Spinal nucleus and tract of the trigeminal nerve	Loss of sensation of pain and temperature over the ipsilateral half of the head and face
	Nucleus ambiguus	Difficulty in swallowing (dysphagia) and in speech (dysarthria)
	Vestibular nuclei	Vomiting, nystagmus and vertigo
	Descending autonomic fibres	Ipsilateral Horner's syndrome characterized by ptosis, miosis, enophthalmos, anhydrosis and loss of ciliospinal reflex

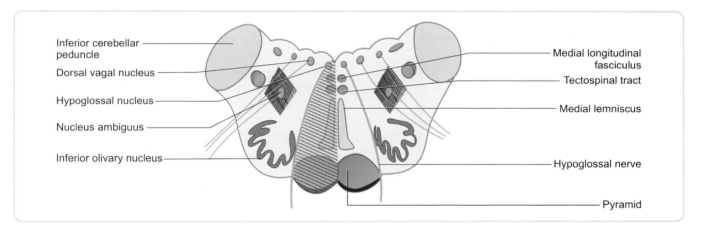

Figure 5.6: Occlusion of medullary branches of anterior spinal artery which causes medial medullary syndrome (shaded area)

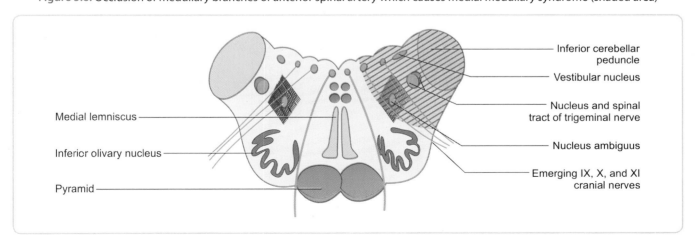

Figure 5.7: Occlusion of posterior inferior cerebellar artery which causes lateral medullary syndrome (shaded area)

pathway, i.e. between the cerebral cortex and contralateral cerebellar hemisphere. They receive corticopontine fibres from the frontal, temporal, parietal and occipital lobes of the cerebrum.

Their efferents form the transverse fibres of the pons known as pontocerebellar fibres which pass through middle cerebellar peduncle and terminate in the cerebellum of opposite side. It has been estimated that there are about 20 million neurons in pontine nuclei. Most of them are glutaminergic (excitatory).

Descending Longitudinal Fibres

The descending longitudinal fibres (Figure 5.8) consist of:
- **Corticospinal fibres** as they traverse the pons and converge again to form pyramid in medulla
- **Corticonuclear fibres** terminate in the contralateral (and to some ipsilateral and some bilateral) motor nuclei of the cranial nerves

Transverse Pontine Fibres

Transverse fibres arise in the pontine nuclei and cross to the opposite side to form the middle cerebellar peduncle. These are pontocerebellar fibres.

Trapezoid Body

Trapezoid body separates the basilar and the tegmental parts of the pons. It consists of decussating fibres of

cochlear nuclei and thus is a part of auditory pathway. The fibres which cross in the trapezoid body ascend up as lateral lemniscus.

Structure of the Tegmental Part of Pons

The dorsal part (or tegmentum) of the pons is an upward continuation of the part of the medulla behind the pyramids. Superiorly, it is continuous with the tegmentum of the midbrain. It is bounded posteriorly by the fourth ventricle. Laterally, it is related to the inferior cerebellar peduncles in its lower part (Figure 5.9) and to the superior cerebellar peduncles in its upper part (Figure 5.12).

The region adjoining the ventral part (of the pons) is occupied by important ascending tracts. The medial lemniscus occupies a transversely elongated oval area next to the midline. The cervical fibres lie medially and sacral fibres lie laterally. Lateral to this are the trigeminal and the spinal lemniscus. The fibres of the spinotectal tract run along with the spinal lemniscus, while those of the anterior spinothalamic tract join the medial lemniscus. Still more laterally, there is lateral lemniscus.

The ventral spinocerebellar tract lies ventromedial to the inferior cerebellar peduncle in the lower part of the pons (Figure 5.9). In the upper part of the pons, it joins the superior cerebellar peduncle (Figure 5.12).

Descending tracts passing through the dorsal part of the pons are the tectospinal tract and the rubrospinal tract. The medial longitudinal fasciculus lies dorsally near the midline.

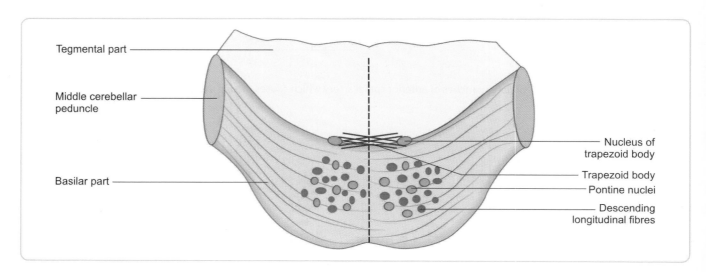

Figure 5.8: Diagrammatic representation of lower part of the pons showing the basilar part of pons lying ventral to the trapezoid body and the tegmental part of the pons lying dorsal to it

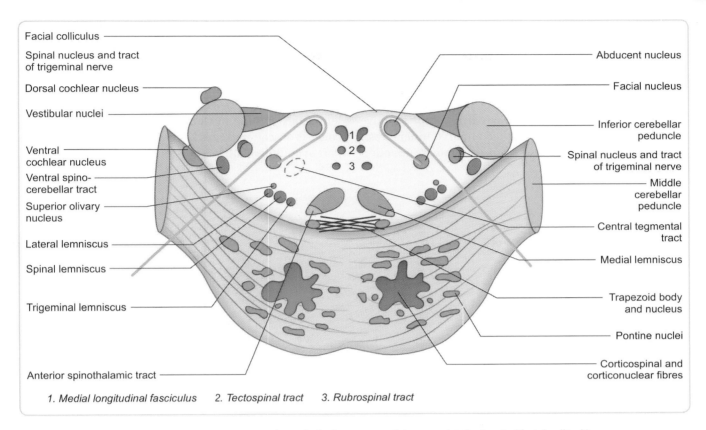

Facial colliculus

Spinal nucleus and tract of trigeminal nerve

Dorsal cochlear nucleus

Vestibular nuclei

Ventral cochlear nucleus

Ventral spino-cerebellar tract

Superior olivary nucleus

Lateral lemniscus

Spinal lemniscus

Trigeminal lemniscus

Anterior spinothalamic tract

Abducent nucleus

Facial nucleus

Inferior cerebellar peduncle

Spinal nucleus and tract of trigeminal nerve

Middle cerebellar peduncle

Central tegmental tract

Medial lemniscus

Trapezoid body and nucleus

Pontine nuclei

Corticospinal and corticonuclear fibres

1. Medial longitudinal fasciculus   2. Tectospinal tract   3. Rubrospinal tract

Figure 5.9: Transverse section through the lower part of the pons (at the level of facial colliculi)

The cranial nerve nuclei of the tegmentum are different in the upper and lower parts of pons. Hence, it is customary to study the internal structure of pons at two different levels—lower part, transverse section passing through the facial colliculi and upper part, transverse section passing through trigeminal nuclei (Levels D and E in Figure 5.1).

This section (Figure 5.9) shows the **abducent** and the **vestibular** nuclei lying in the floor of the fourth ventricle. At a deeper level in the lateral part of the reticular formation, two additional nuclei are seen. These are the **spinal nucleus** of the trigeminal nerve (along with its tract) and the **facial** nucleus. The **dorsal and ventral cochlear** nuclei lie dorsal and ventral, respectively to the inferior cerebellar peduncle.

┌─ **Clinical Anatomy** ─────────────

Pontine Haemorrhage
Haemorrhage into the pons leads to coma (and is often fatal). The reticular formation and the autonomic fibres from hypothalamus are affected. Apart from coma, the condition is marked by pin point pupils and hyperpyrexia. Bilateral facial paralysis and paralysis of all four limbs can occur if the haemorrhage is extensive. (**PPP-P**inpoint pupils, **P**yrexia and **P**aralysis).

SECTION THROUGH LOWER PART OF PONS (AT THE LEVEL OF FACIAL COLLICULI)

The transverse section through the lower part of pons corresponds to the level of facial colliculi (Level D in Figure 5.1).

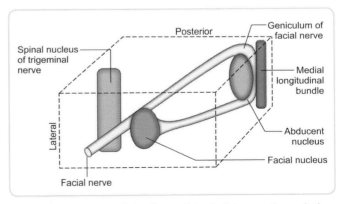

Spinal nucleus of trigeminal nerve

Posterior

Geniculum of facial nerve

Medial longitudinal bundle

Abducent nucleus

Facial nucleus

Lateral

Facial nerve

Figure 5.10: Course of the fibres of the facial nerve through the pons and formation of the facial colliculus

The facial nerve fibres loop around the abducent nucleus **(internal genu of facial nerve).** These together form a surface elevation, the **facial colliculus** (Figure 5.10), in the floor of the fourth ventricle. The unusual course of the facial nerve fibres is an example of neurobiotaxis. Facial nucleus communicates with trigeminal nucleus to complete the reflex arc. (Trigeminal carries proprioceptive fibres from facial muscles that facial nerve innervates.) The facial nerve fibres also want to retain connection with medial longitudinal fasciculus. (Medial longitudinal fasciculus coordinates lip movements and tongue movements during articulation.)

Other masses of grey matter to be seen in the lower part of the pons are the **superior olivary complex** (made up of several nuclei), which lies dorsomedial to the lateral lemniscus and the nuclei of the **trapezoid body,** which consists of scattered cells lying within this body. These are part of auditory pathway and reflexes.

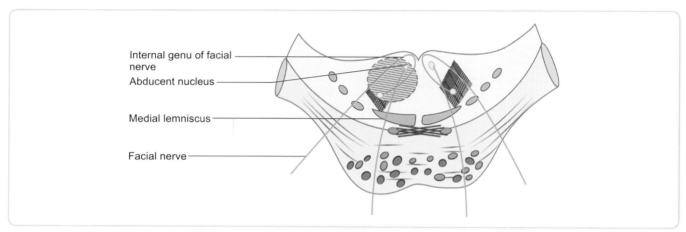

Figure 5.11: Schematic diagram to show Foville syndrome (shaded area)

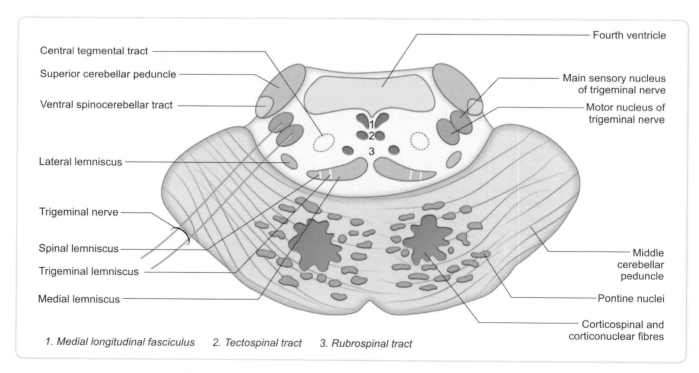

1. *Medial longitudinal fasciculus*   2. *Tectospinal tract*   3. *Rubrospinal tract*

Figure 5.12: Transverse section through the upper part of the pons

Foville Syndrome (Figure 5.11)
- The lesion is in dorsomedial pons involving facial nerve nucleus and fibres, abducent nucleus, and (close to abducent nucleus) paramedian pontine reticular formation for horizontal conjugate gaze.
- It results in ipsilateral facial paralysis, ipsilateral conjugate gaze paralysis (ipsilateral lateral rectus and contralateral medial rectus). Convergence for accommodation by both medial recti are normal.

SECTION THROUGH UPPER PART OF PONS (AT THE LEVEL OF TRIGEMINAL NERVE)

The transverse section through the upper part of pons passes through **the motor and principal sensory nuclei** of the trigeminal nerve (Level E in Figure 5.1).

At this level (Figure 5.12), main sensory nucleus of the trigeminal nerve lies laterally and the motor nucleus lies medially.

Raymond Syndrome (Figure 5.13A)
Basal pontine vascular occlusions involving abducent nerve fibres (ipsilateral lateral rectus palsy) and descending corticospinal fibres (contralateral hemiplegia).

Millard-Gubler Syndrome (Fig. 5.13B)
- Basal pontine vascular occlusions involving facial nerve fibres (ipsilateral facial palsy) and descending corticospinal fibres (contralateral hemiplegia)
- In Millard-Gubler syndrome, if lesion is **extensive**, it will also include abducent nerve fibres (ipsilateral lateral rectus palsy).

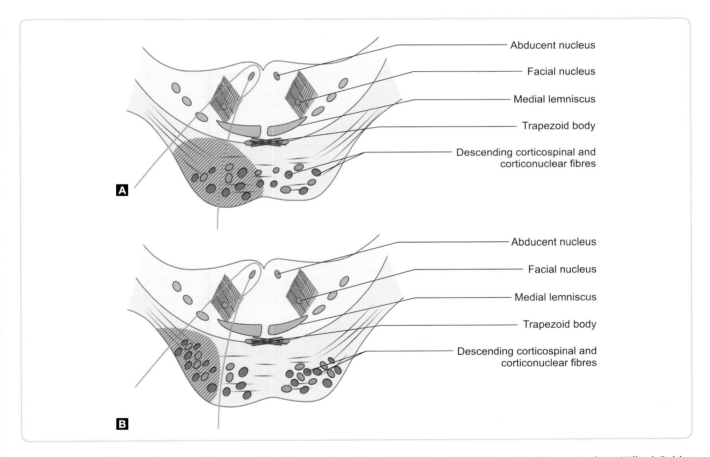

Figures 5.13A and B: (A) Schematic diagram to show Raymond syndrome (shaded area); (B) Schematic diagram to show Millard-Gubler syndrome (shaded area)

MIDBRAIN

For convenience of description, the midbrain may be divided as follows (Flowchart 5.1 and Figure 5.14).

The part lying dorsal to a transverse line drawn through the cerebral aqueduct is called the **tectum.** It consists of the **superior and inferior colliculi** of the two sides. Therefore, it is also called **corpora quadrigemina.** The part lying ventral to the transverse line is made up of right and left halves called the **cerebral peduncles.** Each peduncle consists of three parts. From anterior to posterior, these are the **crus cerebri** (also called **basis pedunculi**), the **substantia nigra,** and the **tegmentum.**

Crus Cerebri

The crus cerebri consists of a large mass of vertically running fibres, which descend from the cerebral cortex. The fibres in the crus cerebri consist of the following:

- Corticopontine fibres
- Corticospinal fibres
- Corticonuclear fibres

Flowchat 5.1: Parts of midbrain

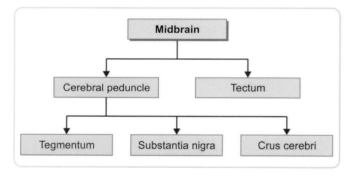

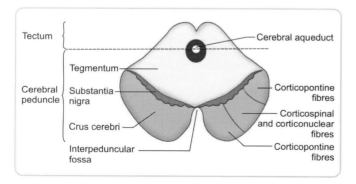

Figure 5.14: Transverse section of the midbrain showing its main subdivisions

Its medial one-sixth is occupied by frontopontine fibres and the lateral one-sixth is occupied by tempopontine, parietopontine and occipitopontine fibres. The intermediate two-thirds of the crus cerebri are occupied by corticospinal and corticonuclear fibres (Figure 5.14). The fibres for the head are most medial and those for the leg are most lateral.

Substantia Nigra

The substantia nigra lies immediately behind and medial to the crus cerebri (Figure 5.14). It appears dark in unstained sections, as neurons within it contain a pigment (**neuromelanin**). The substantia nigra is divisible into a dorsal part, the **pars compacta** and a ventral part, the **pars reticularis**. The substantia nigra is closely connected, functionally, with the corpus striatum.

Connections of Substantia Nigra

The main connections (both afferent and efferent) of substantia nigra are with the striatum (i.e. caudate nucleus and putamen). Dopamine produced by neurons in the substantia nigra (pars compacta) passes along their axons to the striatum (**mesostriatal dopamine system**).

> **Clinical Anatomy**
>
> Dopamine is much reduced in patients with a disease called **Parkinsonism,** in which there is degeneration of the substantia nigra. It is characterized by akinesia, rigidity, and tremors.

The midbrain is traversed by the cerebral aqueduct, which is surrounded by central grey matter. Ventrally, the central grey matter is related to cranial nerve nuclei (oculomotor and trochlear) and dorsolaterally to the mesencephalic nucleus of trigeminal nerve (Figure 5.15). The region between the substantia nigra and the central grey matter is occupied by the reticular formation.

Tegmentum

The tegmentum is the region of midbrain that lies between substantia nigra and tectum (Figure 5.14).

The tegmentum contains important masses of grey matter as well as fibre bundles. The largest of the nuclei is the **red nucleus** (Figure 5.17) present in the upper half of the midbrain. The tegmentum also contains the **reticular formation,** which is continuous below with that of the pons and medulla.

The internal structure of tegmentum and tectum varies at different levels of midbrain; hence, the internal structure of midbrain is studied by transverse sections at two different levels—lower part, transverse section passing through the inferior colliculi and upper part, transverse section passing through superior colliculi (Levels F and G in Figure 5.1).

SECTION THROUGH MIDBRAIN AT THE LEVEL OF INFERIOR COLLICULI (LEVEL F IN FIGURE 5.1)

A section through the midbrain at the level of the inferior colliculus shows the following features (Figure 5.15).

The **trochlear nucleus** lies in the ventral part of the central grey matter. Fibres arising in this nucleus follow an unusual course. They run dorsally and decussate (in the superior medullary velum) before emerging on the dorsal aspect of the brainstem.

The **mesencephalic nucleus of the trigeminal nerve** lies in the lateral part of the central grey matter.

A compact bundle of fibres lies in the tegmentum dorsal to the substantia nigra. It consists of the medial lemniscus, the trigeminal lemniscus, and the spinal lemniscus in that order from medial to lateral side. The lateral lemniscus merges with the inferior colliculus.

Important fibre bundles are also located near the midline of the tegmentum. The medial longitudinal fasciculus lies ventral to the trochlear nucleus, followed by tectospinal tract, decussation of superior cerebellar peduncle and rubrospinal tracts.

The **inferior colliculus** is a large mass of grey matter lying in the tectum. It forms a cell station in the auditory pathway and is probably concerned with reflexes involving the auditory stimuli.

Connections of Inferior Colliculus

The inferior colliculus is an important relay centre in the auditory pathway and auditory reflexes.

Afferent Fibres

It receives fibres of the lateral lemniscus and from superior olivary complex (Flowchart 5.2 and Figure 5.16). Each colliculus receives auditory impulses from both the ears.

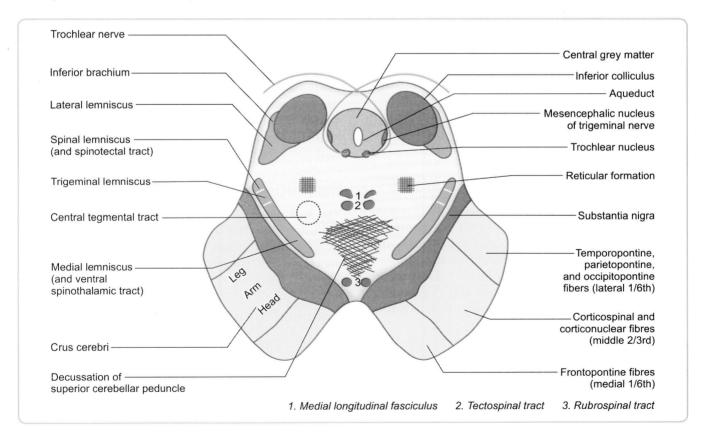

1. *Medial longitudinal fasciculus*   2. *Tectospinal tract*   3. *Rubrospinal tract*

Figure 5.15: Transverse section through the lower part of the midbrain at the level of inferior colliculus

Flowchart 5.2: Depicting connections of inferior colliculus

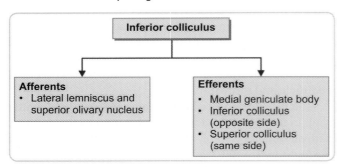

Figure 5.16: Connections of the inferior colliculus

SECTION THROUGH MIDBRAIN AT THE LEVEL OF SUPERIOR COLLICULI (LEVEL G IN FIGURE 5.1)

A section through the upper part of the midbrain (Figure 5.17) shows two large oval masses of grey matter not seen at lower levels. These are the **red nuclei** in the tegmentum.

The **oculomotor** nucleus lies in relation to the ventral part of the central grey matter. The nuclei of the two sides lie close together forming a single complex. The **Edinger-Westphal (accessory oculomotor)** nucleus (which supplies the sphincter pupillae and ciliaris muscle) forms part of the oculomotor complex. The oculomotor complex is related ventrally to the medial longitudinal fasciculus (Figure 5.17).

Closely related to the cranial part of the superior colliculus, there is a small collection of neurons that constitute the **pretectal nucleus.** This nucleus is concerned with the pathway for the pupillary light reflex. It receives retinal fibres through the optic tract. The main efferents of the nucleus reach the oculomotor nuclei (of both sides).

The bundle of ascending fibres consisting of the medial lemniscus, the trigeminal lemniscus and the spinal lemniscus lies more laterally than at lower levels (because of the presence of the red nucleus). The lateral lemniscus has already ended in the inferior colliculus.

The region of the tegmentum near the midline shows two groups of decussating fibres. The **dorsal tegmental decussation** starts from superior colliculus to form tectospinal tract. The **ventral tegmental decussation** starts from red nucleus and form rubrospinal tract.

Red Nucleus

The **red nucleus** contains an iron oxide giving it a reddish colour. It is an important motor nucleus of the extrapyramidal system. The connections of the red nucleus are considered below and are shown in Flowchart 5.3 and Figure 5.18.

Connections of Red Nucleus

Afferent Fibres

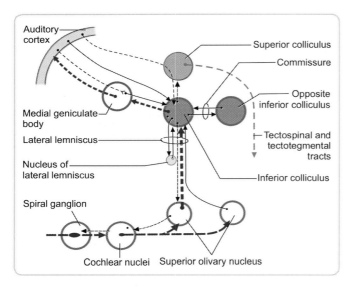

Efferent Fibres

Auditory impulses from inferior colliculus are relayed to the medial geniculate body (the fibres passing through the inferior brachium) and from there, to the auditory (acoustic) area of the cerebral cortex. Some efferents from the inferior colliculus terminate in the contralateral inferior colliculus (Flowchart 5.2 and Figure 5.16).

Efferents from the inferior colliculus also project to the superior colliculus of the same side. The superior colliculus, in turn, sends these auditory signals to the spinal cord via tectospinal tracts.

Clinical Anatomy

Lesions of the inferior colliculus produce defects in appreciation of tones, localization of sound, and reflex movements in response to sound.

- Motor and premotor cortex
- Cerebellum
- Corpus striatum
- Tectum

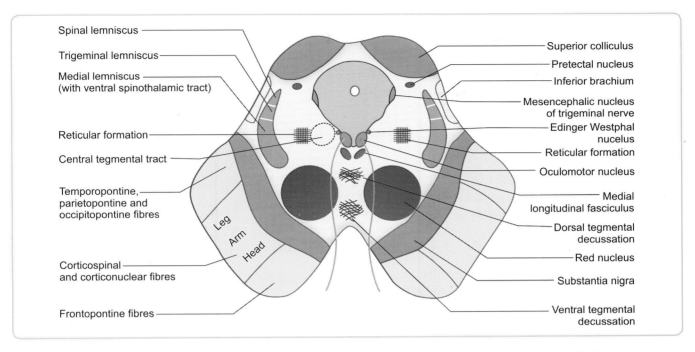

Figure 5.17: Transverse section through the upper part of the midbrain at the level of superior colliculi

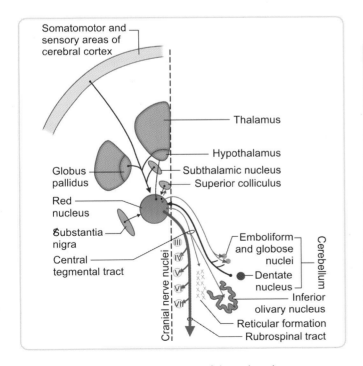

Figure 5.18: Connections of the red nucleus

Flowchart 5.3: The connections of the red nucleus

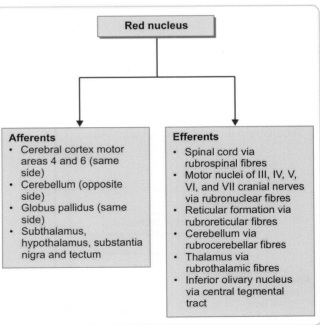

Red nucleus

Afferents
- Cerebral cortex motor areas 4 and 6 (same side)
- Cerebellum (opposite side)
- Globus pallidus (same side)
- Subthalamus, hypothalamus, substantia nigra and tectum

Efferents
- Spinal cord via rubrospinal fibres
- Motor nuclei of III, IV, V, VI, and VII cranial nerves via rubronuclear fibres
- Reticular formation via rubroreticular fibres
- Cerebellum via rubrocerebellar fibres
- Thalamus via rubrothalamic fibres
- Inferior olivary nucleus via central tegmental tract

Efferent Fibres

- Spinal cord (rubrospinal tract)
- Cranial nerve motor nuclei III, IV, V, VI, and VII (rubronuclear)
- Inferior olivary nucleus (through central tegmental tract)
- Reticular formation (rubroreticular)
- Thalamus (rubrothalamic)

Superior Colliculus

The **superior colliculus** is a centre concerned with visual reflexes. Its connections are shown in Flowchart 5.4 and 5.19.

Connections of Superior Colliculus

The superior colliculus has a complex laminar structure, being made up of alternating layers of white and grey matter.

Afferent Fibres (Flowchart 5.4 and Figure 5.19)

- Retina
- Spinal cord (pain and tactile fibres) through spinotectal tract
- Frontal and occipital visual cortex (for conjugate eye movements)
- Inferior colliculus

Efferent Fibres

- Tectospinal tract and tectobulbar tract to the nuclei of cranial nerves, responsible for moving the eyes and head
- Tectotegmental tract to the brainstem (red nucleus, substantia nigra and reticular formation)
- Tectocerebellar tract to cerebellar cortex

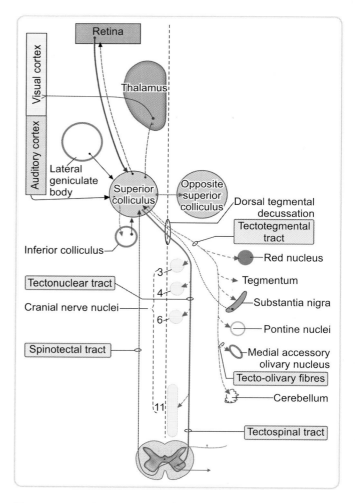

Figure 5.19: Connections of the superior colliculus—the connections to the visual cortex through the thalamus provide an extrageniculate retinocortical pathway

MEDIAL LONGITUDINAL FASCICULUS

The medial longitudinal fasciculus (MLF) consists of fibres arising mainly from vestibular nuclei in the medulla. The fasciculus is closely related and connected to the motor nuclei of:

- Third, fourth, sixth (vestibulo-ocular reflex—doll's eye movement)
- Seventh, twelfth (lip and tongue coordination for articulation)
- Eleventh and upper cervical nerves (head righting reflex)

Fibres of medial longitudinal fasciculus of each side cross the midline at the posterior commissure.

Flowchart 5.4: Connections of the superior colliculus

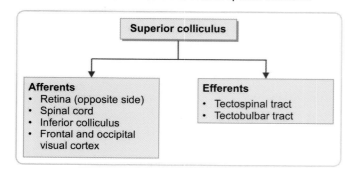

Clinical Anatomy

The anatomical basis of clinical syndromes affecting midbrain are seen in Table 5.5.

TABLE 5.5: Anatomical basis of clinical syndromes affecting midbrain

Name of the syndrome	Structures affected	Clinical effects produced
Weber syndrome (Fig. 5.20)	Corticospinal tract	Contralateral hemiplegia
	Oculomotor nerve	Ipsilateral lower motor neuron type oculomotor nerve palsy with lateral squint
Benedikt syndrome (Fig. 5.21)	Oculomotor nerve rootlets	Ipsilateral lower motor neuron type oculomotor nerve palsy with lateral squint
	Red nucleus	Contralateral coarse tremors
	Medial lemniscus	Contralateral hemianaesthesia
Parinaud syndrome	Nucleus of posterior commissure	Upward gaze palsy

Clinical Anatomy

Alternating Hemiplegias
These occur when the descending corticospinal fibres along with the cranial nerve fibres get affected due to vascular occlusion. Such a lesion, seen in the brainstem vascular occlusions, results in contralateral hemiplegia and ipsilateral paralysis of the cranial nerve. These are called **alternating hemiplegias** or **crossed hemiplegias** (Table 5.6).

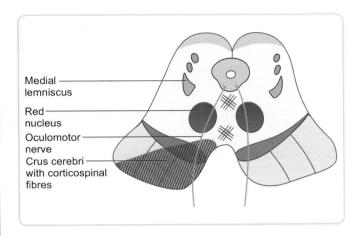

Figure 5.20: Weber syndrome (shaded area)

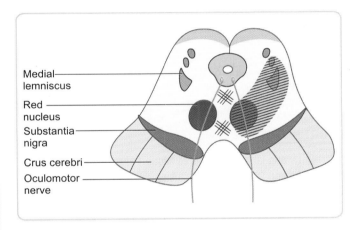

Figure 5.21: Benedikt syndrome (shaded area)

TABLE 5.6: Alternating hemiplegias

Site of lesion	Clinical effects produced	Name of the syndrome
Medial part of medulla	Ipsilateral hypoglossal nerve paralysis and contralateral hemiplegia	Dejerine's anterior bulbar syndrome
Medial basal pons	Ipsilateral abducent nerve paralysis and contralateral hemiplegia	Raymond syndrome
Lateral basal pons	Ipsilateral facial nerve paralysis and contralateral hemiplegia	Millard-Gubler syndrome
Crus cerebri of midbrain	Ipsilateral oculomotor nerve paralysis and contralateral hemiplegia	Weber syndrome

MULTIPLE CHOICE QUESTIONS

Q1. Which of the following tracts decussates at the level of superior colliculus of midbrain?
- A. Dentatothalamic
- B. Cerebellorubral
- C. Tectospinal
- D. Medial longitudinal fasciculus

Q2. If a patient presents with left sided hemiplegia and right-sided lateral squint, the lesion is likely to be at the level of:
- A. Right lower pons
- B. Left upper midbrain
- C. Right upper midbrain
- D. Left lower pons

Q3. The structure separating the basilar and tegmental parts of the pons is:
- A. Substantia nigra
- B. Trapezoid body
- C. Vestibular nucleus
- D. Striae medullares

Q4. The fibres that decussate in the trapezoid body originate from which of the following nuclei?
- A. Arcuate
- B. Vestibular
- C. Inferior olivary
- D. Cochlear

Q5. The fibres passing through the middle cerebellar peduncle originate from:
- A. Pontine nuclei
- B. Tectum
- C. Spinal cord
- D. Spinal trigeminal nucleus

Q6. Frontopontine fibres pass through which part of midbrain?
- A. Dorsal tegmentum
- B. Medial part of crus cerebri
- C. Ventral tegmentum
- D. Lateral part of crus cerebri

Q7. Which type of sensations is carried by the spinal lemniscus?
- A. Pain
- B. Unconscious proprioception
- C. Vibration
- D. Tactile localization

ANSWERS

1. C   2. C   3. B   4. D   5. A   6. B   7. A

SHORT NOTES

1. Draw and label a transverse section of medulla oblongata at the level of motor/pyramidal decussation
2. Draw and label a transverse section of medulla oblongata at the level of sensory decussation
3. Draw and label a transverse section of medulla oblongata at the mid-olivary level
4. Draw and label a transverse section of pons at the level of facial colliculi
5. Draw and label a transverse section of upper part of pons
6. Draw and label a transverse section of midbrain at the level of inferior colliculi
7. Draw and label a transverse section of midbrain at the level of superior colliculi

Clinical Cases

5.1: A 45-year-old male developed inability to move his left upper limb and left lower limb. His tongue deviated to right side on putting out.
- A. Specify the anatomical basis of these clinical features.
- B. Specify the level and the side of lesion.

5.2: A 35-year-old male developed (i) inability to move his right upper and right lower limbs, (ii) loss of wrinkles on left half of face, (iii) deviation of mouth to right side
- A. Specify the anatomical basis of these clinical features.
- B. Specify the level of lesion and name the condition.

5.3: A 50-year-old female developed (i) loss of pain and temperature sensation on right half of the body, (ii) loss of pain and temperature sensation on left half of the face, (iii) had giddiness
- A. Specify the anatomical basis of these clinical features.
- B. Specify the site and side of lesion.

5.4: A 40-year-old female suddenly developed (i) inability to move her left upper limb and left lower limb, (ii) double vision and right divergent (lateral) squint
- A. Specify the anatomical structures involved.
- B. Specify the level of lesion and name the condition.

Chapter 6 | Cranial Nerves

Specific Learning Objectives

At the end of learning, the student shall be able to:
- Describe the location of nuclei and functional components of twelve cranial nerves
- Describe the cortical control of cranial nerve nuclei supplying skeletal muscles
- Describe course, distribution, and clinical anatomy of the cranial nerves

INTRODUCTION

A peripheral nerve may be motor (efferent), sensory (afferent), or mixed (efferent and afferent). They may supply soma (somatic) or viscera (visceral). Thus, functionally, a spinal nerve has four functional components—(1) somatic efferent, (2) visceral efferent, (3) somatic afferent and (4) visceral afferent.

Cranial nerves, in addition, supply muscles of pharyngeal arches (**special visceral efferent**), and carry **visceral and somatic special senses**, making a total of seven functional components (four general, mentioned earlier, and three special). No spinal nerve carries special functional components.

There are 12 pairs of cranial nerves (Figures 6.1A and B)

I	–	Olfactory
II	–	Optic
III	–	Oculomotor
IV	–	Trochlear
V	–	Trigeminal
VI	–	Abducent
VII	–	Facial
VIII	–	Vestibulocochlear
IX	–	Glossopharyngeal

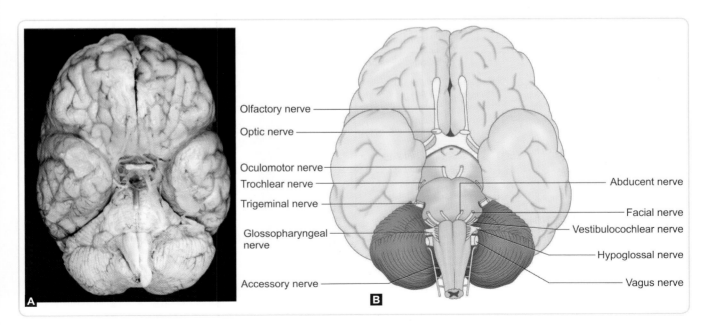

Olfactory nerve
Optic nerve
Oculomotor nerve
Trochlear nerve
Trigeminal nerve
Glossopharyngeal nerve
Accessory nerve
Abducent nerve
Facial nerve
Vestibulocochlear nerve
Hypoglossal nerve
Vagus nerve

Figures 6.1A and B: Cranial nerves at the base of the brain: (A) Specimen; (B) Diagrammatic presentation

X   – Vagus (Vagoaccessory)
XI*   – Spinal accessory
XII – Hypoglossal

*The eleventh cranial nerve is traditionally described as "accessory" which has a cranial part and spinal part. The cranial accessory is the motor (branchiomotor) part of vagus (hence, the tenth nerve should be correctly called vagoaccessory). The spinal accessory is an independent nerve.

Developmental Aspects

In the embryo, the nuclei related to the various components are arranged in vertical rows (or columns) in a definite sequence in the grey matter related to the floor of the fourth ventricle (Figure 6.2). The sequence is easily remembered, if the following facts are kept in mind:

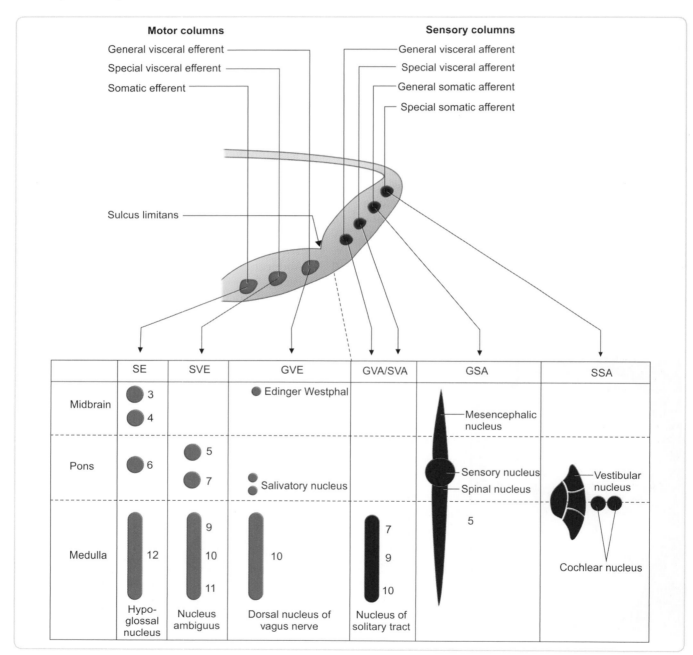

Figure 6.2 : Functional classification of cranial nerve nuclei. The upper figure shows the arrangement of nuclear columns in the brainstem of the embryo. The lower figure shows the nuclei derived from each column. Numbers indicate the cranial nerves connected to the nuclei (*Abbreviations*: SVE, special visceral efferent; GVE, general visceral efferent; GVA, general visceral afferent; SVA, special visceral afferent; GSA, general somatic afferent; SSA, special somatic afferent; SE, somatic efferent)

TABLE 6.1: Nuclear columns in basal and alar lamina	
Nuclear columns of basal lamina	**Nuclear columns of alar lamina**
Somatic efferent	General visceral afferent
Special visceral efferent	Special visceral afferent
General visceral efferent	General somatic afferent
	Special somatic afferent

- Each half of the floor of the ventricle is divided into a medial part and a lateral part by the **sulcus limitans. Efferent nuclei** lie in the medial part (called the **basal lamina**) and **afferent nuclei** in the lateral part (called the **alar lamina**) (Table 6.1).
- In each part (medial or lateral), **visceral nuclei** lie nearer the sulcus limitans than **somatic nuclei.**
- Within each category (for example, visceral efferents, somatic afferents, etc.), the **general nucleus** lies nearer the sulcus limitans than the **special nucleus.**
- Thus, in proceeding laterally from the midline, the sequence of nuclear columns is as follows:
  - Somatic efferent: This column is **not subdivided** into general and special parts
  - Special visceral (or branchial) efferent
  - General visceral efferent
  - General visceral afferent
  - Special visceral afferent
  - General somatic afferent
  - Special somatic afferent

Each functional component has its own nuclei of origin (in the case of efferent fibres) or termination (in the case of afferent fibres).

As development proceeds, parts of these columns disappear, so that each of them no longer extend to the whole length of the brainstem, but is represented by one or more discrete nuclei. These nuclei are shown schematically in the lower half of Figure 6.2. Some nuclei retain their original positions in relation to the floor of the fourth ventricle, but some others migrate deeper into the brainstem. The position of the nuclei relative to the posterior surface of the brainstem is illustrated in Figure 6.3. The positions of the nuclei as seen in transverse sections of the brainstem are shown in Figures 6.4A to F.

The olfactory and the optic nerves are not true nerves. They are extensions of telencephalon and diencephalon, respectively. They carry the cavity of the brain (which secondarily gets obliterated) and the meninges with them. They are not covered by Schwann cells. The myelinated parts of the pathways are formed by oligodendrocytes.

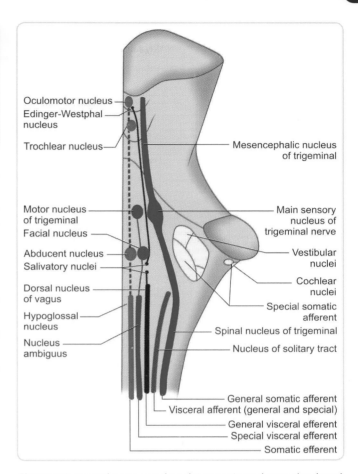

Figure 6.3: Cranial nerves and nuclei as projected onto the dorsal aspect of the brainstem

In the description that follows, the nuclei of the third to twelfth cranial nerves are considered as they are located in the brainstem. The cranial nerves **III and IV belong to the midbrain; V, VI, VII, and part of VIII to the pons;** and **IX, X, XI, XII to the medulla.**

ORGANIZATION OF FUNCTIONAL COMPONENTS OF CRANIAL NERVE NUCLEI

The functional components of cranial nerve nuclei are shown in Table 6.2. It should be noted that some of these **nuclei contribute fibres for more than one nerve.** Similarly, some of the cranial nerves consist of fibres arising from more than one nucleus.

The motor cranial nerve nuclei are under cortical control through corticonuclear fibres (Table 6.3).

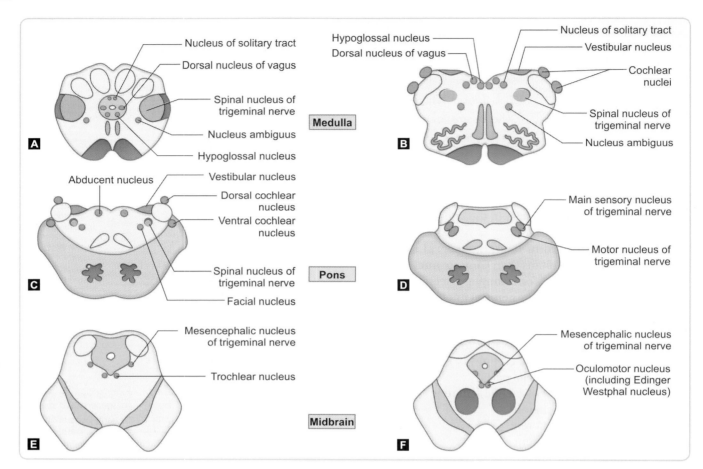

Figures 6.4A to F: Location of cranial nerve nuclei as seen in transverse sections at various levels of the brainstem

Location	Motor (Efferent)			Sensory (Afferent)		
	SE	SVE	GVE	GVA/SVA	GSA	SSA
Midbrain	Oculomotor (III) Trochlear (IV)		Edinger–Westphal nucleus (III)		Mesencephalic nucleus of trigeminal nerve (V)	
Pons	Abducent (VI)	Motor nucleus of trigeminal nerve (V) Facial (VII)	Salivatory nuclei (VII, IX)		Sensory nucleus of trigeminal nerve (V)	Vestibulo-cochlear nuclei (VIII)
Medulla	Hypoglossal nucleus (XII)	Nucleus ambiguus (IX, X, Cr XI)	Dorsal nucleus of vagus (X)	Nucleus of the solitary tract (VII, IX, X)	Nucleus of the spinal tract of the trigeminal nerve (V)	Vestibulo-cochlear nuclei (VIII)
Spinal cord		Spinal accessory (Sp XI)				

TABLE 6.2: The functional nuclear columns and cranial nerve nuclei

Abbreviations: SE, somatic efferent; SVE, special visceral efferent; GVE, general visceral efferent; GVA, general visceral afferent; SVA, special visceral afferent; GSA, general somatic afferent; SSA, special somatic afferent; Cr, cranial; Sp, spinal

TABLE 6.3: Cortical control of nuclei supplying skeletal muscles

S. No.	Nucleus	Cortical control*
1	Oculomotor (all muscles except medial rectus)	Bilateral
2	Oculomotor (medial rectus)†	Ipsilateral
3	Trochlear	Bilateral
4	Trigeminal	Bilateral
5	Abducent	Contralateral
6	Facial (supplying upper face)	Bilateral
7	Facial (supplying lower face)	Contralateral
8	Glossopharyngeal	Bilateral
9	Vagus (including cranial accessory)	Bilateral
10	Spinal accessory (supplying sternocleidomastoid)‡	Ipsilateral
11	Spinal accessory (supplying trapezius)	Contralateral
12	Hypoglossal	Bilateral

* Cortical/capsular hemiplegia, normally, does not paralyze eye movements, jaw movements, soft palate, pharynx, larynx, and tongue. If they do get affected, then there would be a history of an earlier hemiplegia/hemiparesis of the opposite side which had subsequently resolved. The new lesion suddenly unmasks the loss of cortical control for the bilaterally-controlled cranial nerve nuclei concerned.

† Medial rectus acts conjugately with opposite lateral rectus to cause the eye to move to the opposite side. However, during convergence (for accommodation), medial rectus is controlled by the cortex bilaterally.

‡ The apparent contradiction of cortical control for sternocleidomastoid is evident in capsular hemiplegia. Sternocleidomastoid turns the head to the opposite side. If the sternocleidomastoid were controlled by the opposite cortex (like limb muscles), then during hemiplegia, the unopposed pull of the normal sternocleidomastoid would cause the head to turn away from the (only) normal side! Also, in convulsions originating from frontal lobe, the eyes and the head look (turn) towards the affected limbs!

FUNCTIONAL COMPONENTS, NUCLEI, BRIEF COURSE, AND DISTRIBUTION OF INDIVIDUAL CRANIAL NERVES

I. Olfactory Nerve

This is the nerve of smell. As the olfactory mucosa is derived from ectoderm (of the nasal placodes), this nerve is classified, developmentally, as **special somatic afferent** (along with vision and hearing). However, in view of the close relationship between the sensations of smell and taste, this nerve is functionally classified as **special visceral afferent.**

The olfactory nerves arise from **olfactory receptor cells,** which are bipolar cells. The peripheral processes end as olfactory hairs in the roof of nose. The central processes form **olfactory nerve fibres,** which pass through cribriform plate of ethmoid bone to enter **olfactory bulb.** The detail course of this cranial nerve is considered under olfactory pathway in Chapter 7.

> **Clinical Anatomy**
>
> The olfactory nerve is tested by asking the patient to recognize various odors (coffee, tea, etc.). The right and left nerves are tested separately by closing one nostril and putting the substance near the open nostril. Irritants such as ammonia should not be used, since they would stimulate the trigeminal nerve that supplies the nasal mucosa. Loss of sense of smell is called **anosmia.** Block of the respiratory tract due to excessive secretion of mucus, in common cold, is the most frequent cause. If there is damage to olfactory epithelium (which is a neuroepithelium), it regenerates. This is the only example of neuronal cell body, when damaged, is capable of regeneration.

II. Optic Nerve

This is the nerve of vision. Its fibres are **special somatic afferent.** From the point of view of its structure and development, this nerve is to be regarded as a tract of the brain rather than as a peripheral nerve.

The detail of the course of optic nerve is given under visual/optic pathway in Chapter 7.

Clinical Anatomy

- **Acuity (sharpness) of vision** can be tested by making the patient read letters of various sizes printed on a chart (Snellen's chart) from a fixed distance (6 meters). Near vision can be tested by Jaeger charts. Loss of acuity of vision can be caused by errors of refraction, or by the presence of opacities in the cornea or the lens (cataract). Opacities need to be corrected surgically.

  In **hypermetropia** (far-sightedness), a biconvex lens corrects the diverging rays, from near objects, so that they are brought to a focus on the retina.

  In **myopia** (near-sightedness), a biconcave lens in front of the eye causes the parallel light rays, from far objects, to diverge slightly before striking the eye.

  If the curvature of the cornea is not uniform, it is called **astigmatism**. It is corrected with cylindrical lenses placed in such a way that they equalize the refraction in all meridians.

  With advancing age, due to increasing hardness of the lens, there is loss of accommodation, which is known as **presbyopia**. It is corrected by wearing reading glasses with convex lenses.
- Colour vision can be tested by Ishihara charts. **Red-green colour blindness** is an X-linked recessive disorder (both, red cone and green cone genes are encoded on X chromosome, but not the cone gene), while **blue-yellow colour blindness** is autosomal recessive.
- Field of vision can be tested by perimetry. Field of vision is tested clinically by keeping the patient's gaze fixed while presenting objects at various places within his visual field. A chart is plotted depicting the patient's field of vision in each eye.

III. Oculomotor Nerve

Functional Components and Nuclei (Figure 6.5)

- **Somatic efferent** fibres arise in the **oculomotor nucleus**, at the level of superior colliculus of the midbrain and **supply all extrinsic muscles of the eyeball** except the lateral rectus and the superior oblique.
- **General visceral efferent** fibres (preganglionic) arise in the **Edinger-Westphal nucleus** and relay in the **ciliary ganglion**. Postganglionic fibres arising in this ganglion supply the sphincter pupillae and the ciliaris muscle via **short ciliary nerves**.

The general visceral efferent component of the oculomotor nerve is involved in **accommodation of lens** (for the near vision) and **constriction of pupil**. The accommodation of lens is due to contraction of ciliary muscles and the constriction of pupils is due to contraction of sphincter pupillae muscle of iris.

Course and Distribution (Figure 6.6 and Table 6.4)

Intracranial course: The nerve emerges from the ventral aspect of the midbrain. It passes forwards into the middle cranial fossa and lies in the lateral wall of cavernous sinus. It divides into superior and inferior divisions and enters the orbital cavity through the **superior orbital fissure**.

Extracranial course: It supplies the extrinsic muscles of the eye i.e. levator palpebrae superioris, superior rectus, inferior rectus, medial rectus and inferior oblique.

Clinical Anatomy

Paralysis of Oculomotor Nerve

All movements of the eyeball are lost in the affected eye. When the patient is asked to look directly forwards, the affected eye is directed laterally (by the lateral rectus) and downwards (by the superior oblique). There is lateral squint (external strabismus) and it results in diplopia or double vision. As the levator palpebrae superioris is paralyzed, there is drooping of the upper eyelid (ptosis).

As **parasympathetic fibres** to the sphincter pupillae pass through the oculomotor nerve, the sphincter pupillae is paralyzed. Unopposed action of dilator papillae produces a dilated pupil.

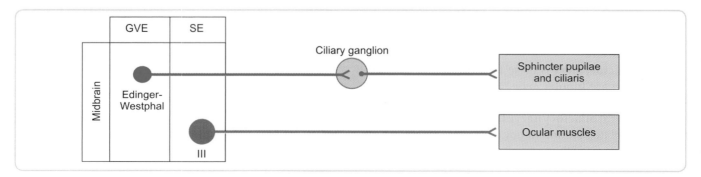

Figure 6.5: Functional components of the oculomotor nerve (*Abbreviations*: GVE, general visceral efferent; SE, somatic efferent)

TABLE 6.4: Branches and distribution of oculomotor nerve

Branches	Distribution
Superior division	Levator palpebrae superioris, superior rectus
Inferior division	Medial rectus, inferior rectus, inferior oblique

IV. Trochlear Nerve

Functional Components and Nuclei

This nerve is made up of **somatic efferent** fibres arising in the **trochlear nucleus** from the midbrain at the level of inferior colliculus and supplies the superior oblique muscle of the eyeball.

Course and Distribution (Figure 6.7 and Table 6.5)

Intracranial course: The trochlear nerve emerges from the dorsal aspect of the midbrain at the level of inferior colliculus and immediately decussates with the nerve

TABLE 6.5: Branches and distribution of trochlear nerve

Nerve	Distribution
Trochlear nerve	Superior oblique

of the other side. In the middle cranial fossa it lies in the lateral wall of cavernous sinus. The nerve enters the orbit through **superior orbital fissure.**

Extracranial course: In the orbit it supplies the superior oblique muscle that helps to turn the eye downward and laterally.

Clinical Anatomy

Paralysis of Trochlear Nerve
The superior oblique muscle (supplied by the trochlear nerve) moves the eyeball downward and laterally, and the inferior rectus (supplied by the oculomotor nerve) moves it downward and medially. For direct downward movement synchronized action of both muscles is required. When the superior oblique muscle is paralyzed the eyeball deviates medially on trying to look downward.

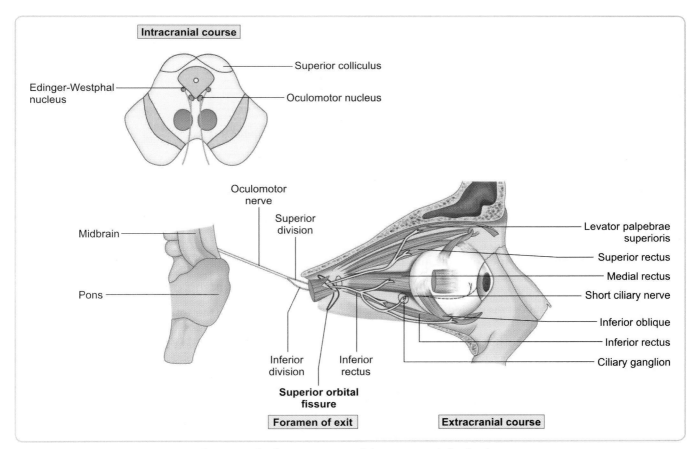

Figure 6.6: Oculomotor nerve: origin, course and distribution

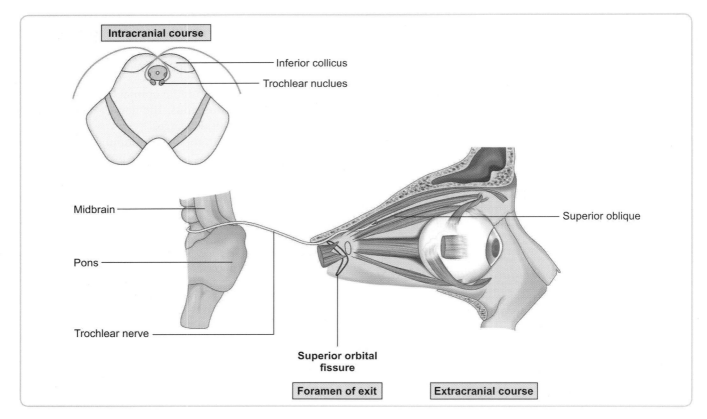

Figure 6.7: Trochlear nerve: origin, course and distribution

VI. Abducent Nerve

Functional Components and Nuclei

This nerve consists of **somatic efferent** fibres that arise from the **abducent nucleus** in lower pons and supply the lateral rectus muscle of the eyeball.

Course and Distribution (Figure 6.8 and Table 6.6)

Intracranial course: The abducent nerve emerges in the groove between lower border of pons and medulla oblongata. It traverses forward in the medial wall of the cavernous sinus, lying below, and lateral to internal carotid artery. The nerve enters the orbit through **superior orbital fissure.**

Extracranial course: In the orbit, it supplies the lateral rectus muscle which turns the eye laterally.

TABLE 6.6: Branches and distribution of abducent nerve	
Nerve	**Distribution**
Abducent	Lateral rectus

> **Clinical Anatomy**
>
> **Paralysis of Abducent Nerve**
> This nerve supplies the lateral rectus muscle which moves the eyeball laterally. In looking forwards the lateral pull of the lateral rectus is counteracted by the medial pull of the medial rectus and so the eye is maintained in the centre. When the lateral rectus is paralyzed the affected eye deviates medially **(medial squint, or internal strabismus).**

V. Trigeminal Nerve

Functional Components and Nuclei

This nerve contains the following components (Figure 6.10):

- **Special visceral efferent** fibres arise from the **motor nucleus** of the nerve located at the level of upper pons and supply the muscles of mastication.
- **General somatic afferent** fibres of the nerve are peripheral processes of unipolar neurons in the trigeminal ganglion. They carry exteroceptive sensations from the skin of the face and the mucous

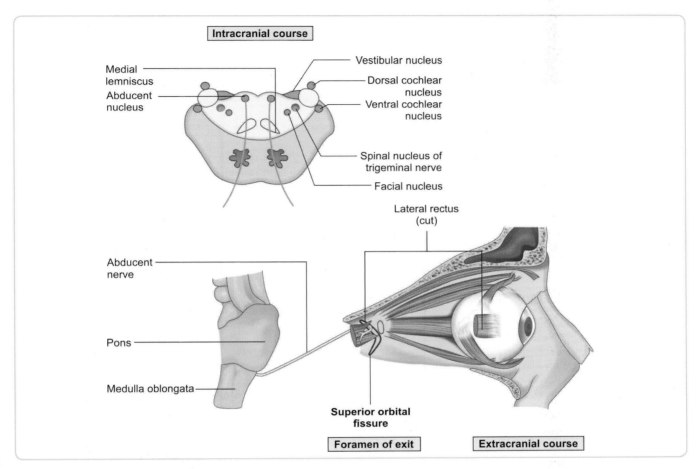

Figure 6.8: Abducent nerve: origin, course and distribution

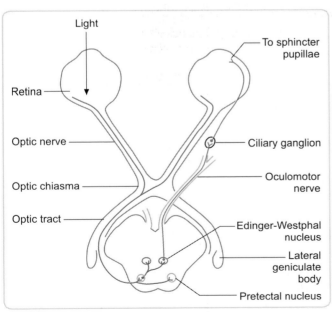

Figure 6.9: Pathway for the light reflex

membrane of the mouth and nose. The central processes of the neurons in the ganglion constitute the sensory root of the nerve. They terminate in the **main sensory nucleus** in upper pons and **in the spinal nucleus of the nerve** extending up to spinal cord.

Another group of general somatic afferent neurons carry proprioceptive impulses from the muscles of mastication (and possibly from ocular, facial, and lingual muscles). These fibres are believed to be peripheral processes of unipolar neurons located in the **mesencephalic nucleus** of this nerve located in the midbrain. The central processes of this nucleus terminate in the main sensory nucleus.

Course and Distribution

Intracranial course: The trigeminal nerve is attached to the ventrolateral surface of the pons by two roots, a very large lateral sensory root, and a small medial motor root. The sensory root contains a ganglion **(trigeminal/ Gasserian ganglion)** which lies at the apex of petrous part

---

Clinical Anatomy

Oculomotor, Trochlear, and Abducent Nerves

These three nerves are responsible for movements of the eyeball. In a routine clinical examination, the movements are tested by asking the patient to keep his head fixed and to move his eyes in various directions, i.e. upward, downward, inward, and outward. An easy way is to ask the patient to keep his head fixed and to follow the movements of your finger with his eyes. Such an examination can detect a gross abnormality in movement of the eyes.

Parasympathetic fibres of oculomotor nerve can be tested by examining the pupils for their equality and constriction to light and accommodation.

Reflexes in relation to Oculomotor Nerve

Normally, both pupils contract when exposed to light in one eye **(pupillary light reflex)**. Constriction of ipsilateral pupil is called **direct light reflex**, while constriction of contralateral pupil is called **consensual light reflex**. The pupil also contracts when the relaxed eye is made to concentrate on a near object **(accommodation reflex)**.

Accommodation reflex involves convergence (voluntary), pupillary constriction and accommodation (involuntary). Both these reflexes are lost in oculomotor nerve damage. The power of accommodation is lost because of paralysis of the ciliaris muscle.

The neural pathway for **pupillary light reflex** is as follows (Figure 6.9):

Retina → optic nerve → optic chiasma → optic tract → superior brachium → midbrain at level of superior colliculus → **pretectal nucleus** (midbrain) → both Edinger-Westphal nuclei → oculomotor nerve → ciliary ganglion → short ciliary nerves → sphincter pupillae

The neural pathway for **convergence** reaction is as follows:

Retina → optic nerve → optic chiasma → optic tract → lateral geniculate body → optic radiation → visual cortex → corticonuclear tract → both oculomotor nuclei → **medial recti contraction**

(Since this neural pathway involves the cerebral cortex and requires voluntary participation of the patient, it is called convergence reaction. Convergence of the eyeball causes pupillary constriction and contraction of ciliaris, which is called accommodation reflex)

The neural pathway for **accommodation reflex** is as follows:

Medial recti contraction → proprioception from medial recti → **nucleus of Perlia** (midbrain) → both Edinger-Westphal nuclei → oculomotor nerve → ciliary ganglion → short ciliary nerves → sphincter pupillae and ciliaris

Damage to the dorsal aspect of rostral midbrain causes loss of constriction of pupils due to pupillary light reflex but not due to accommodation reflex (*Argyll-Robertson* pupils). (Remember: **A**rgyll-**R**obertson **p**upils = **a**ccommodation **r**eflex **p**resent).

Squint (Strabismus) and Diplopia

Squint is a condition in which the two eyes do not look in the same direction. In this condition, the optical axes are not parallel. Hence, there are two images formed which is called diplopia. The squint becomes obvious when the eye movement involves a muscle that is paralyzed or weak, because the weak muscle cannot keep up with the muscle of the normal side.

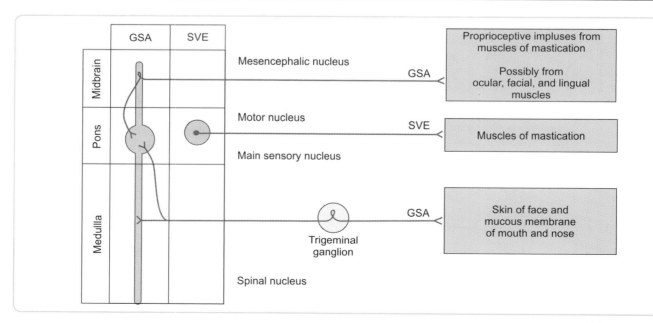

Figure 6.10: Functional components of the trigeminal nerve (*Abbreviations*: GSA, general somatic afferent; SVE, special visceral efferent)

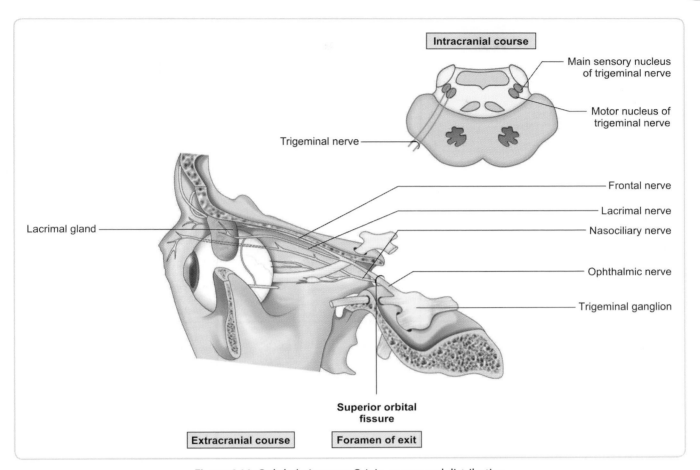

Figure 6.11: Ophthalmic nerve: Origin, course and distribution

TABLE 6.7: Branches and distribution of ophthalmic nerve

	Branches	Distribution
Frontal	Supratrochlear	Skin of lower forehead
	Supraorbital	Skin of scalp up to vertex, frontal sinus
Lacrimal		Lateral conjunctiva
Nasociliary	Anterior ethmoidal	Anterior ethmoidal air cells, middle ethmoidal air cells, anterosuperior quadrant of lateral wall of nose, anterosuperior part of septum of nose
	Posterior ethmoidal	Posterior ethmoidal air cells, sphenoidal air sinus
	Infratrochlear	Conjunctiva over medial aspect, skin of root of nose
	External nasal	Skin of external aspect of nose

of the temporal bone in the **Meckel's cave.** The trigeminal ganglion divides into three branches: (1) ophthalmic, (2) maxillary, and (3) mandibular nerves. The ophthalmic and maxillary nerves are sensory nerves, while the mandibular nerve has both motor and sensory fibres.

Extracranial course: The **foramen of exit** of the ophthalmic nerve is **superior orbital fissure** (Table 6.7 and Figure 6.11).

The **foramen of exit** of the maxillary nerve is **foramen rotundum** (Table 6.8 and Figure 6.12).

TABLE 6.8: Branches and distribution of maxillary nerve

Branches			Distribution
Posterior superior alveolar			Molar teeth of upper jaw
Ganglionic	Palatine		Palatine mucosa
	Nasal		Nasal mucosa
	Pharyngeal		Mucosa of nasopharynx
Zygomatic	Zygomaticofacial		Skin of the prominence of cheek
	Zygomaticotemporal		Skin of the temporal region of scalp, Postganglionic fibres of lacrimal gland
Infraorbital	Palpebral		Skin and conjunctiva of lower eyelid
	Middle superior alveolar		Premolar teeth of upper jaw
	Anterior superior alveolar		Canine and incisor teeth of upper jaw
	Superior labial		Skin of upper lip including philtrum

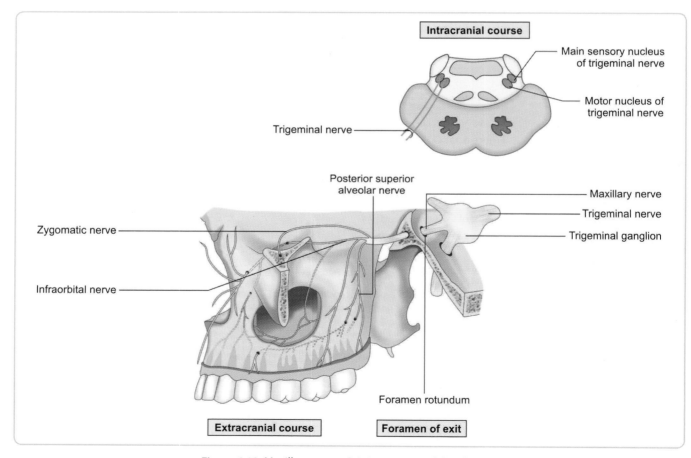

Figure 6.12: Maxillary nerve: Origin, course and distribution

TABLE 6.9: Branches and distribution of mandibular nerve

Branches		Distribution
Nervus spinosus		Dura of middle cranial fossa
Nerve to medial pterygoid		Medial pterygoid, tensor veli palatini, tensor tympani
Anterior division	Buccal	Skin over buccinator, mucosa of the vestibule of mouth
	Deep temporal	Temporalis
	Masseteric	Masseter
	Nerve to lateral pterygoid	Lateral pterygoid
Posterior division	Auriculotemporal	Temporomandibular joint, skin over pinna, external acoustic meatus, tympanic membrane, skin of temporal region of scalp
	Lingual	Mucosa of anterior two-thirds of tongue, gums of lower jaw, mucosa of floor of mouth
	Inferior alveolar	Mylohyoid muscle and anterior belly of digastric muscle, all teeth of lower jaw, skin of chin and lower lip, mucosa of lower lip

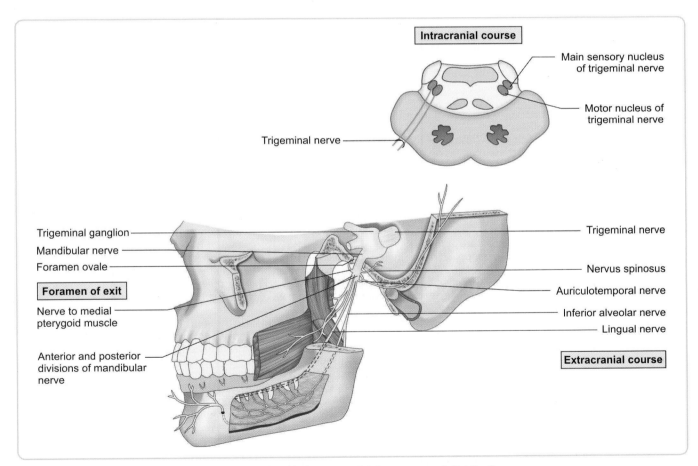

Figure 6.13: Mandibular nerve: Origin, course and distribution

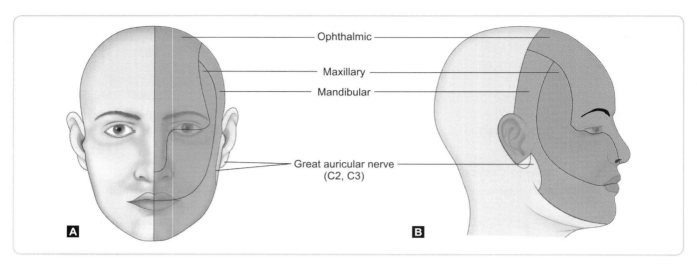

Figures 6.14A and B: Cutaneous territory of three divisions of the trigeminal nerve: (A) Frontal view; (B) Lateral view

---

Clinical Anatomy

The trigeminal nerve has a wide sensory distribution. It also supplies the muscles of mastication.

The sensation of touch in the area of distribution of the nerve can be tested by touching different areas of skin with a wisp of cotton wool. The sensation of pain can be tested by gentle pressure with a pin.

Motor function is tested by asking the patient to clench his teeth firmly. Contraction of the masseter can be felt by palpation when the teeth are clenched.

Effects of Injury or Disease

Injury to the trigeminal nerve causes paralysis of the muscles supplied and loss of sensations in the area of supply. Some features of special importance are as follows:

- Apart from their role in opening and closing the mouth, the muscles of mastication are responsible for side-to-side movements of the mandible. Contraction of these muscles on one side moves the chin to the opposite side. Normally, the chin is maintained in the midline by the balanced tone of the muscles of the right and left sides. In paralysis of the pterygoid muscles of one side, the chin is pushed to the paralyzed side by muscles of the opposite side.
- Loss of sensation in the ophthalmic division (especially the nasociliary nerve) is of great importance. Normally, the eyelids close as soon as the cornea is touched (corneal reflex). Loss of sensation in the cornea abolishes this reflex leaving the cornea unprotected. This can lead to the formation of ulcers on the cornea, which can in turn lead to blindness.
- Pain arising in a structure supplied by one branch of the nerve may be felt in an area of skin supplied by another branch. This is called **referred pain**. Some examples are as follows:
  - Caries of a tooth in the lower jaw (supplied by the inferior alveolar nerve) may cause pain in the ear (auriculotemporal).
  - If there is an ulcer or cancer on the tongue (lingual nerve), the pain may again be felt over the ear and temple (auriculotemporal).
  - In frontal sinusitis (Frontal sinus is supplied by a branch from the supraorbital nerve), the pain is referred to the forehead (skin supplied by supraorbital nerve). In fact, headache is a common symptom when any structure supplied by the trigeminal nerve is involved (e.g. eyes, ears, and teeth).
- A source of irritation in the distribution of the nerve may cause severe persistent pain in the area of cutaneous distribution (Figures 6.14A and B) of the nerve (**trigeminal neuralgia**). Removal of the cause can cure the pain. However, in some cases, no cause can be found. In such cases, pain can be relieved by injection of alcohol into the trigeminal ganglion, into one of the divisions of the nerve, or into its sensory root. In some cases, it may be necessary to cut fibres of the sensory root. In this connection, it is important to know that the fibres for the maxillary and mandibular divisions can be cut without destroying those for the ophthalmic division. This is possible as the fibres for the ophthalmic division lie separately in the upper medial part of the sensory root. Finally, it may be noted that trigeminal pain can also be relieved by cutting the spinal tract of the trigeminal nerve. This procedure is useful, especially for relieving pain in the distribution of the ophthalmic division as pain can be abolished without loss of the sense of touch and, therefore, without the abolition of the corneal reflex.
- **Mandibular nerve block:** This is used for anaesthesia of the lower jaw for extraction of teeth. Palpate the anterior margin of the ramus of the mandible. Just medial to it, you will feel the pterygomandibular raphe (ligament). The needle is inserted in the interval between the ramus and the raphe. The tip of the needle is now very near the inferior alveolar nerve, just before it enters the mandibular canal. Anaesthetic drug is injected here to block the nerve.
- The lingual nerve lies very close to the medial side of the third molar tooth, just deep to the mucosa. The nerve can be injured in careless extraction of a third molar tooth. In cases of cancer of the tongue, having intractable pain, the lingual nerve can be cut at this site to relieve pain.

The **foramen of exit** of the mandibular nerve is **foramen ovale** (Table 6.9 and Figure 6.13).

Reflexes Mediated by Trigeminal Nerve

The trigeminal nerve is involved in a number of reflexes summarized in Table 6.10.

VII. Facial Nerve

Functional Components and Nuclei

The components of this nerve are as follows (Figure 6.15):

- **Special visceral efferent** fibres begin from the **motor nucleus** at the level of lower pons and supply the muscles of facial expression.

- **General visceral efferent** fibres (preganglionic) arise in the superior salivatory nucleus. They relay in the submandibular ganglion from which postganglionic fibres arise to supply the submandibular and sublingual salivary glands.
The facial nerve also carries general visceral efferent fibres for the lacrimal gland. The preganglionic neurons concerned are said to be located in the lacrimatroy nucleus which is a part of superior salivatory nucleus. Their axons terminate in the pterygopalatine ganglion, from which postganglionic fibres arise to supply the gland.

- **Special visceral afferent** fibres are peripheral processes of cells in the geniculate ganglion of the nerve. They supply taste buds in the anterior

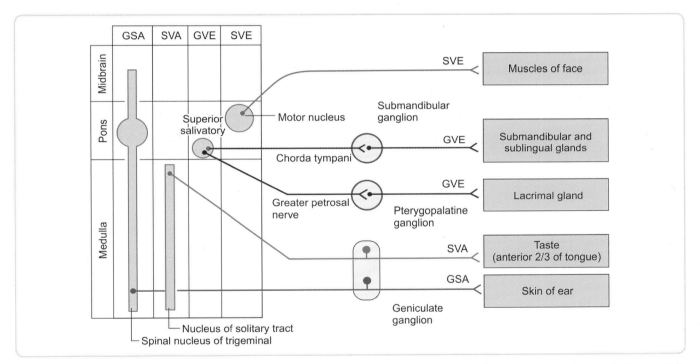

Figure 6.15: Functional components of the facial nerve (*Abbreviations*: GSA, general somatic afferent; SVA, special visceral afferent; GVE, general visceral efferent; SVE, special visceral efferent)

TABLE 6.10: Important reflexes mediated by the trigeminal nerve

Reflex	Afferent limb	Efferent limb
Corneal reflex	Ophthalmic nerve	Facial nerve
Conjunctival reflex	Ophthalmic/maxillary nerve	Facial nerve
Lacrimation reflex	Ophthalmic nerve	Facial nerve
Sneezing reflex	Maxillary nerve	Vagus nerve
Jaw-jerk (masseteric) reflex	Mandibular nerve	Mandibular nerve

two-thirds of the tongue (and some in the soft palate). The central processes of the ganglion cells carry these sensations to the upper part of the **nucleus of the solitary tract.**

- **General somatic afferent** fibres are also peripheral processes of some cells of the geniculate ganglion. They innervate a part of the skin of the external ear. The central processes of these cells end in the **spinal nucleus of the trigeminal nerve.**

Course and Distribution (Figure 6.16 and Table 6.11)

Intracranial course:

- *Intraneural course:* Fibres of facial nerve which emerge from the motor nucleus first run dorsally within the

pons and wind around the nucleus of abducent nerve (**internal genu of facial nerve**) and then run forward and laterally to emerge at the pontomedullary junction medial to vestibulocochlear nerve. The sensory root of facial nerve is between the motor root of facial nerve and vestibulocochlear nerve.

- *Extraneural course:* The facial nerve and the vestibulocochlear nerve pass through the cerebellomedullary cistern and enter the internal acoustic meatus. Facial nerve runs along the roof of the inner ear and enters the facial canal in the middle ear. In the facial canal, the facial nerve traverses forward and laterally, forms a bend, the **(external) genu of facial nerve where geniculate ganglion is located**.

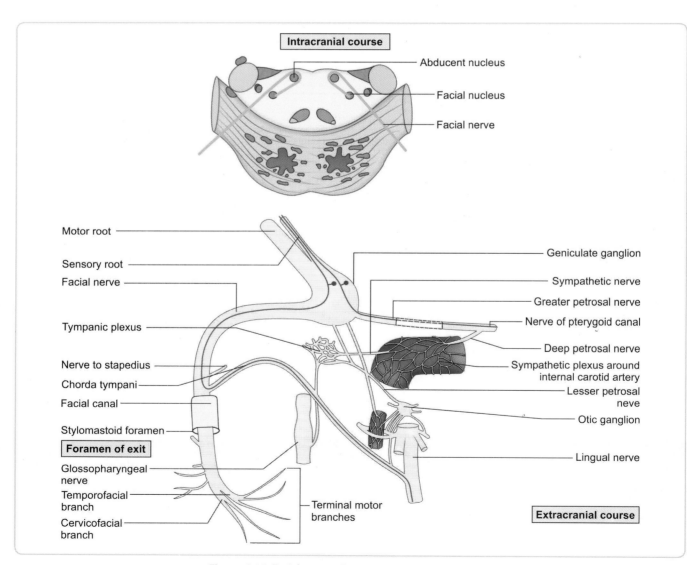

Figure 6.16: Facial nerve: Origin, course and distribution

TABLE 6.11: Branches and distribution of facial nerve

Branches		Distribution
Greater petrosal (preganglionic)		Lacrimal gland, nasal and palatine glands
Nerve to stapedius		Stapedius
Chorda tympani (preganglionic)		Submandibular, sublingual and anterior lingual glands, taste sensations from anterior two-thirds of tongue
Posterior auricular		Occipital belly of occipitofrontalis
Nerve to posterior belly of digastric		Posterior belly of digastric
Nerve to stylohyoid		Stylohyoid
Temporofacial	Temporal	Frontal belly of occipitofrontalis
	Zygomatic	Orbicularis oculi
	Buccal	Buccinator, muscles of upper lip
Cervicofacial	Marginal mandibular	Muscles of lower lip, mentalis
	Cervical	Platysma

> ## Clinical Anatomy
>
> The facial nerve supplies the muscles of the face, including the muscles that close the eyelids and the mouth. The nerve is tested as follows:
> - Ask the patient to close his eyes firmly. In complete paralysis of the facial nerve, the patient will not be able to close the eye on the affected side. In partial paralysis, the closure is weak and the examiner can easily open the closed eye with his fingers (which is very difficult in a normal person).
> - Ask the person to smile. In smiling, the normal mouth is more or less symmetrical, the two angles moving upward and outward. In facial paralysis, the angle fails to move on the paralyzed side and the angle is pulled to the normal side.
> - Ask the patient to fill his mouth with air. Press the cheek with your finger and compare the resistance (by the buccinator muscle) on the two sides. The resistance is less on the paralyzed side. On pressing the cheek, air may leak out of the mouth because the muscles closing the mouth are weak.
> - Sensations of taste can be tested by applying substances that are salty (salt), sweet (sugar), sour (lemon), or bitter (quinine) to the anterior two-thirds of the tongue. The mouth should be rinsed and the tongue dried before each substance is applied.
>
> **Paralysis of Facial Nerve**
> Paralysis of the facial nerve is fairly common. It can occur due to injury or disease of the facial nucleus (*nuclear* paralysis) or of the nerve anywhere along its course (**infranuclear** paralysis). Both are together called as Lower Motor Neuron (LMN) type of paralysis. In the most common type of infranuclear paralysis called **Bell's palsy** the nerve is affected near the stylomastoid foramen **(Table 6.12)**. Facial muscles can also be paralyzed by interruption of corticonuclear fibres running from the motor cortex to the facial nucleus: this is referred to as **supranuclear** paralysis (Upper Motor Neuron type of paralysis) **(Table 6.13, and Figures 6.17A and B)**.
> The effects of paralysis are due to the failure of the muscles concerned to perform their normal actions. Some effects are as follows:
> - The normal face is more or less symmetrical. When the facial nerve is paralyzed on one side the most noticeable feature is the loss of symmetry.
> - Normal furrows on the forehead are lost because of paralysis of the frontal belly of occipitofrontalis.
> - The palpebral fissure is wider on the paralyzed side because of paralysis of the orbicularis oculi. The corneal and conjunctival reflexes are lost for the same reason.
> The neural pathway for corneal/conjunctival reflex:
>   Touch of cornea (nasociliary nerve)/conjunctiva (ophthalmic/maxillary) → trigeminal ganglion → main sensory nucleus of trigeminal in pons → motor nucleus of facial → facial nerve → orbicularis oculi
> - There is marked asymmetry of the mouth because of paralysis of the orbicularis oris and of muscles inserted into the angle of the mouth. This is most obvious when a smile is attempted. **When the patient attempts to smile, the angle of the mouth deviates to the normal side.**
> - During mastication food tends to accumulate between the cheek and the teeth (This is normally prevented by the buccinator).

TABLE 6.12: Lower motor neuron lesion of facial nerve

S. No.	Site of lesion	Effect
1.	Stylomastoid foramen	Ipsilateral loss of movement of all facial muscles (Bell's palsy)
2.	Geniculate ganglion	As in 1 + hyperacusis, decreased taste from anterior two-thirds of the tongue, decreased salivary secretion, decreased lacrimation
3.	Internal acoustic meatus/cerebellopontine angle	As in 2 + involvement of vestibulocochlear nerve which will result in deafness and loss of equilibrium
4.	Facial nucleus (nuclear paralysis)	As in 2

TABLE 6.13: Differences between supranuclear lesion and infranuclear lesion of facial nerve

S. No.	Supranuclear lesion of facial nerve	Infranuclear lesion of facial nerve
1.	Lesion is usually in internal capsule	Lesion is usually at stylomastoid foramen
2.	Accompanied by hemiplegia, on the same side as facial paralysis	Hemiplegia, seen only in nuclear paralysis in lower pons, will be contralateral
3.	Movements of the lower part of the face affected because the upper part of the face is under bilateral cortical control	Movements of the entire half of face affected
4.	Voluntary movements are affected, emotional expressions appear to be normal since different pathways are involved	Both voluntary and emotional movements are affected since it is final common pathway

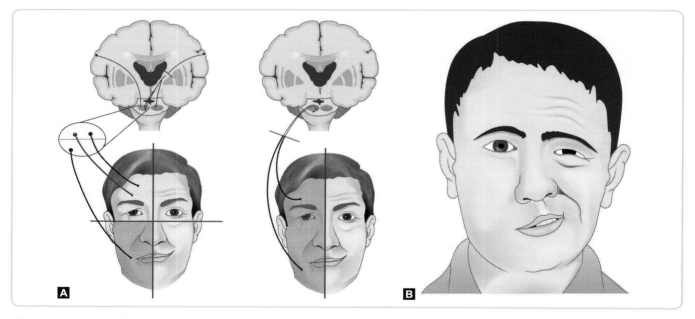

Figures 6.17A and B: (A) Effects of upper motor neuron and lower motor neuron lesions of the facial nerve; (B) Infranuclear paralysis of the facial nerve on the right side

The greater petrosal nerve arises from the geniculate ganglion. The nerve is then directed backward and is related to medial wall of the middle ear, above lateral semicircular canal. The second turn is downward, in the posterior wall of middle ear. In this segment it gives rise to the nerve to stapedius and chorda tympani nerve. The facial nerve leaves the middle ear through the **stylomastoid foramen.**

Extracranial course

Upon emerging from stylomastoid foramen, it gives the posterior auricular branch, nerve to posterior belly of digastric and nerve to stylohyoid and then enters the

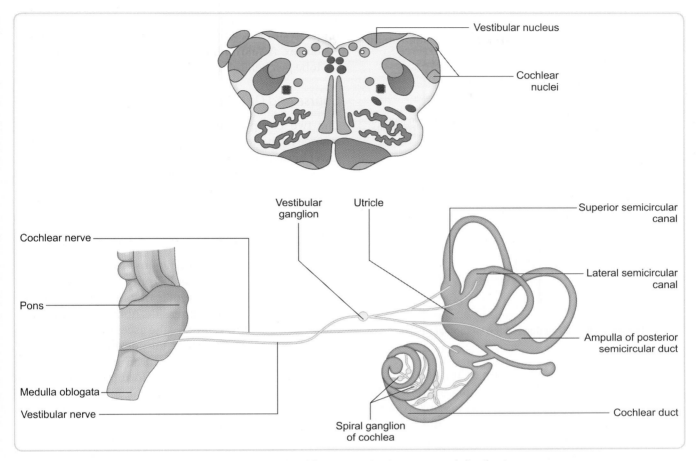

Figure 6.18: Vestibulocochlear nerve: Origin, course and distribution

substance of parotid salivary gland where it divides into five terminal branches supplying the muscles of facial expression.

VIII. Vestibulocochlear Nerve

Functional Components and Nuclei

Both the cochlear and vestibular divisions of this nerve are made up of **special somatic afferent** fibres. The fibres of the cochlear nerve are central processes of bipolar cells in the spiral ganglion. The peripheral processes of these neurons supply the organ of Corti. The fibres of the vestibular nerve are central processes of bipolar neurons in the vestibular ganglion. The peripheral processes of these neurons innervate the semicircular ducts, the utricle, and the saccule of the internal ear. The detail course of cochlear nerve is given as auditory pathway in Chapter 7.

Vestibular Nuclei

The vestibular nuclei lie in the grey matter underlying the lateral part of the floor of the fourth ventricle (Figure 6.18). They lie partly in the medulla and partly in the pons. Four distinct nuclei are recognized. These are medial, lateral, inferior, and superior. The lateral nucleus is also called **Deiters' nucleus.**

Connections of Vestibular Nuclei

The vestibular nuclei receive the following afferents (Figure 6.19)**:**
- The main afferents are central processes of bipolar neurons of the vestibular ganglion. These fibres constitute the vestibular part of the vestibulocochlear nerve. They convey impulses from end organs in the semicircular ducts, utricle, and saccule. These are necessary for maintenance of equilibrium.

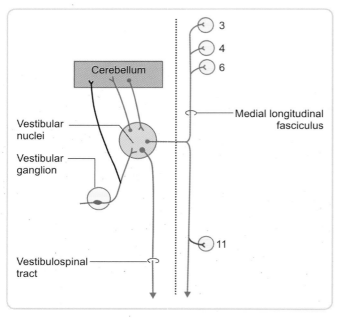

Figure 6.19: Connections of the vestibular nuclei

After entering the medulla, the fibres of the vestibular nerve divide into ascending and descending branches. The descending branches end in the medial, lateral, and inferior vestibular nuclei. The ascending branches reach the superior vestibular nucleus.

- The vestibular nuclei also receive fibres from some parts of the cerebellum.

The efferents from the vestibular nuclei are as follows:

- Vestibulocerebellar fibres pass through the inferior cerebellar peduncle. The vestibulocerebellar fibres form a separate bundle, the **juxtarestiform body**, within the peduncle. Some fibres of the vestibular nerves bypass the vestibular nuclei and go straight to the cerebellum.
- Fibres arising in the vestibular nuclei establish connections with cranial nerve nuclei responsible for movements of the eyes (third, fourth, and sixth) and of the neck (eleventh). These fibres form the **medial longitudinal fasciculus (or bundle).**
- Fibres from the lateral vestibular nucleus descend to the spinal cord as the vestibulospinal tract. Fibres from the medial (and other) nuclei descend to the spinal cord through the medial longitudinal fasciculus. These fibres are sometimes named the **medial vestibulospinal tract.** Some fibres reach the pontine reticular formation.
- Some fibres from the vestibular nuclei enter the lateral lemniscus.

- Some vestibular impulses reach the thalamus (ventro-posterior nucleus) and are relayed to the cerebral cortex. A **vestibular centre** is present in the parietal lobe just behind the postcentral gyrus.

Course and Distribution

The two components of the vestibulocochlear nerve emerge from the ventral aspect of the brainstem between lower border of pons and medulla, in the cerebellopontine angle. They traverse the posterior cranial fossa and then enter the internal acoustic meatus. The distribution is shown in Figure 6.18.

MEDIAL LONGITUDINAL FASCICULUS

The medial longitudinal fasciculus (MLF) consists of a bundle of fibres, arising mainly from right and left medial vestibular nuclei in the medulla, that lie near the midline of the brainstem, one on either side. Above, it reaches up to the level of the third ventricle. The ascending fibres end in the interstitial nucleus of Cajal, the nucleus of the posterior commissure, and the nucleus of Darkschewitsch. Fibres of this bundle cross the midline forming the **posterior commissure** which is located in the inferior lamella of the pineal stalk. Through this commissure, the vestibular nuclei of both sides are connected.

Below, the medial longitudinal bundle becomes continuous with the anterior intersegmental tract of the spinal cord.

The fasciculus is closely related to the nuclei of the **third, fourth, sixth and twelfth** cranial nerves (all of the **somatic efferent column** and lying next to the midline). It is also related to the fibres of the **seventh** nerve (as they wind around the abducent nucleus), the **spinal accessory** nerve (for head movements) and to some fibres arising from the cochlear nuclei. In the spinal cord it establishes connections with ventral horn cells that innervate the muscles of the neck (Figure 6.20).

The **functions of the MLF** are:

- Fibres arise in the vestibular nuclei of the same side as well as those of the opposite side. These fibres ascend or descend in the fasciculus to reach nuclei supplying the muscles of the eyeball and neck. These connections ensure harmonious movements of the eyes and head in response to vestibular stimulation.
- Some fibres of the fasciculus are connected to some nuclei of the auditory pathway. These are the nucleus of the trapezoid body and the nucleus of the lateral lemniscus. Through these connections movements of

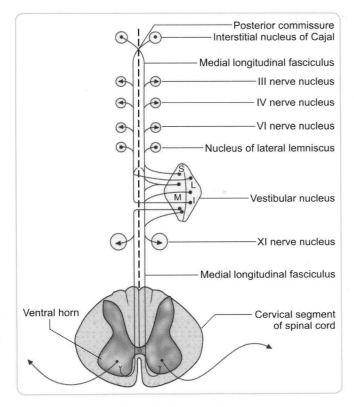

Figure 6.20: Medial longitudinal fasciculus

the head and of the eyes can take place in response to auditory stimuli.

- The medial longitudinal fasciculus affords a pathway for fibres interconnecting the nuclei related to it. Connections between the facial and hypoglossal nuclei facilitate simultaneous movements of the lips and tongue as in speech.

Clinical Anatomy

The cochlear part is tested as follows:

- The hearing of the patient can be tested by the ticking of a watch. The distance at which the sounds are first heard should be compared with the other ear.
- Air conduction and bone conduction can be compared by using a tuning fork. Strike the tuning fork against an object so that it begins to vibrate producing sound. Place the tuning fork near the patient's ear and then immediately put the base of the tuning fork on the mastoid process. Ask the patient where he hears the sound better. This is called **Rinne's test**. (Air conduction should be better than bone conduction). Bone conduction is better than air conduction in **conductive** deafness.
- In another test the base of a vibrating tuning fork is placed on the forehead. The sound should be heard equally in both ears. This is **Weber's test.** Sound is localized to affected ear in conductive deafness; but to the normal ear in **sensorineural** deafness.

IX. Glossopharyngeal Nerve

Functional Components and Nuclei

The components of this nerve are as follows:

- **Special visceral efferent** fibres arise in the **nucleus ambiguus** and supply the stylopharyngeus muscle.
- **General visceral efferent** fibres (preganglionic) begin from the **inferior salivatory nucleus** and travel to the otic ganglion. Postganglionic fibres arising in the ganglion supply the parotid gland.
- **General visceral afferent** fibres are peripheral processes of neurons in the inferior ganglion of the nerve. They carry general sensations (touch, pain, and temperature) from the pharynx and the posterior part of the tongue to the ganglion. They also carry inputs from the carotid sinus and carotid body. Central processes of the neurons carry these sensations to the **nucleus of the solitary tract.** Some fibres from the carotid sinus and body reach the paramedian reticular formation of the medulla.
- **Special visceral afferent** fibres are also peripheral processes of neurons in the inferior ganglion. They carry sensations of taste from the posterior one-third of the tongue to the ganglion. The central processes carry these sensations to the **nucleus of the solitary tract.**

Course and Distribution
(Figure 6.21 and Table 6.14)

Intracranial course: The glossopharyngeal nerve emerges from medulla as a series of rootlets between the olive and inferior cerebellar peduncle. It traverses the posterior cranial fossa and exits through the **jugular foramen.**

Extracranial course: The superior and inferior sensory ganglia are situated on the nerve at the exit.

TABLE 6.14: Branches and distribution of glossopharyngeal nerve

Branches		Distribution
Tympanic (preganglionic)	Lesser petrosal (preganglionic)	Parotid gland, mucosa of tympanic cavity
Carotid		Carotid sinus, carotid body
Pharyngeal		Mucosa of pharynx
Muscular		Stylopharyngeus
Tonsillar		Mucosa of tonsillar fossa
Lingual		Taste and general sensations from mucosa of posterior one-third of tongue

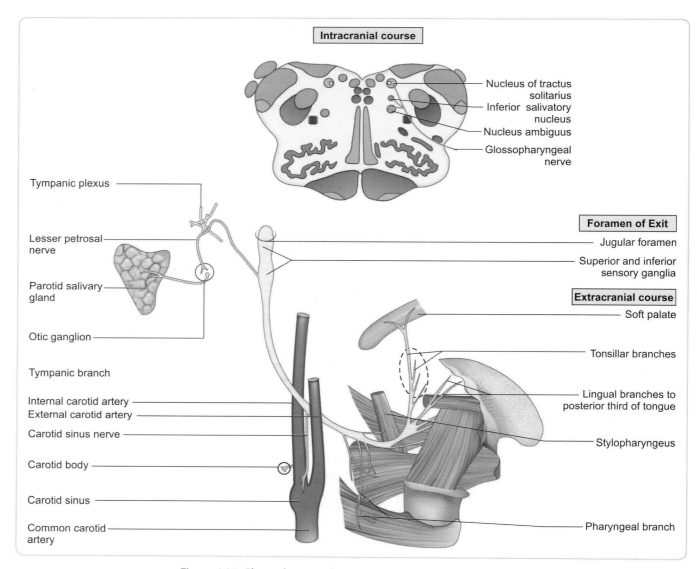

Figure 6.21: Glossopharyngeal nerve: Origin, course and distribution

The glossopharyngeal nerve descends in the neck and supplies stylopharyngeus muscle. The nerve then passes between superior and middle constrictors of pharynx and supply the mucosa of the pharynx and posterior one-third of tongue.

The important reflexes mediated by glossopharyngeal nerve are shown in Table 6.15.

TABLE 6.15: Important reflexes mediated by glossopharyngeal nerve

Reflex	Afferent limb	Efferent limb
Gag reflex	Glossopharyngeal nerve	Vagus nerve
Carotid sinus reflex	Glossopharyngeal nerve	Vagus nerve

Clinical Anatomy

Testing of this nerve is based on the fact that the nerve carries fibres of taste from the posterior one-third of the tongue and that it provides sensory innervation to the pharynx.

- Sensations of taste can be tested by applying substances that are salty (salt), sweet (sugar), sour (lemon), or bitter (quinine) to the posterior one-third of the tongue. The mouth should be rinsed and the tongue dried before the substance is applied.
- Touching the pharyngeal mucosa causes reflex constriction of pharyngeal muscles. The glossopharyngeal nerve provides the afferent part of the pathway for gag reflex.

The lesion of the glossopharyngeal nerve is associated with the following:
- Loss of taste and general sensation from the posterior third of tongue
- Loss of gag reflex, due to interruption of the afferent limb
- The neural pathway for gag reflex: Touch of posterior wall of oropharynx → glossopharyngeal nerve → inferior glossopharyngeal ganglion → nucleus of tractus solitarius → nucleus ambiguus → vago-accessory nerve → constrictors of pharynx
- Loss of carotid sinus reflex due to interruption of the afferent limb
- Loss of general sensations in pharynx, tonsils, and fauces.

X. Vagus Nerve and Cranial Part of Accessory Nerve

Functional Components and Nuclei

The components of this nerve are as follows (Figure 6.22):

- **Special visceral efferent** fibres are processes of neurons in the **nucleus ambiguus** in the medulla and supply the muscles of the pharynx and larynx.

- **General visceral efferent** fibres arise in the **dorsal (motor) nucleus of the vagus.** These are preganglionic parasympathetic fibres. They are distributed to thoracic and abdominal viscera. The postganglionic neurons concerned are situated in ganglia close to or within the walls of the viscera supplied.

- **General visceral afferent** fibres are peripheral processes of neurons located in the inferior ganglion of the nerve. They bring sensations from the pharynx, larynx, trachea, oesophagus, and abdominal and thoracic viscera. These are conveyed by central processes of the ganglion cells to the **nucleus of the solitary tract.** According to some authorities, some of these fibres terminate in the dorsal nucleus of the vagus.

- **Special visceral afferent** fibres are also peripheral processes of neurons in the inferior ganglion. They carry sensations of taste from the posterior most part of the tongue and the epiglottis. The central processes of the neurons concerned terminate in the upper part of the **nucleus of the solitary tract.**

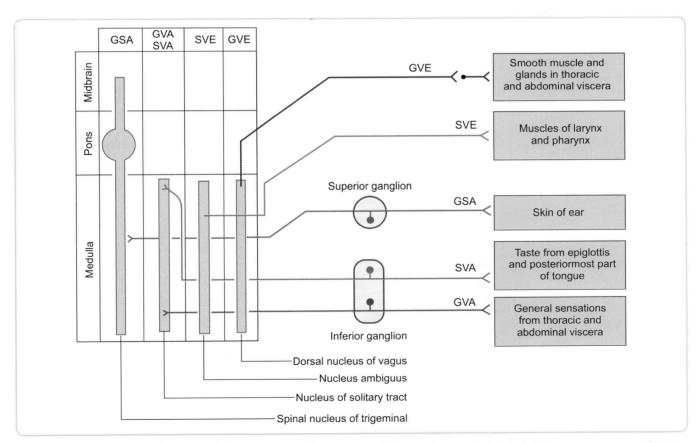

Figure 6.22: Functional components of the vagus nerve (*Abbreviations*: GSA, general somatic afferent; GVA, general visceral afferent; SVA, special visceral afferent; SVE, special visceral efferent; GVE, general visceral efferent)

- **General somatic afferent** fibres are peripheral processes of neurons in the superior ganglion and are distributed to the skin of the external ear. The central processes of the ganglion cells terminate in relation to the **spinal nucleus of the trigeminal nerve.**

Course and Distribution (Figure 6.23 and Table 6.16)

Intracranial course: The vagus nerve emerges as a series of rootlets in a groove between the olive and inferior cerebellar peduncle. It traverses the posterior cranial fossa and exits the skull through **jugular foramen.** The superior

sensory ganglion of the nerve is located in the jugular foramen.

Extracranial course: The inferior ganglion of vagus lies just below the jugular foramen. Just below the inferior ganglion, the cranial root of accessory nerve joins the vagus nerve to be distributed along its pharyngeal and laryngeal branches. In the neck, the vagus lies in the carotid sheath along with the internal jugular vein and common carotid arteries. The right vagus passes posterior to the root of right lung, contributes to pulmonary plexus, and then runs on the posterior surface of oesophagus, contributing to the oesophageal plexus. It enters the

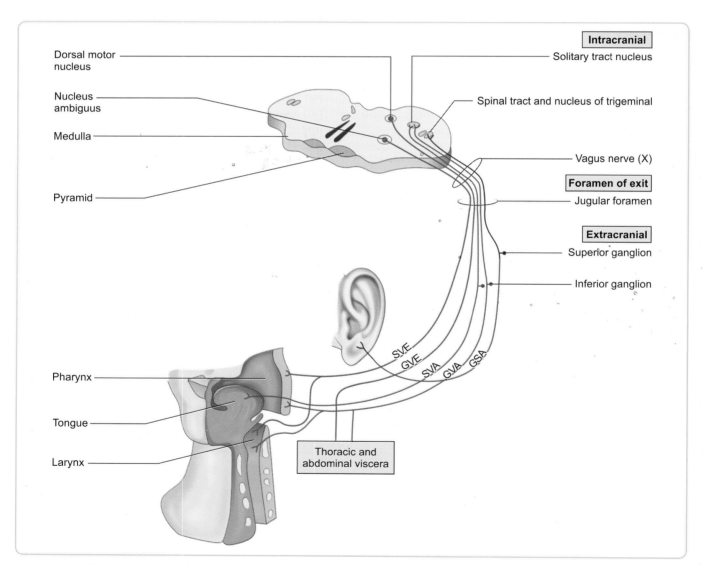

Figure 6.23: Vagus nerve: Origin, course and distribution (*Abbreviations*: SVE, special visceral efferent; GVE, general visceral efferent; SVA, special visceral afferent; GVA, general visceral afferent; GSA, general somatic afferent)

TABLE 6.16: Branches and distribution of vago-accessory nerve

Branches		Distribution
Auricular		Skin of external acoustic meatus
Pharyngeal		Muscles of pharynx
Superior laryngeal	External laryngeal	Cricothyroid
	Internal laryngeal	Mucosa of larynx—supraglottic part
Cardiac		Heart
Recurrent laryngeal		Muscles of larynx except cricothyroid and mucosa of larynx—infraglottic part
Pulmonary		Lungs
Oesophageal		Oesophagus
Gastric		Stomach, liver, gallbladder, pancreas, small intestine, large intestine up to right two-thirds of transverse colon

abdomen by passing through the oesophageal opening in the diaphragm. It supplies stomach, duodenum, liver, kidneys, small and large intestine up to the junction of proximal two-thirds and distal third of transverse colon. It has a wide distribution in the abdomen via coeliac, superior mesenteric and renal plexuses. The left vagus enters thorax, contributes to pulmonary and oesophageal plexuses, then enters abdomen supplies stomach, liver, duodenum and head of pancreas.

Clinical Anatomy

This nerve has an extensive distribution, but testing is based on its motor supply to the soft palate and to the larynx.
- Ask the patient to open the mouth wide and say "aah". Observe the movement of the soft palate. In a normal person, the soft palate is elevated. When one vagus nerve is paralyzed, the palate is pulled toward the normal side. When the nerve is paralyzed on both sides, the soft palate does not move at all.
- In injury to the superior laryngeal nerve, the voice is weak due to paralysis of the cricothyroid muscle.
- Injury to the recurrent laryngeal nerve also leads to hoarseness, but this hoarseness is permanent. On examining the larynx through a laryngoscope, it is seen that on the affected side the vocal fold does not move. It is fixed in a position midway between adduction and abduction. In cases where the recurrent laryngeal nerve is pressed upon by a tumour, it is observed that nerve fibres that supply abductors are lost first (Semon's law).
- In paralysis of both recurrent laryngeal nerves, voice is lost as both vocal folds are immobile (cadaveric position).
- It may be remembered that the left recurrent laryngeal nerve runs part of its course in the thorax. It can be involved in bronchial or oesophageal carcinoma or by secondary growths in mediastinal lymph nodes.

XI. Spinal Accessory Nerve

Functional Components and Nuclei

This nerve consists of **special visceral efferent** fibres which arise from the **lateral part of the anterior grey column of the upper five cervical segments** of the spinal cord, to supply the trapezius and sternocleidomastoid muscles.

Course and Distribution (Figure 6.24 and Table 6.17)

The spinal root is from the axons of nerve cells in the spinal nucleus, from the upper five cervical segments. The nerve ascends into the skull through foramen magnum, traverses a short distance with the cranial root as they pass through **jugular foramen**. It then enters deep surface of sternocleidomastoid muscle, and supplies it. Thereafter, it crosses the posterior triangle of the neck and ends by supplying trapezius muscle.

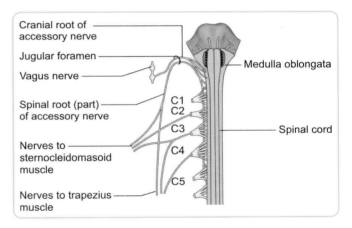

Figure 6.24: Spinal accessory nerve

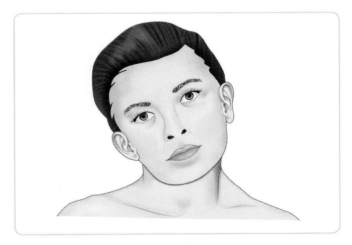

Figure 6.25: Torticollis

Clinical Anatomy

This nerve is tested as follows:
- Put your hands on the right and left shoulders of the patient and ask him/her to elevate (shrug) his/her shoulders. In paralysis, the movement will be weak on one side (due to paralysis of the trapezius).
- Ask the patient to turn his/her face to the opposite side (against resistance offered by your hand). In paralysis, the movement is weak on the affected side (due to paralysis of the sternocleidomastoid muscle).

Lesion of the Spinal Accessory Nerve
Unilateral peripheral lesion of spinal accessory nerve leads to paralysis of sternocleidomastoid and trapezius muscles.
- Paralysis of sternocleidomastoid leads to wry neck, i.e. difficulty in turning of head to the opposite side.
- The paralysis of trapezius results in the inability to shrug the shoulder towards the side of injury. As the lower part of trapezius is also supplied by C3 and C4 segments, an injury to the accessory nerve will not result in complete paralysis of trapezius.

Irritation of the Spinal Accessory Nerve
Results in the condition called "torticollis" (Figure 6.25). In this condition, there is a spasmodic contraction of sternocleidomastoid and trapezius.

TABLE 6.17: Branches and distribution of spinal accessory nerve

Branches	Distribution
Muscular	Sternocleidomastoid, trapezius

XII. Hypoglossal Nerve

Functional Components and Nuclei

This nerve is made up of the **somatic efferent** fibres which are processes of neurons in the **hypoglossal nucleus** in the medulla. They supply the muscles of the tongue (except palatoglossus).

The general somatic afferent fibres carrying proprioceptive impulses from muscles of the eyeball, face and tongue are carried by communicating fibres of trigeminal nerve (ophthalmic nerve from eyeball, cutaneous branches of ophthalmic, maxillary and mandibular nerves from facial muscles, and lingual branch of mandibular nerve from tongue).

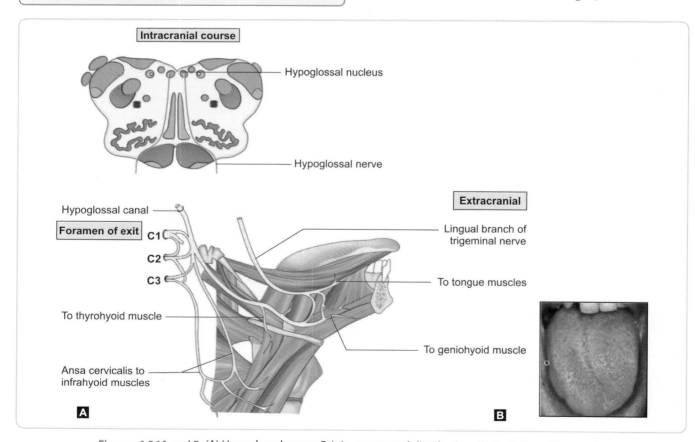

Figures 6.26A and B: (A) Hypoglossal nerve: Origin, course and distribution; (B) Deviation of tongue in paralysis of left hypoglossal nerve

Course and Distribution (Figures 6.26A and B and Table 6.18)

Intracranial course: The hypoglossal nerve emerges as rootlets from the ventral aspect of the medulla between pyramid and olive. It traverses the posterior cranial fossa and exits through hypoglossal canal.

Extracranial course: In the neck, it is closely associated with IX, X and XIth cranial nerves, internal carotid artery and internal jugular vein. It descends, crosses the loop of lingual artery, and ends by supplying the muscles of the tongue.

TABLE 6.18: Branches and distribution of hypoglossal nerve

Branches	Distribution
Muscular	Genioglossus, hyoglossus, styloglossus and intrinsic muscles of tongue

The cranial nerve nuclei with their functional components are summarized in Table 6.19.

Clinical Anatomy

This nerve supplies both intrinsic and extrinsic muscles of the tongue. To test the nerve, ask the patient to protrude the tongue. In a normal person the protruded tongue lies in the midline. If the nerve is paralyzed, the **tongue deviates to the paralyzed side.**
The explanation for this is as follows:
Protrusion of the tongue is produced by the pull of the right and left genioglossus muscles. The origin of the right and left genioglossus muscles lies anteriorly (on the mandible), and the insertion lies posteriorly (on to the posterolateral part of the tongue). Each muscle draws the posterior part of the tongue forward and medially. Normally, the medial pull of the two muscles cancels out, but when one muscle is paralyzed it is this medial pull of the intact muscle that causes **the tongue to deviate to the paralyzed side (Figure 6.26B).**

TABLE 6.19: Summary of cranial nerve nuclei with their functional components

Cranial nerve	Somatic efferent	Special visceral efferent	General visceral efferent	General visceral afferent	Special visceral afferent	General somatic afferent	Special somatic afferent
Olfactory					Olfactory epithelium*		Olfactory epithelium*
Optic							Bipolar cells of retina
Oculomotor	Oculomotor		Edinger-Westphal				
Trochlear	Trochlear						
Trigeminal		Motor				Mesencephalic, main sensory and spinal	
Abducent	Abducent						
Facial		Motor	Superior salivatory		Tractus solitarius	Belonging to trigeminal	
Vestibulo-cochlear							Vestibular and Cochlear
Glosso-pharyngeal		Ambiguus	Inferior salivatory	Tractus solitarius	Tractus solitarius	Belonging to trigeminal	
Vago-accessory		Ambiguus	Dorsal vagal	Tractus solitarius	Tractus solitarius	Belonging to trigeminal	
Spinal accessory		Accessory					
Hypoglossal	Hypoglossal						

*Olfactory mucosa develops from nasal placode (ectodermal in origin), hence it is considered as somatic, developmentally. However, due to the close relationship between the sensations of smell and taste, this nerve is functionally classified as visceral.

MULTIPLE CHOICE QUESTIONS

Q1. Which one of the following nuclei belongs to the general visceral efferent column?
A. Motor nucleus of facial
B. Motor nucleus of trigeminal
C. Dorsal nucleus of vagus
D. Nucleus ambiguus

Q2. The cranial nerve that emerges from dorsal surface of brain is:
A. II
B. IV
C. VI
D. VII

Q3. The axons that supply the ciliaris muscle of the eye are located in the:
A. Oculomotor nucleus
B. Superior cervical ganglion
C. Edinger-Westphal nucleus
D. Ciliary ganglion

Q4. The mesencephalic nucleus of the trigeminal nerve receives:
A. Pain sensations from the scalp
B. Proprioceptive impulses from the muscles of mastication
C. Sensations from the cornea
D. Tactile impulses from the face

Q5. The nerves belonging to the somatic efferent column supply the muscles developed from:
A. Somites
B. Intermediate mesoderm
C. Pharyngeal arches
D. Somatopleuric mesoderm

Q6. Which one of the following nuclei belong to the special visceral efferent column?
A. Oculomotor
B. Trochlear
C. Abducent
D. Facial

Q7. Which one of the following functional components is represented by the accessory nerve?
A. Somatic efferent
B. Special visceral efferent
C. General visceral efferent
D. General somatic afferent

Q8. The functional component of the taste sensations carried by glossopharyngeal nerve is:
A. General somatic afferent
B. Special somatic afferent
C. General visceral efferent
D. Special visceral afferent

Q9. The nucleus ambiguus is associated with which one of the following cranial nerves:
A. Facial
B. Glossopharyngeal
C. Spinal accessory
D. Hypoglossal

Q10. The nucleus that carries the parasympathetic fibres of the facial nerve begins from:
A. Motor nucleus of facial nerve
B. Inferior salivatory nucleus
C. Nucleus of tractus solitarius
D. Superior salivatory nucleus

ANSWERS

1. C   2. B   3. D   4. B   5. A   6. D   7. B   8. D   9. B   10. D

SHORT NOTES

1. Nuclei of facial nerve
2. Nuclei of trigeminal nerve

LONG QUESTIONS

1. Describe the oculomotor nerve under the following headings: nuclei, functional components, course and relations, branches and distribution, clinical anatomy.
2. Describe the trochlear nerve under the following headings: nuclei, functional components, course and relations, branches and distribution, clinical anatomy.
3. Describe the mandibular nerve under the following headings: nuclei, functional components, course and relations, branches and distribution, clinical anatomy.

4. Describe the abducent nerve under the following headings: nuclei, functional components, course and relations, branches and distribution, clinical anatomy.
5. Describe the extracranial course of facial nerve under the following headings: nuclei, functional components, course and relations, branches and distribution, clinical anatomy.
6. Describe the glossopharyngeal nerve under the following headings: nuclei, functional components, course and relations, branches and distribution, clinical anatomy.
7. Describe the vagus nerve in neck, under the following headings: nuclei, functional components, course and relations, branches and distribution, clinical anatomy.
8. Describe the hypoglossal nerve under the following headings: nuclei, functional components, course and relations, branches and distribution, clinical anatomy.

Clinical Cases

6.1: Supranuclear or Infranuclear?
One person had paralysis of the muscles of the lower and upper half of the right face. There were no other symptoms. Another person had similar complaints, but in addition, he had hyperacusis, tinnitus and vertigo.
A. Specify the type of facial paralysis in these two persons.
B. Localize the site of lesion in them.

6.2: Nerve Lesion: Left or Right?
One person had deviation of tongue to the right side on protrusion. Another person had deviation of jaw to the left side on opening the mouth.
A. Localize the lesion in both the cases.
B. Specify the muscles responsible for the deviation in both the cases.

6.3: Two patients presented with lower motor neuron (LMN) type of facial paralysis of the right side with loss of lacrimation. Of these, one of them also had tinnitus.
A. Localize the lesion in the patient with tinnitus.
B. Which nerve carries the preganglionic fibres for lacrimation and where do they relay?

6.4: A 40-year-old lady was diagnosed to suffer from trigeminal neuralgia which is also known as tic douloureux. She had severe stabbing pain on the right side of her face but surprisingly there was no pain near the angle of mandible and below.
A. Explain the anatomical basis of her not feeling the pain of trigeminal neuralgia over the angle of mandible
B. What does the word "dolor" mean in tic douloureux?

6.5: A 25-year-old man had developed ptosis of his right eye, divergent squint and crossed diplopia. He also had loss of direct light reflex and accommodation reflex.
A. Specify the nerve affected and its side.
B. Name the nerve that forms the afferent limb of accommodation reflex.

6.6: An 18-year-old girl had to undergo root canal therapy and her dental surgeon wanted to block the inferior alveolar nerve and lingual nerve by injecting local anaesthetic drug. After the block, the patient did not feel any sensation over the tongue and surprisingly, she had also lost the taste sensation.
A. What is the site where inferior alveolar nerve is easily accessible intraorally?
B. Explain the anatomical basis of loss of taste sensation.

Chapter 7

Pathways of Special Senses

INTRODUCTION

The special sensory pathways consist of a specialized receptor (epithelial receptor), a peripheral neuron (ganglion) whose central process relays on to a central neuron (nucleus). From here, secondary pathways cross the midline and carry the impulses to the thalamus and from there to the appropriate sensory areas of cerebral cortex.

The special sensory pathway of vision and audition are special somatic afferents. The gustatory sense is special visceral afferent. Olfaction, although developmentally ectodermal in origin, functionally, is closely related to gustation. Hence functionally it is also special visceral afferent. The olfactory pathway is also the only pathway that distinctly stands out as an exception to the above general rule.

The olfactory receptors are different from the other receptors, in the fact, that they are neuronal receptors. These are bipolar neurons and the only neuronal cell bodies that are capable of regeneration when damaged. Olfactory pathway is functionally a part of limbic system. Olfaction is the only sense that is directly projected to the cerebral cortex and then relayed to the thalamus. Olfactory pathway also is the only sensory pathway where second order neurons do not cross the midline.

OLFACTORY PATHWAY

The peripheral end organ for smell is the **olfactory epithelium** that lines the upper and posterior parts of the nasal cavity. Nerve fibres arising in this mucosa collect to form about 20 bundles that together constitute **olfactory nerve** (cranial nerve I). The bundles pass through foramina in the cribriform plate of the ethmoid bone to enter the cranial cavity, where they terminate in the **olfactory bulb** (Flowchart 7.1 and Figure 7.1).

The components of olfactory pathway are shown in Flowchart 7.1.

Olfactory Epithelium

The fibres of the olfactory nerves are processes of **olfactory receptor cells,** lying in the epithelium lining the olfactory mucosa (Figure 7.1). These receptor cells are homologous to sensory neurons located in sensory ganglia. In other words, the first order sensory neurons of the olfactory pathway are located within the olfactory epithelium itself. In the course of evolution, all neurons have arisen by modification of epithelial cells and their migration, in most cases, into deeper tissues. The olfactory receptor cells retain their position in the epithelium and are, therefore, regarded as primitive.

Each receptor cell consists of a cell body and of two processes, i.e. it is a bipolar cell. The peripheral process (dendrite) reaches the surface of the olfactory epithelium.

Flowchart 7.1: Parts of the olfactory pathway

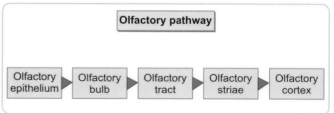

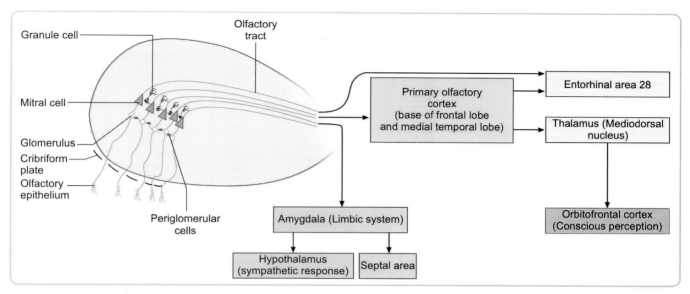

Figure 7.1: Main features of the olfactory pathway

The central process (axon) enters the submucosa and forms one fibre of the olfactory nerve. These fibres are nonmyelinated. The olfactory nerve fibres terminate in the olfactory bulb.

Olfactory Bulb

The olfactory bulb receives fibres of the olfactory nerves, arising from olfactory sensory neurons. These incoming fibres synapse with neurons within the bulb.

Several types of cells are present in the olfactory bulb. Out of these the mitral cells give origin to the fibres of olfactory tract. Granule cells are interneurons .

A small group of cells in the posterior part of olfactory tract constitute the **anterior olfactory nucleus**.

Connections of Olfactory Bulb

The axons of mitral cells run in the olfactory tract. The olfactory bulb is continuous posteriorly with the olfactory tract. They send collateral branches to the anterior olfactory nucleus. Fibres from the anterior olfactory nucleus pass through the anterior commissure to the opposite olfactory bulb. Olfactory bulb also receives fibres from basal forebrain, midbrain reticular formation and locus coeruleus. (Figure 7.2).

Olfactory Tract

The olfactory tract is predominantly made up of axons of mitral cells of the olfactory bulb.

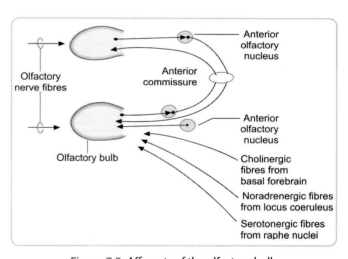

Figure 7.2: Afferents of the olfactory bulb

When traced posteriorly, the olfactory tract flattens to form olfactory trigone.

Olfactory Striae

From the trigone, arise medial, intermediate, and lateral olfactory striae (Figures 7.3 and 7.4).

- When traced backwards, the lateral olfactory stria reaches the limen insulae (in the depth of the stem of the lateral sulcus). Here, it bends sharply to the medial side and becomes continuous with a small area of grey matter called the gyrus semilunaris (or periamygdaloid area). The lateral olfactory stria is

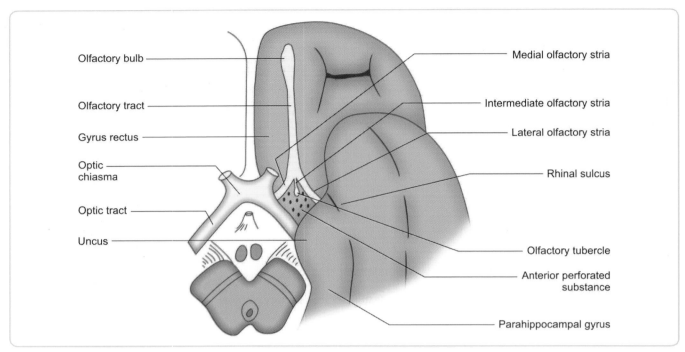

Figure 7.3: Olfactory pathway: olfactory bulb, olfactory tract, olfactory striae, olfactory tubercle

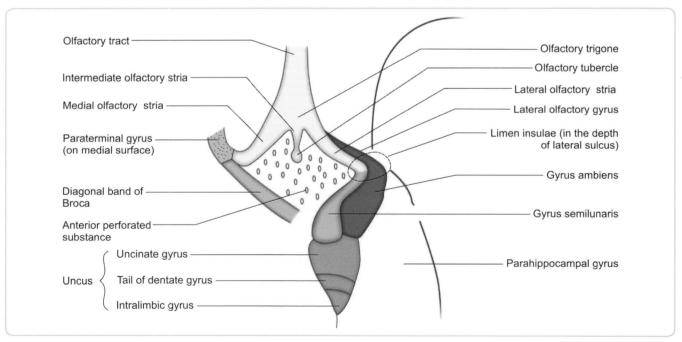

Figure 7.4: Olfactory pathway: olfactory striae, olfactory tubercle, olfactory cortices

covered by a thin layer of grey matter called the lateral olfactory gyrus. When traced backwards, this gyrus becomes continuous with a part of the cortex called the gyrus ambiens. The lateral olfactory gyrus and the gyrus ambiens collectively form the prepiriform region (or area).

- The lateral olfactory stria also projects to the amygdala. It is concerned with emotional reactions.
- The medial olfactory stria, reaches the medial surface of the hemisphere, where it ends near the paraterminal gyrus (which lies just in front of the lamina terminalis).
- The intermediate olfactory stria ends in the olfactory tubercle in the anterior perforated substance. The olfactory tubercle is a sensory processing centre and plays a role in reward function.

Primary Olfactory Cortex (Figure 7.1)

The primary olfactory cortex or piriform lobe lies between anterior perforated substance and the uncus. It receives direct afferents from the lateral olfactory stria.

The main regions receiving direct fibres from the olfactory bulb are:

- The prepiriform cortex (including the lateral olfactory gyrus and the gyrus ambiens)
- The gyrus semilunaris (periamygdaloid area).
- Anterior part of entorhinal area (Brodmann area 28) of parahippocampal gyrus and the uncus

Secondary Olfactory Cortex

The entorhinal area (Brodmann area 28) receives only a few fibres directly from lateral olfactory stria. The posterior part of entorhinal area is secondary olfactory cortex because it receives fibres from primary olfactory cortex. The entorhinal cortex is concerned with processing information about odours.

Entorhinal area projects to the amygdala and from there to the hippocampus which is involved in memory. Fibres also reach hypothalamus for autonomic responses and to integrate olfaction with visceral functions.

The piriform cortex projects to the medial dorsal nucleus of the thalamus, which then projects to the orbitofrontal cortex. The orbitofrontal cortex is also secondary olfactory cortex. It mediates conscious perception of the odour.

> ### Clinical Anatomy
>
> - Olfactory epithelium is a neuroepithelium, the only example of neuronal cell body which regenerates when damaged. This feature makes them behave like stem cells. Hence, these cells have been used in clinical trials for treating spinal cord injuries.
> - Disorders of olfaction can result due to lesions of olfactory pathway. Loss of smell is known as anosmia and altered sense of smell is parosmia. Irritative lesions of uncus can result in olfactory hallucinations (uncinate fits).

VISUAL PATHWAY

The peripheral receptors for light are situated in the **retina**. Nerve fibres arising in the retina constitute the **optic nerve**. The right and left optic nerves join to form the **optic chiasma,** in which many of their fibres cross to the opposite side. The uncrossed fibres of the optic nerve, along with the fibres that have crossed over from the opposite side, form the **optic tract**.

The optic tract terminates predominantly in the **lateral geniculate body**. Fibres arising in this body form the **geniculocalcarine tract** or **optic radiation,** which ends in the visual areas of the cerebral cortex (Figure 7.5).

The Retina

The retina has a complex structure. It contains photoreceptors that convert the stimulus of light into nervous impulses. These receptors are of two kinds, **rods** and **cones** (Figure 7.6). There are about seven million cones in each retina. The rods are far more numerous around more than a hundred million.

The cones respond best to bright light. They are responsible for sharp vision and for discrimination of colour. They are most numerous in the central region of the retina, which is responsible for sharp vision. This area is about 6 mm in diameter. Within this region, there is an yellowish area called the **macula lutea**. The centre of the macula shows a small depression called the **fovea centralis** (Figure 7.7).

Medial to the macula lutea, there is a circular area called the **optic disc**. This area is devoid of photoreceptors and is, therefore, called the **blind spot**. The fibres of the optic nerve leave the eyeball through the region of the optic disc.

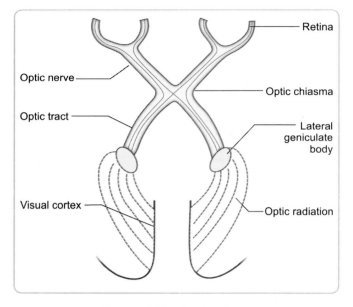

Figure 7.5: The visual pathway

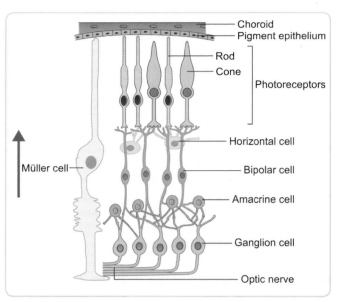

Figure 7.6: Neurons within the retina—the red arrow indicates the direction of light falling on the retina

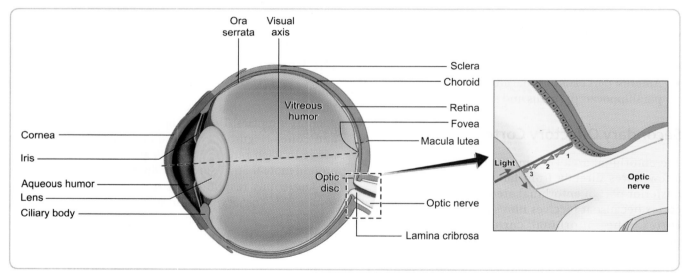

Figure 7.7: Passage of light through retina. Inset: 1- Rod & cone; 2-Bipolar cell; 3 - Ganglion cell

The macula lies in the visual axis of the eyeball. When any object is viewed critically, its image is formed on the macula. The fovea centralis contains cones only. Rods, on the other hand, predominate in the peripheral parts of the retina. They respond to poor light and especially to movement across the field of vision.

Each rod or cone is a modified sensory neuron. It consists of a cell body, a peripheral process, and a central process. The cell body contains a nucleus. The peripheral process is rod-shaped, in the case of rods and cone-shaped, in the case of cones (hence, the names rods and cones). The ends of these peripheral processes are separated from one another by processes of pigment cells. The central processes of rods and cones are like those of neurons. They end by synapsing with other neurons within the retina.

The basic neuronal arrangement within the retina is shown in Figure 7.6. The central processes of rods and cones synapse with the peripheral processes of **bipolar**

cells. The central processes of bipolar cells synapse with dendrites of **ganglion cells**. Axons arising from ganglion cells form the **fibres of the optic nerve**.

The various elements mentioned above form a series of layers within the retina. The outermost layer (towards the choroid) is formed by the pigment cells, followed in sequence by the rods and cones, the bipolar cells, the ganglion cells, and a layer of optic nerve fibres. The layer of optic nerve fibres is apposed to the vitreous. It is obvious that light has to pass through several of the layers of the retina to reach the rods and cones. This 'inverted' arrangement of the retina is necessary, as passage of light in the reverse direction would be obstructed by the layer of pigment cells.

The pigment cells are important in spacing the rods and cones and providing them with mechanical support. They absorb light and prevent back reflection. A nutritive and phagocytic role has also been attributed to them.

Visual Field and Retinal Quadrants

When the head and eyes are maintained in a fixed position and one eye is closed, the area seen by that eye constitutes the **visual field** for that eye. Now, if the other eye is also opened, the area seen is more or less the same as was seen with one eye. In other words, the visual fields of the two eyes overlap to a very great extent. On either side, however, there is a small area seen only by the eye of that side (Figure 7.8). Although the two eyes view the same area, the relative position of objects within the area appears somewhat dissimilar to the two eyes, as they view the object from slightly different angles. The difference, though slight, is of considerable importance, as it forms the basis for the perception of depth (**stereoscopic vision**).

For the convenience of description, the visual field is divided into right and left halves. It may also be divided into upper and lower halves so that the visual field can be said to consist of four quadrants (Figure 7.9). In a similar manner, each retina can also be divided into quadrants. Images of objects in the field of vision are formed on the retina by the lens of the eyeball. As with any convex lens, the image is inverted. If an object is placed in the **right** half of the field of vision, its image is formed on the **left** half of the retina and **vice versa**. The two halves of the retina are usually referred to as **nasal** (= medial) and **temporal** (= lateral) halves. This introduces a complication as the left half of the left eye is the temporal half, while in the case of the right eye, it is the nasal half. Thus, the image of an object placed in the right half of the field of vision falls on the temporal half of the left retina and on the nasal half of the right retina.

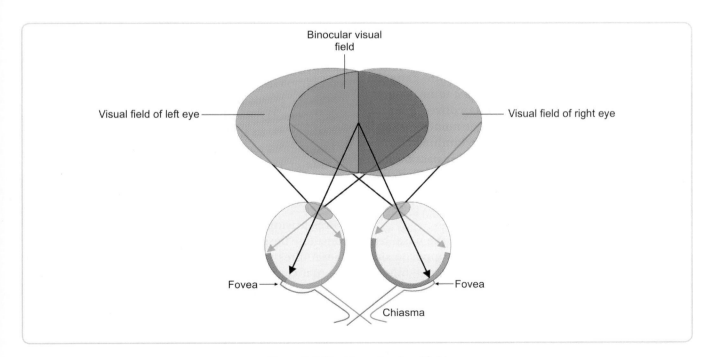

Figure 7.8: The binocular visual field

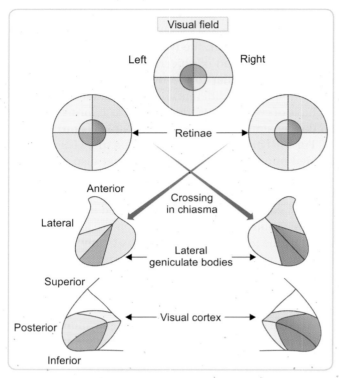

Figure 7.9: Scheme to show the representation of the visual field in the retinae, the lateral geniculate bodies, and the visual cortex of the two sides—the peripheral parts of the visual field are represented by light colours, while the corresponding macular areas are represented by dark colours

Optic Nerve, Optic Chiasma, and Optic Tract

The optic nerve is made up of axons of the ganglion cells of the retina. These axons are at first unmyelinated. The fibres from all parts of the retina converge on the optic disc. In this region, the sclera has numerous small apertures and is, therefore, called the **lamina cribrosa** (**crib = sieve**). Bundles of optic nerve fibres pass through these apertures. Each fibre acquires a myelin sheath as soon as it pierces the sclera. The fibres of the nerve arising from the four quadrants of the retina maintain the same relative position within the nerve.

The fibres of the optic nerve arising in the nasal half of each retina enter the optic tract of the opposite side after crossing in the chiasma. Fibres from the temporal half of each retina enter the optic tract of the same side (Figure 7.5). Thus, the right optic tract comes to contain fibres from the right halves of both retinae and the left tract from the left halves. In other words, all optic nerve fibres carrying impulses relating to the left half of the field of vision are brought together in the right optic tract and **vice**

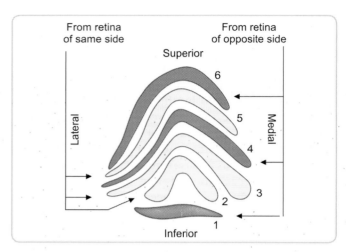

Figure 7.10: Laminae of lateral geniculate body

versa. Each optic tract carries these fibres to the lateral geniculate body of the corresponding side.

Lateral Geniculate Body

The grey matter of this body is split into six laminae. Fibres from the eye of the same side end in laminae 2, 3, and 5; while those from the opposite eye end in laminae 1, 4, and 6 (Figure 7.10). The macular fibres end in the central and posterior part of the lateral geniculate body, and this area is relatively large (Figure 7.9). Fibres from the peripheral parts of the retina end in the anterior part of the lateral geniculate body. The upper half of the retina is represented laterally and the lower half of the retina is represented medially. Specific points on the retina project to specific points in the lateral geniculate body. In turn, specific points of this body project to specific points in the visual cortex. In this way, a point-to-point relationship is maintained between the retinae and the visual cortex (retinotopy).

Geniculocalcarine Tract and Visual Cortex

Fibres arising from cells of the lateral geniculate body constitute the **geniculocalcarine tract** or **optic radiation**. These fibres pass through the retrolentiform part of the internal capsule. The optic radiation ends in the visual area of the cerebral cortex (area 17) (Figure 7.11). Fibres of the optic radiation, from the lower half of the retina (upper field of vision) loop forward and downward into the temporal lobe (to swerve around the atrium and inferior horn of lateral ventricle) before turning backward to the occipital lobe. This is called **Meyer's loop** (Figure 7.12).

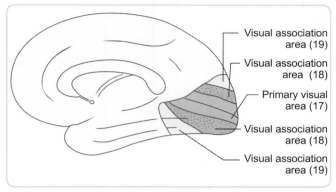

Figure 7.11: Medial aspect of cerebral hemisphere showing visual cortex

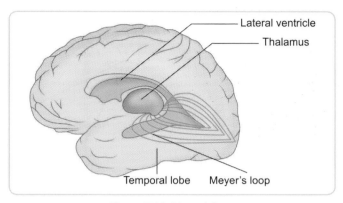

Figure 7.12: Meyer's loop

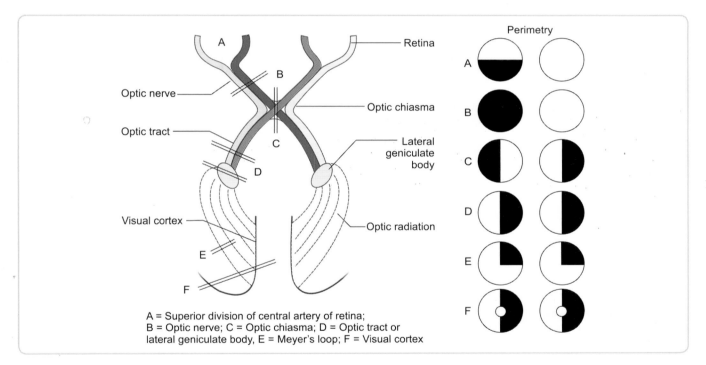

A = Superior division of central artery of retina;
B = Optic nerve; C = Optic chiasma; D = Optic tract or
lateral geniculate body, E = Meyer's loop; F = Visual cortex

Figure 7.13: Sites of lesion in the visual pathway and the corresponding field defects detected by perimetry

The optic radiation ends in the primary visual area of the cerebral cortex **(Brodmann's area 17)**. The cortex of each hemisphere receives impulses from the retinal halves of the same side (i.e. from the opposite half of the field of vision). The upper quadrants of the retina are represented above the calcarine sulcus, and the lower quadrants below it. The cortical area for the macula is larger than that for peripheral areas. It occupies the posterior part of the visual area. The macular area has dual blood supply (posterior cerebral artery and branches of middle cerebral artery). The cortical area for the peripheral part of the retina is situated anterior to the area for the macula.

Neural Pathway for Vision

The first-order sensory neurons carrying visual sensations are bipolar cells of retina. Their dendrites synapse with rods and cones (photoreceptor) and their axons with the dendrites of ganglion cells.

The second-order sensory neurons are the ganglion cells. Axons arising from ganglion cells form the **fibres of the optic nerve**. The right and the left optic nerves join to form the **optic chiasma**, where fibres from nasal half of retina cross to the opposite side and travel through the opposite optic tract to terminate in the opposite lateral

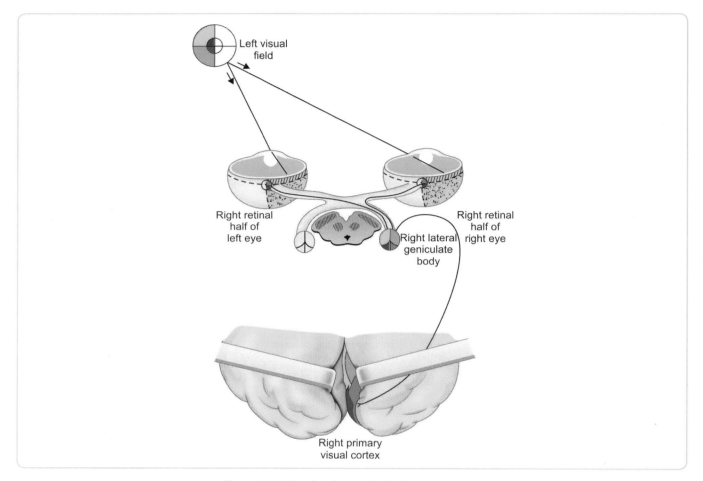

Figure 7.14: Visual pathway: Cortical representation

Clinical Anatomy

Lesions of Visual Pathway

Injuries to different parts of the visual pathway can produce various kinds of defects. Loss of vision in one half (right or left) of the visual field is called **hemianopia**. If the same half of the visual field is lost in both eyes the defect is said to be **homonymous** and if different halves are lost the defect is said to be **heteronymous**.

An **ophthalmoscope** will show the central artery of retina enter the eye through the optic disc and divides into an upper division and a lower division to supply the upper and lower halves of retina. If one of the divisions gets blocked, e.g. superior division, the perimetry of that eye will show lower **hemianopia** (half loss of lower field of vision) **with a sharp horizontal separation of upper or lower halves**. (This is in complete contrast to hemianopia, with lesions in the posterior parts of visual pathway, where there is sharp vertical separation between left and right halves) (Figure 7.13). **Glaucoma** (increased intraocular pressure) compresses the peripheral fibres of optic nerve when they curve and enter the optic disc resulting in **peripheral loss of field of vision**.

Injury to the optic nerve will obviously produce total blindness in the eye concerned, i.e. **amblyopia**. Damage to the central part of the optic chiasma (e.g. by pressure from an enlarged hypophysis) interrupts the crossing fibres derived from the nasal halves of the two retinae resulting in **bitemporal heteronymous hemianopia** (also called **tunnel vision**). Complete destruction of the optic tract, the lateral geniculate body, the optic radiation or the visual cortex of one side, results in loss of the opposite half of the field of vision (Figure 7.14). A lesion on the left side leads to right **homonymous hemianopia**. A lesion in the lower part of optic radiation called **Meyer's loop**, (more susceptible due to its longer course and being more superficial in the temporal lobe), results in superior **quadrantic anopia** (quarter loss of field of vision). Vascular lesions of visual cortex results in macular sparing, because of the dual vascular supply of macular region by posterior cerebral and middle cerebral arteries. A compressive lesion, e.g. meningioma, glioma, will not produce macular sparing.

geniculate body. The fibres from temporal half of each retina enter the optic tract of the same side to terminate in the ipsilateral geniculate body.

The cell bodies of **third-order sensory neurons** are located in the lateral geniculate body. Their axons form the optic radiation, which projects to the visual cortex.

AUDITORY PATHWAY

The internal ear contains the organ of hearing called the cochlea. The cochlea has a central bony core called the modiolus, and a spiral canal runs around it. The organ of Corti, which is the sensory epithelium of hearing, sits on the inner surface of the basilar membrane (Figure 7.15).

The **first order neurons** of this pathway (**primary auditory pathway**) are located in the **spiral ganglion**. These neurons are bipolar (like first order neurons of olfactory and optic nerves, and unlike any other sensory nerves). Their peripheral processes reach the hair cells in the spiral organ of Corti (which is the end organ for hearing). The central processes of the neurons form the cochlear nerve, and terminate in the **dorsal and ventral cochlear nuclei in the medulla.** The neurons in these nuclei are, therefore, second order neurons. Neurons receiving fibres from different parts of the spiral organ are arranged in a definite sequence according to the frequency of sound waves in the ventral nucleus (**tonotopic arrangement**).

The axons of the **second order neurons** pass medially in the dorsal part of the pons. It has some peculiarities that are as follows:

- Most of them cross to the opposite side, (but **some remain uncrossed**), and form the lateral lemniscus.

The crossing fibres of the two sides form a conspicuous mass of fibres called the **trapezoid body**.

- A few fibres from the cochlear nuclei terminate in the **superior olivary complex** (made up of a number of nuclei). The **medial superior olivary nucleus** receives fibres from both cochleae and plays a role in localizing the direction of sound (by calculating the time difference in arrival of inputs from the right and left cochleae).

- Some cochlear fibres that do not relay in the superior olivary nucleus join the lateral lemniscus after relaying in scattered groups of cells lying within the trapezoid body. These cells constitute the **trapezoid nucleus (nucleus of the trapezoid body)**.

- Still other cochlear fibres relay in cells that lie within the lemniscus itself, which form the **nucleus of the lateral lemniscus**.

- Some fibres of the lateral lemniscus ascend to the midbrain and terminate in the **inferior colliculus**. Fibres arising in the colliculus enter the inferior brachium to reach the medial geniculate body.

- Most of the fibres of the lateral lemniscus reach the **medial geniculate body** without relay in the inferior colliculus (Figure 7.16).

Fibres of the **third order neurons** arising in the medial geniculate body form the auditory radiation which ends tonotopically in the auditory area of the cerebral cortex (**anterior and posterior transverse temporal gyri**, Brodmann's areas 41, 42). Since each lateral lemniscus carries impulses arising in the right and left cochlea, lesions of temporal lobe will not cause complete deafness in either ear (Flowchart 7.2).

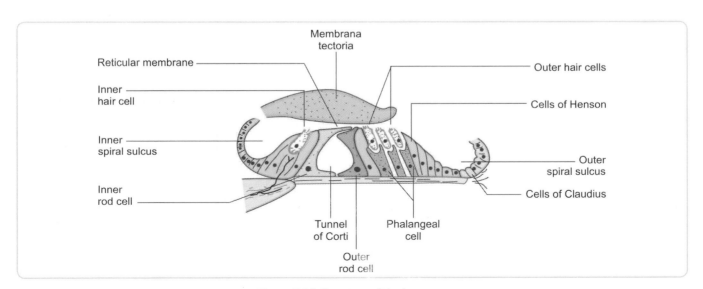

Figure 7.15: Structure of the inner ear

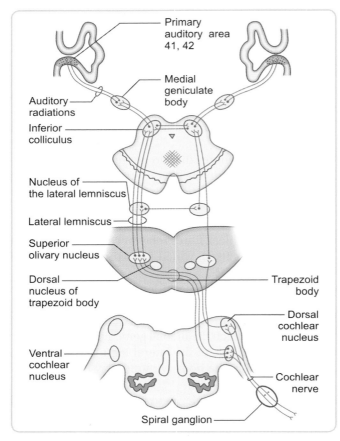

Figure 7.16: The auditory pathway

Flowchart 7.2: Flow diagram showing the neurons involved in auditory pathway

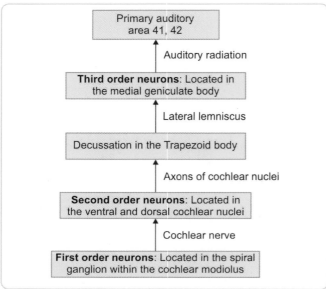

Clinical Anatomy

Unilateral lesions of organ of Corti, cochlear nerve or cochlear nuclei will result in **ipsilateral hearing loss**.

Lesions of central auditory pathway, i.e. lateral lemniscus, medial geniculate body or auditory cortex, will result in **diminution in hearing on both sides but more so on the contralateral side**. This is because auditory sensation is represented bilaterally in the cortex (but predominantly on the contralateral side).

GUSTATORY PATHWAY

The gustatory receptors, or taste buds, are microscopic barrel-shaped epithelial chemoreceptors. These receptors are in synaptic contact with the dendrites of gustatory nerves (Figure 7.17).

- **From the anterior two-thirds of the tongue (excluding the circumvallate papillae)**: Cell bodies of the first order neurons lie in the geniculate ganglion of facial nerve. The peripheral processes (dendrites) pass via the chorda tympani nerve, lingual nerve, and reach the anterior two-thirds of the tongue. The central processes end in the upper part of the nucleus of the solitary tract which is sometimes called the gustatory nucleus (second order neurons).
- **From the posterior one-third of the tongue (including the circumvallate papillae)**: Cell bodies of the first order neurons lie in the inferior ganglion of glossopharyngeal nerve (petrous ganglion). The peripheral processes pass through the terminal

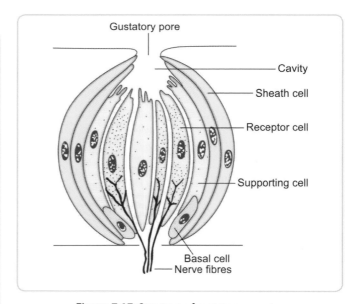

Figure 7.17: Structure of gustatory receptor

Flowchart 7.3: Primary gustatory pathway

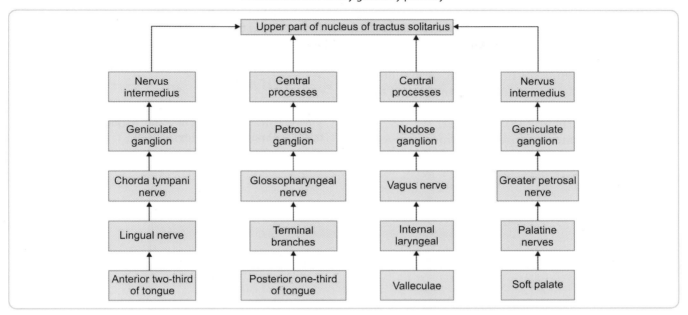

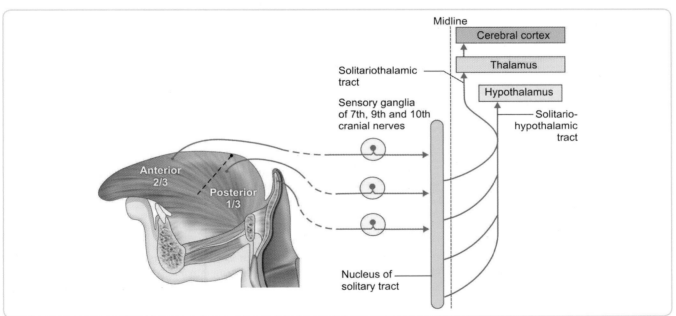

Figure 7.18: Connections of the nucleus of the solitary tract

branches of glossopharyngeal nerve to the posterior one-third of the tongue. The central processes end in the upper part of the nucleus of the solitary tract.

- **From the valleculae**: Cell bodies of the first order neurons lie in the inferior ganglion of vagus nerve (nodose ganglion). The peripheral processes pass through the internal laryngeal branch of superior laryngeal nerve to the valleculae. The central processes end in the upper part of the nucleus of the solitary tract.

- **From the soft palate**: Cell bodies of the first order neurons lie in the geniculate ganglion of facial nerve. The peripheral processes pass via the greater petrosal nerve to the pterygopalatine fossa and from there through the palatine nerves to the soft palate. The central processes end in the upper part of the nucleus of the solitary tract (Flowchart 7.3).

Second order gustatory axons start from the **nucleus of the solitary tract** and carry visceral impulses to the hypothalamus and the thalamus through the **solitario-hypothalamic** and **solitariothalamic tracts**, respectively. The fibres going to thalamus cross the midline and terminate in the ventral posteromedial nucleus (along with the trigeminal lemniscus). The nucleus of the solitary tract also sends fibres to the reticular formation, the general visceral efferent cranial nerve nuclei and to the autonomic nuclei (in the intermediolateral grey column) of the spinal cord (Figure 7.18).

Tertiary gustatory axons start from the ventral posteromedial nucleus of thalamus and radiate through the posterior limb of internal capsule to the inferior part of the postcentral gyrus of cerebral cortex and the insula. The ascending fibres ending in the hypothalamus, reach the limbic system, which allow autonomic reactions to taste.

> **Clinical Anatomy**
>
> Lesions of cranial nerves VII, IX, and X can affect taste sensation and result in **ageusia (loss of taste), hypogeusia (decreased taste)** or **abnormal taste (dysgeusia)**.

MULTIPLE CHOICE QUESTIONS

Q1. Which one of the following cells forms fibres of olfactory tract?
A. Bipolar
B. Granule
C. Mitral
D. Periglomerular

Q2. Where does the medial olfactory stria terminate?
A. Gyrus semilunaris
B. Anterior perforated substance
C. Gyrus ambiens
D. Paraterminal gyrus

Q3. Which of the following acts as a reflex and integration centre of the visual system?
A. Lateral geniculate body
B. Oculomotor nucleus
C. Pontine paramedian reticular formation
D. Superior colliculus

Q4. Which of the following is the centre for pupillary light reflex?
A. Lateral geniculate body
B. Oculomotor nucleus
C. Pretectal nucleus
D. Superior colliculus

Q5. The cells present in retina in its outer nuclear layer are:
A. Amacrine cells
B. Bipolar cells
C. Pigment epithelium
D. Rods and cones

Q6. Lesion of which part of the optic pathway results in bitemporal hemianopia?
A. Optic chiasma
B. Lateral geniculate body
C. Optic tract
D. Superior part of optic radiation

Q7. The primary auditory neurons terminate in:
A. Cochlear nucleus
B. Inferior colliculus
C. Superior olivary nucleus
D. Trapezoid body

Q8. Auditory radiations commence from:
A. Inferior colliculus
B. Medial geniculate body
C. Transverse temporal gyrus
D. Trapezoid body

Q9. Dendrites of geniculate ganglia reach the gustatory receptors located in the:
A. Circumvallate papillae
B. Posterior one-third of tongue
C. Soft palate
D. Vallecular region

Q10. Axons from the inferior vagal ganglion, carrying taste sensations, terminate in:
A. Dorsal nucleus of vagus
B. Nucleus ambiguus
C. Nucleus of tractus solitarius
D. Ventral posteromedial nucleus of thalamus

ANSWERS

1. C   2. D   3. D   4. C   5. D   6. A   7. A   8. B   9. C   10. C

SHORT NOTES

1. Applied anatomy of visual pathway
2. Visual/optic pathway and effects of damage to optic tract

LONG QUESTIONS

1. Describe the auditory pathway and illustrate with suitable diagrams
2. Describe the visual pathway. Add a note on the effects of lesions at different sites on it

---

Clinical Cases

7.1: A person suffers from right-sided homonymous superior quadrantic anopia due to a lesion of temporal lobe.
   A. Specify the vessel affected in the above person
   B. Name the fibres of the visual pathway affected

7.2: A 16 years old boy was found to be
   • Too tall for his age
   • He was not able to see properly on the extreme right and extreme left because of a neurological deficit
   A. Specify the name of the neurological deficit
   B. Correlate the neurological deficit with the tall stature of the boy

Chapter 8 | Cerebellum

Specific Learning Objectives

At the end of learning, the student shall be able to:
➢ Describe the gross features and subdivisions of cerebellum
➢ Enumerate the deep nuclei, afferent and efferent connections of cerebellum and the fibres in the cerebellar peduncles
➢ Describe and correlate the morphological, functional and developmental subdivisions of cerebellum
➢ Explain the anatomical basis of clinical features of cerebellopontine angle tumour and the symptoms of cerebellar disease

INTRODUCTION

The cerebellum (or small brain) lies in the posterior cranial fossa. In an adult, the weight of the cerebellum is about 150 g. This is about 10% of the weight of the cerebral hemispheres. Like the cerebrum, the cerebellum has a superficial layer of grey matter, the cerebellar cortex. Because of the presence of numerous fissures, the cerebellar cortex is much more extensive than the size of this part of the brain would suggest. It has been estimated that the surface area of the cerebellar cortex is about 50% of the area of the cerebral cortex.

The cerebellum lies behind the pons and the medulla. It is separated from the cerebrum by a fold of dura mater called the **tentorium cerebelli.** Anteriorly, the fourth ventricle intervenes between the cerebellum (behind), and the pons and medulla (in front, Figures 8.1A and B). Part of the cavity of the ventricle extends into the cerebellum as a transverse cleft. This cleft is bounded cranially by the superior (or anterior) medullary velum, a lamina of white matter (Figures 8.1A and B).

EXTERNAL FEATURES

Parts of Cerebellum

The cerebellum consists of a part lying near the midline called the **vermis** and two lateral **hemispheres.**

Surfaces of Cerebellum

It has two surfaces, **superior** and **inferior.** On the superior aspect, the vermis merges with the hemispheres. On the

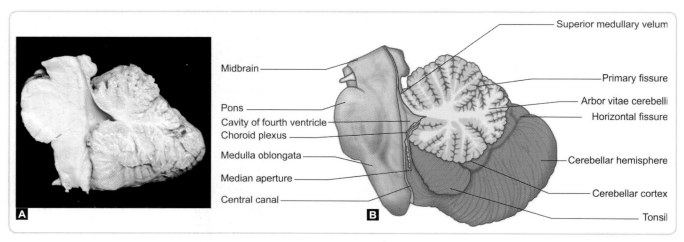

Figures 8.1A and B: Median sagittal section through brainstem and cerebellum: (A) photograph; (B) line diagram

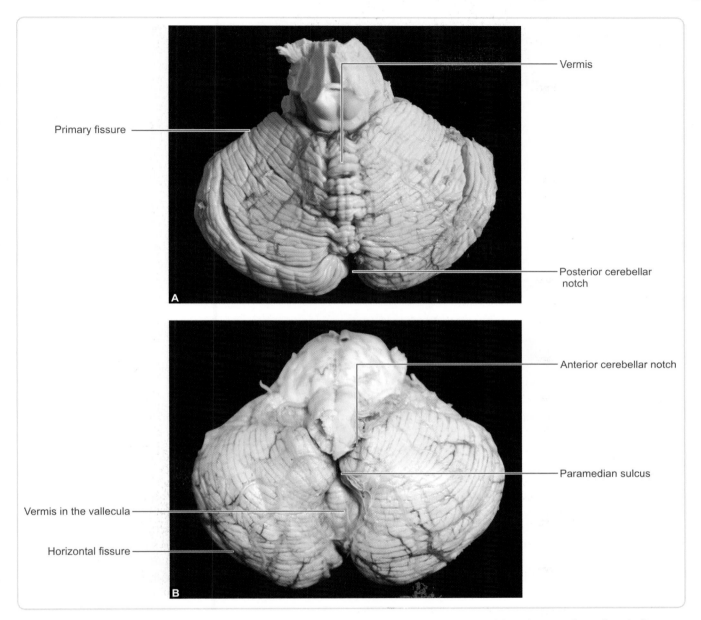

Primary fissure

Vermis

Posterior cerebellar notch

A

Anterior cerebellar notch

Paramedian sulcus

Vermis in the vallecula

Horizontal fissure

B

Figures 8.2A and B: (A) Photograph of the superior surface of cerebellum; (B) Photograph of the inferior surface of cerebellum

inferior aspect, the two hemispheres are separated by a deep depression called the **vallecula** (Figures 8.2A and B). The vermis lies in the depth of this depression. On each side, the vermis is separated from the corresponding cerebellar hemisphere by a **paramedian sulcus**.

Fissures and Lobes of Cerebellum (Figures 8.3 to 8.5)

The surface of the cerebellum is marked by a series of fissures that run more or less parallel to one another.

The fissures subdivide the surface of the cerebellum into narrow leaf-like bands or **folia**. The long axis of the folia is transverse. Sections of the cerebellum cut at right angles to this axis have a characteristic tree-like appearance to which the term **arbor vitae** (tree of life) is applied (Figure 8.1).

Some of the fissures on the surface of the cerebellum are deeper than others. They divide the cerebellum into **lobes** within which smaller **lobules** may be recognized (Figure 8.3).

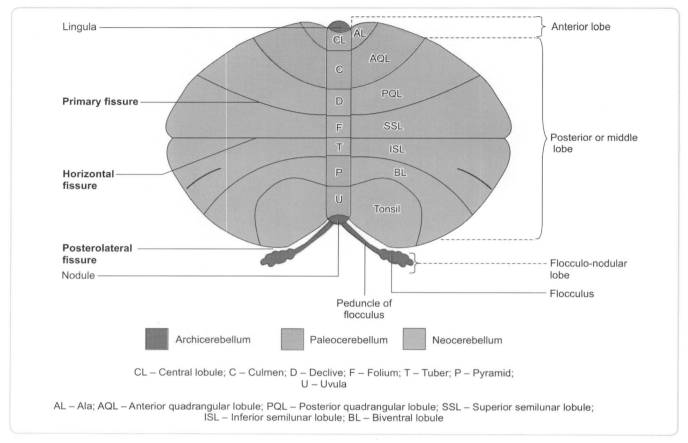

CL – Central lobule; C – Culmen; D – Declive; F – Folium; T – Tuber; P – Pyramid;
U – Uvula

AL – Ala; AQL – Anterior quadrangular lobule; PQL – Posterior quadrangular lobule; SSL – Superior semilunar lobule;
ISL – Inferior semilunar lobule; BL – Biventral lobule

Figure 8.3: Subdivisions of the cerebellum (opened out)

The deepest fissures in the cerebellum are:
- The **primary fissure** (**fissura prima**) running transversely across the superior surface
- The **posterolateral fissure** seen on the inferior aspect
- The **horizontal fissure** (Figures 8.3 and 8.5), which divides the cerebellum into upper and lower halves. The parts seen above the horizontal fissure form the superior surface and those below the fissure form the inferior surface of the cerebellum.

The primary and posterolateral fissures divide the cerebellum into three lobes. The part anterior to the primary fissure is the **anterior lobe.** The part between the two fissures is anatomically, the **posterior lobe** (also called the **middle lobe because of its intermediate position in an "opened out" cerebellum**) (Figure 8.3). The posterior lobe extends on both superior and inferior surfaces. The remaining part is the **flocculonodular lobe,** present in the inferior surface of the cerebellum.

The vermis is so called because it resembles a worm. Proceeding from above downwards (Figure 8.3), it consists of the **lingula, central lobule** and **culmen** (in the anterior lobe); the **declive, folium, tuber, pyramid** and **uvula** (in the middle lobe); and the **nodule** (in the flocculonodular lobe).

With the exception of the lingula, each subdivision of the vermis is related laterally to a part of the hemisphere. In the anterior lobe, the **ala** is lateral to the central lobule and the **anterior quadrangular lobule** is lateral to the culmen. In the middle lobe, the **posterior quadrangular lobule** lies lateral to the declive, the **superior semilunar lobule** is lateral to the folium, the **inferior semilunar lobule** is lateral to the tuber, the **biventral lobule** is lateral to the pyramid, and the **tonsil** lies lateral to the uvula. The nodule is continuous laterally with the flocculus through the inferior medullary velum (Table 8.1).

SUBDIVISIONS OF CEREBELLUM

From developmental, phylogenetic and functional points of view, the cerebellum is often divided into the following subdivisions (Figure 8.3 and Table 8.2):
- **Archicerebellum**: Phylogenetically, it is the oldest part of cerebellum. Anatomically, it consists of flocculonodular lobe and lingula. The connections

TABLE 8.1: Morphological subdivisions of cerebellum

Lobe	Part of vermis	Part of hemisphere
Anterior	Lingula	—
	Central lobule	Ala
	Culmen	Anterior quadrangular lobule
Posterior (or middle)	Declive	Posterior quadrangular lobule
	Folium	Superior semilunar lobule
	Tuber	Inferior semilunar lobule
	Pyramid	Biventral lobule
	Uvula	Tonsil
Flocculonodular	Nodule	Flocculus

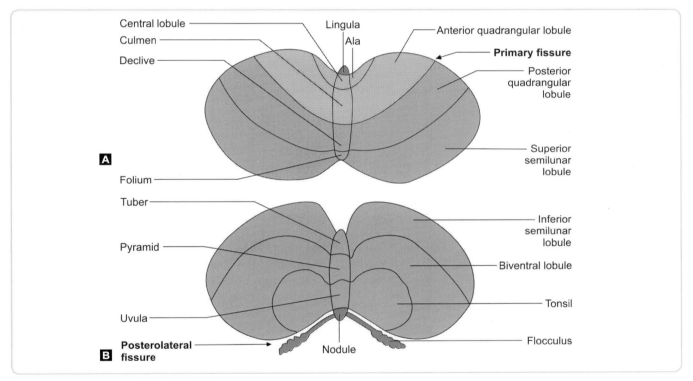

Figures 8.4A and B: Transverse subdivisions of the cerebellum: (A) As seen on superior aspect; (B) As seen on inferior aspect

TABLE 8.2: Components, connections and functions of the phylogenetic subdivisions of cerebellum

Phylogenetic subdivision	Anatomical component	Chief connections	Functions	Functional classification
Archicerebellum (oldest part)	Flocculonodular lobe and lingula	Vestibular apparatus	Maintenance of body equilibrium	Vestibulocerebellum
Paleocerebellum	Anterior lobe, (except lingula), pyramid and uvula	Spinal cord	Maintenance of muscle tone and posture	Spinocerebellum
Neocerebellum	Posterior lobe, except pyramid and uvula	Pons	Responsible for fine coordination of voluntary movements	Cerebrocerebellum

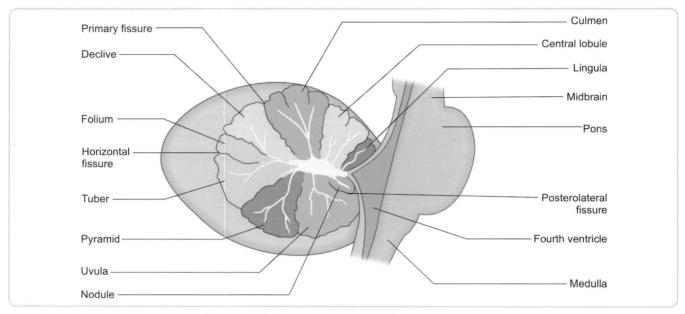

Primary fissure

Declive

Folium

Horizontal
fissure

Tuber

Pyramid

Uvula

Nodule

Culmen

Central lobule

Lingula

Midbrain

Pons

Posterolateral
fissure

Fourth ventricle

Medulla

Figure 8.5: Subdivisions of the vermis of the cerebellum as seen in a median section

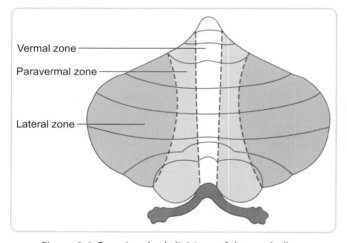

Vermal zone

Paravermal zone

Lateral zone

Figure 8.6: Functional subdivisions of the cerebellum

of the archicerebellum are predominantly vestibular (hence, called vestibulocerebellum), and it is concerned with the maintenance of body equilibrium.
- **Paleocerebellum**: Phylogenetically, it is the next part of cerebellum to arise and is well developed in reptiles and birds. Anatomically, it consists of anterior lobe (except lingula) and pyramid and uvula of the posterior lobe. The paleocerebellum is connected predominantly to the spinal cord (hence, called spinocerebellum). It is concerned mainly with maintenance of muscle tone and posture.

- **Neocerebellum**: It is the most recent part of cerebellum to develop. It is found in mammals only and is the largest in humans. Anatomically, it consists of posterior lobe except pyramid and uvula. The neocerebellum has extensive connections with the cerebral cortex (through pontine nuclei, hence called cerebrocerebellum or pontocerebellum). It is usually regarded as being responsible for fine coordination of voluntary movements.

From the point of view of its connections, the cerebellar cortex may also be divided into a vermal (vermis), paravermal (or paramedian) and lateral parts—longitudinal parcellation (Figure 8.6).

The cerebellum is made-up of a thin surface layer of grey matter, the **cerebellar cortex** and a central core of white matter. Embedded within the central core of white matter are masses of grey matter called **intracerebellar nuclei**.

GREY MATTER OF CEREBELLUM

The grey matter of cerebellum is represented by:
- The cerebellar cortex
- The intracerebellar nuclei

Structure of Cerebellar Cortex

Most of the grey matter of the cerebellum is arranged as a thin layer covering the central core of white matter. This layer is the **cerebellar cortex**.

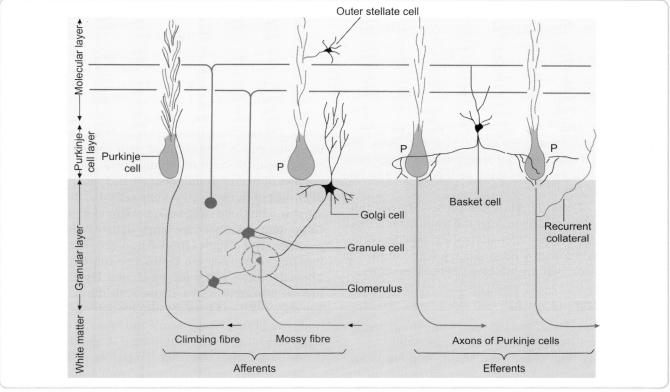

Figure 8.7: Scheme to show the arrangement of neurons in cerebellar cortex

TABLE 8.3: Intrinsic neurons of cerebellar cortex and their location

Intrinsic neurons	Layer of the cerebellar cortex
Stellate cells	Molecular layer
Basket cells	Molecular layer
Purkinje cells	Purkinje cell layer
Granule cells	Granular layer
Golgi cells	Granular layer

Note: All the intrinsic neurons of cerebellar cortex are inhibitory except granule cells.

In striking contrast to the cortex of the cerebral hemispheres, the cerebellar cortex has a uniform structure in all parts of the cerebellum. It is divided into three layers as follows (Figure 8.7):
1. **Molecular layer** (most superficial)
2. **Purkinje cell layer**
3. **Granular layer**, which rests on white matter
The neurons of the cerebellar cortex are of five main types:
1. **Stellate cells**, lying in molecular layer
2. **Basket cells**, lying in the molecular layer
3. **Purkinje cells**, forming the layer named after them
4. **Granule cells**, forming the granular layer
5. **Golgi cells**, present in the granular layer
   Intrinsic neurons of cerebellar cortex and their locations are given in Table 8.3.

Molecular Layer

The molecular layer is the superficial layer of the cortex and situated just below the pia mater.
Two types of cells are found in this layer:
1. **Stellate cells**: Situated in the superficial part of the molecular layer
2. **Basket cells**: Situated in the deeper layer
Stellate cells: These cells and their processes are confined to the molecular layer of the cerebellar cortex. Their dendrites synapse with parallel fibres while their axons synapse with dendrites of Purkinje cells.
Basket cells: These cells lie in the deeper part of the molecular layer of the cerebellar cortex. Their dendrites synapse with parallel fibres. The axons of these cells branch and form networks (or baskets) around the cell bodies of Purkinje cells. Their terminations synapse with Purkinje cells at the junction of the cell body and axon (preaxon).

Purkinje Cell Layer

The Purkinje cell layer contains flask-shaped cell bodies of Purkinje cells. This layer is unusual in that it contains only one layer of neurons. The Purkinje cells are evenly spaced. A dendrite arises from the "neck" of the "flask" and passes "upwards" into the molecular layer. Here, it divides and subdivides to form an elaborate dendritic tree. The branches of this "tree" all lie in one plane (Figure 8.8). This plane is transverse to the long axis of the folium. As a result of this arrangement, the dendritic trees of adjoining Purkinje cells lie in planes more or less parallel to one another.

The axon of each Purkinje cell passes "downwards" through the granular layer to enter the white matter. These axons constitute the only efferents of the cerebellar cortex. They end predominantly by synapsing with neurons in cerebellar nuclei. They are inhibitory to these neurons.

Granular Layer

It is the innermost layer and consists of numerous granule cells and a few Golgi cells and synaptic glomeruli.

Granule cells: These are very small, numerous and spherical neurons that occupy the greater part of the granular layer. The spaces not occupied by them are called **cerebellar islands**. These islands are occupied by special synaptic structures called **glomeruli**.

Each granule cell gives off three to five short dendrites. These end in claw-like endings, which enter the glomeruli where they synapse with the terminals of mossy fibres. The axon of each granule cell enters the molecular layer. Here, it divides into two subdivisions each of which is at right angles to the parent axon (forming a T-junction). These axonal branches of granule cells are called **parallel fibres**. The granule cells being extremely numerous, the parallel fibres are also abundant and almost fill the molecular layer. The parallel fibres run at right angles to the planes of the dendritic trees of Purkinje cells. As a result, each parallel fibre comes into contact and synapses with the dendrites of numerous Purkinje cells. Parallel fibres also synapse with Golgi cells, basket cells and stellate cells.

Golgi neurons: These are large, stellate cells lying in the granular layer (Figures 8.7, 8.8 and 8.9), just deep to the Purkinje cells. They are GABAergic inhibitory neurons. Their dendrites enter the molecular layer, where they branch profusely, and synapse with the parallel fibres. The axons of these neurons also branch profusely. These branches permeate the whole thickness of the granular layer. They take part in the formation of "**glomeruli**". Some dendritic branches also reach the glomeruli.

Each Golgi neuron occupies a definite area there being no overlap between the territories of neighboring Golgi cells. It is interesting to note that the territory of each Golgi cell corresponds to that of about 10 Purkinje cells.

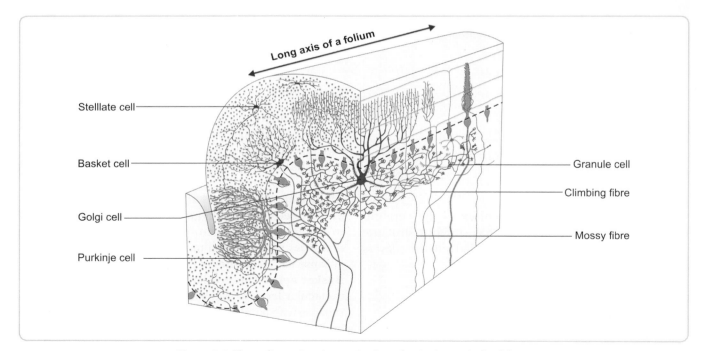

Figure 8.8: Three dimensional organization of a single cerebellar folium

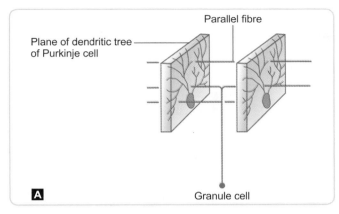

Figure 8.9A: Parallel fibres are at right angles to the plane of dendritic tree of Purkinje cell

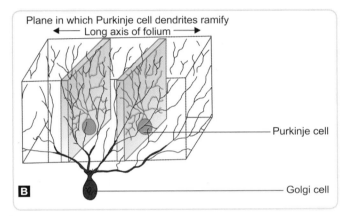

Figure 8.9B: Diagram showing relationship of dendrites of one Golgi neuron to those of Purkinje cells

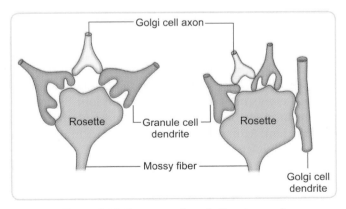

Figure 8.10: Structure of cerebellar glomeruli (the outer capsule is not shown)

Structure of Glomeruli

The glomeruli are complex synaptic structures. The core of each glomerulus is formed by the expanded termination of a mossy fibre (Figure 8.10). This termination is called a **rosette**. Numerous (up to 20) dendrites of granule cells synapse with the rosette. These synapses are axodendritic and excitatory.

The glomerulus also receives axon terminals and dendrites of Golgi cells. These synapses are inhibitory. The entire glomerulus, which is about 10 μm in diameter, is surrounded by a neuroglial capsule.

Intracerebellar Nuclei

Embedded in the central core of white matter there are masses of grey matter, which constitute the **cerebellar nuclei**. From lateral to medial these are as follows (Figure 8.11):

- The **dentate** nucleus lies in the centre of each cerebellar hemisphere. Cross-section through the nucleus shows a thin lamina of grey matter that is folded upon itself, so that it resembles a crumpled purse with the hilum directed medially.
- The **emboliform** and the **globose nuclei** lie medial to dentate nucleus. These two nuclei are together called as **nucleus interpositus** in lower animals.
- The **fastigial** nucleus lies close to the midline in the anterior part of the superior vermis.

These nuclei are close to the roof of fourth (IV) ventricle and hence are also called as "roof nuclei".

The regions of cerebellar cortex from which efferent projections pass to the cerebellar nuclei are arranged in a mediolateral sequence corresponding to the position of the nuclei. The fastigial nucleus receives fibres from the vermis, the globose and emboliform nuclei from paravermal regions, and the dentate nucleus from the lateral region.

WHITE MATTER OF CEREBELLUM

The central core of each cerebellar hemisphere is formed by the white matter. The cerebellar peduncles are continued into this white matter. The white matter of the two sides is connected by a thin lamina of fibres that is closely related to the roof of the fourth ventricle. The upper part of this lamina forms the superior medullary velum, and its lower part forms two crescentic sheets called inferior medullary vela. The white matter consists of two types of fibres—(1) **intrinsic** and (2) **extrinsic.**

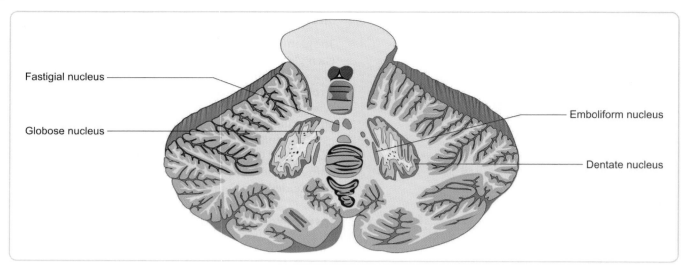

Fastigial nucleus

Globose nucleus

Emboliform nucleus

Dentate nucleus

Figure 8.11: Scheme to show the cerebellar nuclei

- **Intrinsic fibres**: Intrinsic fibres remain confined within the cerebellum. They connect different regions of the cerebellum either in the same hemisphere or of the two cerebellar hemispheres:
  - Projection fibres connect cerebellar cortex to the cerebellar nuclei.
  - Association fibres interconnect different parts of the cerebellar cortex.
  - Commissural fibres connect the two cerebellar hemispheres.
- **Extrinsic fibres**: Extrinsic fibres connect the cerebellum with other parts of the central nervous system, i.e. brain and spinal cord through afferent and efferent fibres. The fibres entering or leaving the cerebellum pass through three thick bundles called the cerebellar peduncles—(1) superior, (2) middle, and (3) inferior.

Afferent Fibres Entering the Cerebellar Cortex

The afferent fibres to the cerebellar cortex are of two different types:
1. Mossy fibres
2. Climbing fibres

Mossy Fibres

All fibres entering the cerebellum, other than through olivocerebellar and par-olivocerebellar tracts, end as mossy fibres. Mossy fibres originate from the vestibular nuclei (vestibulocerebellar), pontine nuclei (pontocerebellar), and spinal cord (spinocerebellar) and terminate in the granular layer of the cortex within the glomeruli. Before terminating, they branch profusely within the granular layer, each branch ends in an expanded terminal called a **rosette** (Figure 8.10).

Afferent inputs through mossy fibres pass through granule cells to reach the Purkinje cells.

Climbing Fibres

These fibres represent terminations of axons reaching the cerebellum from the inferior olivary complex (Olivocerebellar tract and parolivocerebellar tract). They pass through the granular layer and the Purkinje cell layer to reach the molecular layer. Each climbing fibre becomes intimately associated with the proximal part of the dendritic tree of one Purkinje cell, and establishes numerous synapses on them. (These are called climbing fibres as they **climb up** to the molecular layer).

Efferent Fibres

The efferent fibres from the cerebellar cortex are axons of Purkinje cells, which terminate in the cerebellar nuclei. Some efferents from the flocculonodular lobe bypass the cerebellar nuclei and terminate in the vestibular nuclei of brainstem. Axons of the Purkinje cells are inhibitory to cerebellar nuclei.

The fibres from dentate, emboliform and globose nuclei leave the cerebellum through the superior cerebellar peduncle. The fibres from the fastigial nucleus leave the cerebellum through inferior cerebellar peduncle.

The intrinsic neuronal circuit of cerebellum is shown in Figure 8.12.

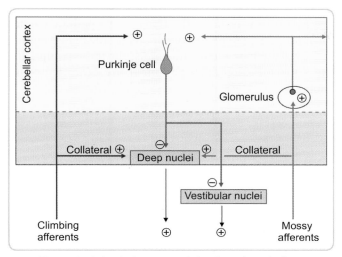

Figure 8.12: Intrinsic neuronal circuitry of cerebellum

CONNECTIONS OF CEREBELLUM

The fundamental points to be appreciated in considering the connections of the cerebellum are, as a rule, as follows:

- Afferent fibres terminate in the cortex.
- Efferent fibres arising in the cortex end in cerebellar nuclei.
- Fibres arising in the nuclei project to centres outside the cerebellum.

The important exception to this rule is that some vestibular fibres project directly to the cerebellar nuclei. Some parts of the cortex give off efferents that bypass the cerebellar nuclei to reach vestibular nuclei outside the cerebellum. That is why, vestibular nucleus is considered as displaced cerebellar nucleus.

The main afferent input, from periphery, received by cerebellum are proprioception, exteroception, vision and from vestibular apparatus. The integrative input comes from cerebral cortex, reticular formation and inferior olivary complex.

The main efferents from cerebellum go via thalamus to the cerebral cortex. Other outputs go to the red nucleus, reticular formation and vestibular nuclei.

> **Clinical Anatomy**
>
> **Disorders of Equilibrium**
> The maintenance of equilibrium and correct posture is dependent on reflex arcs involving various centres including the spinal cord, the cerebellum, and the vestibular nuclei. Afferent impulses for these reflexes are carried by the posterior column tracts (fasciculus gracilis and fasciculus cuneatus), the spinocerebellar tracts, and others. Efferents reach neurons of the ventral grey column (anterior horn cells) through rubrospinal, vestibulospinal, and other "extrapyramidal" tracts. Interruption of any of these pathways or lesions in the cerebellum or the vestibular nuclei can result in various abnormalities involving maintenance of posture and coordination of movements.

CEREBELLAR PEDUNCLES

The various fibres entering or leaving the cerebellum pass through the superior, middle and inferior cerebellar peduncles. These connect the cerebellum to the midbrain, the pons, and the medulla, respectively (Figure 8.13).

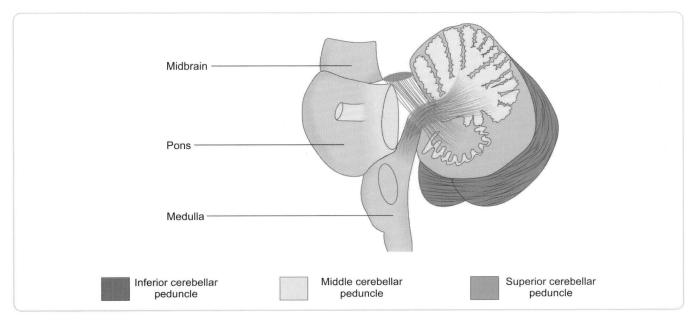

Figure 8.13: Cerebellar peduncles

Superior Cerebellar Peduncle

The superior cerebellar peduncle consists predominantly of efferent fibres arising in cerebellar nuclei (mainly the dentate nucleus). The fibres pass forwards, upwards and medially, lying along the upper and lateral margin of the rhomboid fossa (Fourth ventricle). The fibres of the peduncle enter the midbrain and cross to the opposite side before ending in the red nucleus and the thalamus. The fibres comprising the superior cerebellar peduncle are enumerated in Table 8.4.

S. No.	Tract		Functions
		Superior cerebellar peduncle	
A. *Fibres entering the cerebellum:*			
1.	Ventral spinocerebellar tract		Proprioception and exteroception (lower limb)
2.	Tectocerebellar fibres		Visual input
3.	Trigeminocerebellar fibres		Proprioception from mesencephalic nucleus
4.	Hypothalamocerebellar fibres		Somatic visceral integration
5.	Coerulocerebellar fibres		Noradrenergic modulation of cerebellar learning
B. *Fibres leaving the cerebellum:*			
1.	Cerebellorubral fibres		From the dentate, emboliform and globose nuclei for fine motor coordination and muscle tone
2.	Cerebellothalamic fibres		
3.	Cerebelloreticular		Somatomotor and autonomic modulation
4.	Cerebello-olivary fibres		GABAergic feedback
5.	Cerebellohypothalamic fibres		Cerebellar autonomic modulation
		Middle cerebellar peduncle (Consists of fibres entering the cerebellum only)	
1	Pontocerebellar fibres		Cortico-ponto-cerebellar pathway for motor planning
2	Few serotoninergic fibres		Modulates the responses of other neurotransmitters
		Inferior cerebellar peduncle	
A. *Fibres entering the cerebellum:*			
1	Posterior spinocerebellar tract		Proprioception and exteroception (lower limb)
2	Cuneocerebellar tract (posterior external arcuate fibres)		Proprioception and exteroception (upper limb)
3	Olivocerebellar fibres		Climbing fibres from inferior olivary and accessory olivary nucleus for cerebellar learning
4	Par-olivocerebellar fibres		
5	Reticulocerebellar fibres		Feedback from entire central nervous system: spinal cord to cortex
6	Vestibulocerebellar fibres		Information about head position in its movement
7	Anterior external arcuate fibres		From arcuate nuclei and pontobulbar body, both of which are displaced pontine nuclei (cortico-arcuato-cerebellar pathways and cortico-pontobulbar-cerebellar circumolivary bundle)
8	Fibres of striae medullares		
9	Trigeminocerebellar fibres		Exteroception (main sensory and spinal nuclei)
B. *Fibres leaving the cerebellum:*			
1	Cerebello-olivary fibres		GABAergic feedback
2	Cerebellovestibular fibres		Regulates body equilibrium
3	Cerebelloreticular fibres		Somatomotor modulation
	Fibres in all the above mentioned efferent tracts in inferior cerebellar peduncle arise from the fastigial nucleus		

TABLE 8.4: Tracts in cerebellar peduncles and their functions

Middle Cerebellar Peduncle

The middle cerebellar peduncle is the largest of the three peduncles. It begins as a lateral continuation of the ventral part of the pons (demarcated on the surface by the attachment of trigeminal nerve). Its fibres, which arise in pontine nuclei, cross to the opposite side. The fibres of the peduncle form a thick bundle that passes laterally and backwards to enter the white core of the cerebellum through the horizontal fissure. On entering the cerebellum, the fibres are placed lateral to those of the inferior peduncle (the superior peduncle being still more medial in position).

Middle cerebellar peduncles consist of only afferent fibres, which transmit the impulses mainly from pontine nuclei to the opposite cerebellar hemisphere (pontocerebellar fibres).

Clinical Anatomy

Cerebellopontine Angle
This is a small triangular interval bounded by the pons (anteromedially) and the cerebellum (posteromedially). A tumour in this space produces characteristic symptoms:
- Pressure on the spinal nucleus of the trigeminal nerve leads to loss of sensations of pain and temperature over the face.
- Pressure on fibres and nucleus of the facial nerve results in facial paralysis.
- Pressure on the middle cerebellar peduncle leads to ataxia.
- Pressure on fibres and nucleus of vestibulocochlear nerve results in vertigo, tinnitus, nystagmus and deafness.

Inferior Cerebellar Peduncle

This peduncle is also called the restiform body. This is a thick bundle of fibres that connects the posterolateral part of the medulla with the cerebellum. The peduncle passes upwards and laterally along the inferolateral margin of the rhomboid fossa (Fourth ventricle). Near the upper end of the medulla, the peduncle lies between the superior cerebellar peduncle (on its medial side) and the middle cerebellar peduncle (laterally). The inferior peduncle then turns sharply backwards to enter the while core of the cerebellum.

Over the medial part of the inferior cerebellar peduncle there are fibres that pass through the vestibular nuclei before entering the cerebellum. These fibres constitute the juxtarestiform body.

The fibres comprising the inferior cerebellar peduncle are enumerated in Table 8.4.

CONNECTIONS BETWEEN CEREBELLUM AND SPINAL CORD

From a clinical point of view, the most important connections of the cerebellum are with the spinal cord and with the cerebral cortex. These connections are through various pathways that are summarized below.

Spinocerebellar pathways convey to the cerebellum proprioceptive information necessary for controlling muscle tone and for maintaining body posture. These pathways also carry exteroceptive impulses.
- **Direct pathways from spinal cord to cerebellum**: These are the ventral spinocerebellar and the dorsal spinocerebellar tracts, which convey information from the hindlimb. Information from the forelimb is conveyed by the cuneocerebellar tract. The cuneocerebellar tract begins in the medulla and is functionally equivalent to spinocerebellar tracts.
- **Indirect pathways from spinal cord to cerebellum**: These are as follows:
  - Spino-olivocerebellar
  - Spinoreticulocerebellar
  - Spinovestibulocerebellar
  - Spinotectocerebellar pathways

Although these are not concerned with the spinal cord, it is useful to consider here the pathways that carry impulses from tissues in the head to the cerebellum. Exteroceptive impulses from the head, reach the cerebellum through trigeminocerebellar fibres arising in the main sensory and spinal nuclei of this nerve. Fibres from the mesencephalic nucleus convey proprioceptive information from the muscles of mastication to the cerebellum.
- **Cerebellospinal pathways**: The cerebellum influences the spinal cord through the following pathways:
  - Cerebellorubrospinal
  - Cerebellovestibulospinal
  - Cerebelloreticulospinal
  - Cerebellotectospinal
  - Cerebellothalamocorticospinal

CONNECTIONS BETWEEN CEREBELLUM AND CEREBRAL CORTEX

The connections between the cerebellum and the cerebral cortex are all indirect.
- **Corticocerebellar pathways**: The cerebral cortex influences the cerebellum through various centres in the brainstem through the following pathways:
  - **Cortico-ponto-cerebellar pathway**: This is the most important of the corticocerebellar pathway. The arcuate nuclei and the pontobulbar body represent displaced pontine nuclei. The cortico-arcuato-cerebellar and the cortico-pontobulbar-cerebellar pathways are functionally equivalent to the cortico-ponto-cerebellar pathway.
  - Cortico-olivo-cerebellar
  - Cortico-reticulo-cerebellar

- Cortico-rubro-cerebellar
- Cortico-tecto-cerebellar

Some of the impulses may reach these intermediary centres through the corpus striatum.

- **Cerebellocortical pathways**: The cortex of cerebellum projects upon the cerebellar nuclei from where fibres relay to the thalamus. Thalamocortical fibres then convey these impulses to the cerebral cortex. Cerebellar connection reaches the cerebral cortex through cerebelloreticulo-thalamocortical pathway also.

Connections and functions of cerebellar nuclei are summarized in Table 8.5.

FUNCTIONS OF CEREBELLUM

The cerebellum plays an essential role in the control of movement. It is responsible for ensuring that movement takes place smoothly, in the right direction and to the right extent. Cerebellar stimulation modifies movements produced by stimulation of motor areas of the cerebral cortex. The cerebellar cortex is also important for learning of movements (for example, in learning to write).

Through its vestibular and spinal connections, the cerebellum is responsible for maintaining the equilibrium of the body.

These functions are possible because the cerebellum constantly receives proprioceptive information regarding the state of contraction of muscles and of the position of various joints. It also receives information from the eyes, the ears, the vestibular apparatus, the reticular formation and the cerebral cortex. All this information is integrated and is used to influence movement through motor centres in the brainstem and spinal cord and also through the cerebral cortex.

Functional Localization in Cerebellum

In the cerebellar cortex, it is possible to localize areas that receive afferents from different parts of the body. There is a double representation, one on the superior surface and one on the inferior surface of the cerebellum. Representation on the superior surface is ipsilateral; and that on the inferior surface is bilateral. On either surface, the anteroposterior sequence of parts represented is leg, trunk, arm and head. These areas are located in vermal and paravermal areas (paleocerebellum) and correspond to areas that receive fibres from the spinal cord. Stimulation of these areas produces movements in parts of the body that correspond roughly to those from which sensory impulses are received (Figure 8.14).

In addition to proprioceptive impulses, the cerebellum receives visual impulses, which reach the folium and tuber. A second visual area is located in the biventral lobule and tonsil. These visual areas also receive auditory impulses. Vestibular impulses are received mainly by the uvula, nodule and flocculus (vestibulocerebellum).

TABLE 8.5: Connections and functions of the nuclei of the cerebellum

Nucleus	Afferent	Efferent	Functions
Fastigial nucleus	• Vestibular apparatus through the vestibular nerve • Vestibulocerebellum, i.e. vermis and flocculonodular lobe	• To vestibular nuclei • To reticular formation of the medulla • To thalamus • To midbrain (red nucleus, central grey matter—nucleus of Darkschewitsch) • To visceral centres in brainstem • To medial accessory and main inferior olivary nuclei	Control of muscle action (axial and proximal limb muscles) in response to labyrinthine stimuli
Emboliform and globose nuclei	From the paravermal area or spinocerebellum	• To red nucleus • To thalamus • To reticular formation • To pontine nuclei • To dorsal accessory olivary nucleus	Controls crude movements of the limbs
Dentate nucleus	From neocerebellum or the lateral part of cerebellar hemisphere	• To thalamus • To red nucleus • To oculomotor nucleus • To inferior olivary nucleus • To reticular formation	Controls highly skilled voluntary movements of precision

Cerebellar Syndrome

The cerebellar lesions due to trauma, haemorrhage, tumours, etc. produce a number of signs and symptoms, which together constitute the cerebellar syndrome.

The signs and symptoms produced by cerebellar lesions are as follows:

Ataxia: Inability to maintain the equilibrium of the body, while standing, or while walking, is referred to as **ataxia**. This may occur as a result of the interruption of afferent proprioceptive pathways **(sensory ataxia)**. Lack of proprioceptive information can be compensated to a considerable extent by information received through the eyes. The defects mentioned are, therefore, much more pronounced with the eyes closed **(Romberg's sign positive)**.

However, disease of the cerebellum itself, or of its efferent pathways, results in more severe disability. Coordination of the activity of different groups of muscles is interfered with, leading to various defects. The person is unable to stand with his/her feet close together: the body sways from side to side and the person may fall. While walking, the patient staggers and is unable to maintain progression in the desired direction. Visual input adds little improvement in cerebellar lesions.

Asynergia: Lack of coordination of muscles also interferes with purposeful movements **(asynergia)**. Movements are jerky and lack precision. For example, the patient finds it difficult to touch his nose with a finger, or to move a finger along a line. There is difficulty in performing movements involving rapid alternating action of opposing groups of muscles (for example, tapping one hand with the other; repeated pronation and supination of the forearm). This phenomenon is called **dysdiadokokinesia.**

Dysarthria: Incoordination of the muscles responsible for the articulation of words leads to characteristic speech defect-staccato speech **(dysarthria)**.

Nystagmus: For the same reason, the eyes are unable to fix the gaze on an object for any length of time. Attempts to bring the gaze back to the same point result in repeated jerky movements of the eyes. This is called **nystagmus.**

Hypotonia: Apart from incoordination, cerebellar disease is characterized by diminished muscle tone **(hypotonia)**.

Asthenia: The muscles are soft and tire easily. Joints may lack stability **(flail joints)**.

Reflexes: Tendon reflexes may be diminished. Alternatively, tapping a tendon may result in oscillating movements of the part concerned like a pendulum.

Correlation of the symptoms of cerebellar damage with different regions of the cerebellum is as follows:

When the flocculus, nodule and uvula are damaged **(flocculonodular syndrome)** the main symptom is imbalance. Remember that the connections of the flocculonodular lobe are predominantly vestibular.

Small lesions in the cerebellar cortex may produce no effect. Extensive lesions are marked by hypotonia and incoordination (on the side of the lesion).

Intention tremors and staggering appear when the dentate nucleus or the superior cerebellar peduncle (which carries fibres from the nucleus) is damaged.

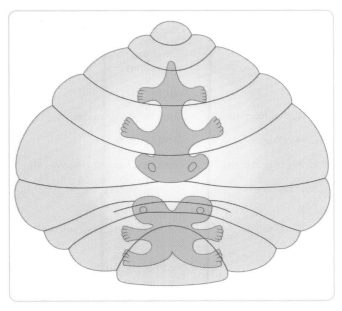

Figure 8.14: Projection areas in the cerebellum

CEREBELLUM AND LEARNING

The cerebellum is concerned with learned adjustments that make coordination easier when a given motor task is performed over and over. As a task is being learned, activity in the brain shifts from the prefrontal areas to the basal nuclei and the cerebellum. The tasks where the neocerebellum, most clearly comes into play, are those where it is necessary to make fine adjustments to the way an action is performed.

The basis of the learning in the cerebellum is through the input via the inferior olivary complex (the only climbing fibre input). Each Purkinje cell receives inputs from 250,000 to 1 million mossy fibres, but each has only a single climbing fibre from the inferior olive, and this fibre makes 2,000–3,000 synapses on the Purkinje cell. Climbing fibre activity is increased when a new movement is being learned, and selective lesions of the olivary complex abolish the ability to produce long-term adjustments in certain motor responses.

During motor learning, climbing fibre activation produces a large, complex spike in the Purkinje cell and this spike produces a long-term modification of the pattern of mossy fibre input to that particular Purkinje cell. This is especially so, when there is a mismatch between an intended movement and the movement that is actually executed. Climbing fibre activity acts as an error signal, and may cause synchronously activated parallel fibre inputs to be weakened. Climbing fibres thus provide a teaching signal that induces synaptic modification in parallel fibre-Purkinje cell synapses. This explains why net practice is so important prior to playing cricket matches at an international level!

ARTERIAL SUPPLY OF CEREBELLUM

The cerebellum is supplied by three pairs of cerebellar arteries (Figure 8.15):
1. **Superior cerebellar artery**: A branch of basilar artery supplies the superior surface of the cerebellum.
2. **Anterior inferior cerebellar artery**: A branch of basilar artery supplies the anterior part of the inferior surface of the cerebellum.

3. **Posterior inferior cerebellar artery**: A branch of vertebral artery supplies the posterior part of the inferior surface of the cerebellum.

CEREBELLUM: THE RULE OF THREE

There are several aspects of cerebellum that run in threes (Table 8.6).

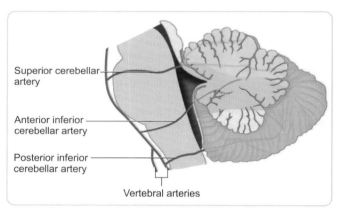

Figure 8.15: Blood supply of cerebellum

	TABLE 8.6: Cerebellum: the rule of three			
1	Subdivisions	Left hemisphere	Vermis	Right hemisphere
2	Fissures	Posterolateral	Primary	Horizontal
3	Lobes	Anterior	Posterior	Flocculonodular
4	Developmental	Archicerebellum	Paleocerebellum	Neocerebellum
5	Connections	Vestibular	Spinal cord	Cerebral cortex
6	Functions	Body equilibrium	Muscle tone	Fine coordination of voluntary movements
7	Longitudinal subdivisions	Vermal	Paravermal	Lateral
8	Core subdivisions	Cerebellar cortex	Cerebellar white matter	Deep cerebellar nuclei
9	Cerebellar cortex	Molecular layer	Purkinje cell layer	Granular layer
10	Cerebellar glomeruli	Axon of a mossy fibre	Dendrites of granule cells	Axon and dendrite of Golgi cell
11	Cerebellar white matter	Commissural fibres	Association fibres	Projection fibres
12	Cerebellar peduncles (old names within brackets)	Superior (brachium conjunctivum)	Middle (brachium pontis)	Inferior (restiform and juxtarestiform body)
13	Brainstem connected	Midbrain	Pons	Medulla oblongata
14	Deep cerebellar nuclei	Dentate	Emboliform and globose (nucleus interpositus)	Fastigial
15	Arterial supply	Posterior inferior cerebellar	Anterior inferior cerebellar	Superior cerebellar

MULTIPLE CHOICE QUESTIONS

Q1. Which one of the following fissures divides the cerebellum into anterior and posterior lobes?
A. Horizontal
B. Primary
C. Posterolateral
D. Secondary

Q2. Which one of the following is a part of the paleo-cerebellum?
A. Flocculus
B. Lingula
C. Nodule
D. Uvula

Q3. The deep furrow separating the cerebellar hemispheres inferiorly is known as:
A. Cerebellar notch
B. Fissura prima
C. Vallecula
D. Vermis

Q4. The neocerebellum is concerned with:
A. Regulation of muscle tone of limbs
B. Maintenance of equilibrium
C. Regulation of muscle tone of trunk
D. Smooth performance of skilled acts

Q5. Most of the efferents of the cerebellum are projected to the:
A. Midbrain
B. Pons
C. Medulla oblongata
D. Spinal cord

Q6. The excitatory neurons of the cerebellar cortex are:
A. Basket
B. Granule
C. Golgi
D. Stellate

Q7. The pathway that passes through the middle cerebellar peduncle is:
A. Anterior spinocerebellar
B. Pontocerebellar
C. Posterior spinocerebellar
D. Tectocerebellar

Q8. The dendrites of Purkinje cells of the cerebellar cortex synapse with the axons of:
A. Deep cerebellar nuclei
B. Golgi cells
C. Mossy fibres
D. Granule cells

Q9. Which one of the following neurons forms the sole output neurons of the cerebellar cortex?
A. Basket
B. Golgi
C. Purkinje
D. Stellate

Q10. The axons of the Purkinje cells end mainly in the:
A. Cerebellar nuclei
B. Midbrain
C. Pons
D. Medulla oblongata

Q11. Flocculonodular lobe receives direct afferent connections from:
A. Spinal cord
B. Vestibular apparatus
C. Reticular formation
D. Inferior olivary nucleus

Q12. Climbing fibres of cerebellum arise from which tract?
A. Anterior spinocerebellar
B. Cuneocerebellar
C. Posterior spinocerebellar
D. Olivocerebellar

Q13. The cells contributing to the efferents of the cerebellar cortex are:
A. Purkinje
B. Basket
C. Granular
D. Golgi

Q14. The nucleus, from which the mossy fibres of cerebellum arise, is:
A. Inferior olivary
B. Dentate
C. Vestibular
D. Fastigius

ANSWERS

1. B	2. D	3. C	4. D	5. A	6. B	7. B	8. D	9. C	10. A
11. B	12. D	13. A	14. C						

SHORT NOTES

1. Inferior cerebellar peduncle
2. Superior cerebellar peduncle
3. Flocculonodular lobe of cerebellum
4. Connections of cerebellum
5. Cerebellar disorders

LONG QUESTION

Describe the cerebellum under the following headings: Gross features, connections, blood supply, applied anatomy

---

Clinical Cases

8.1: A 35-year-old man complained of tinnitus and vertigo, decreased lacrimation in the left eye, and asymmetry of face with deviation of angle of mouth to the right side. Magnetic resonance imaging (MRI) examination revealed a tumour in the cerebellopontine angle.
  A. On which side would the tumour be?
  B. Explain the anatomical basis of all the symptoms mentioned above.

8.2: A 10-year-old female child showed intention tremors, hypotonia and severe ataxia. She was diagnosed to have Friedrich's ataxia (hereditary cerebellar degeneration). Specify the functional part of cerebellum that is affected to cause
  A. Intention tremors
  B. Ataxia

Chapter 9 | Diencephalon

Specific Learning Objectives

At the end of learning, the student shall be able to:
➢ Enumerate the subdivisions of the diencephalon
➢ Describe the structure, nuclei, connections and functions of thalamus
➢ Describe the structure, nuclei, connections and functions of hypothalamus

INTRODUCTION

The diencephalon is the part of the brain between the cerebrum above and midbrain below. It extends from the interventricular foramen to posterior commissure. The hypothalamic sulcus divides the diencephalon into two parts— a dorsal part (**pars dorsalis**) and a ventral part (**pars ventralis**) (Figure 9.1).
- **Pars dorsalis** consists of the thalamus, metathalamus, and epithalamus
- **Pars ventralis** consists of the hypothalamus and subthalamus

The cavity of the diencephalon is the third ventricle. The divisions of diencephalon with important nuclear groups are shown in Table 9.1

The subthalamic nucleus is included with the basal nuclei to which it is closely related functionally.

THALAMUS (DORSAL THALAMUS)

External Features

Anatomically, the thalamus (or dorsal thalamus) is a large egg-shaped mass of grey matter that lies immediately lateral to the third ventricle (Figures 9.2 and 9.3). It has two

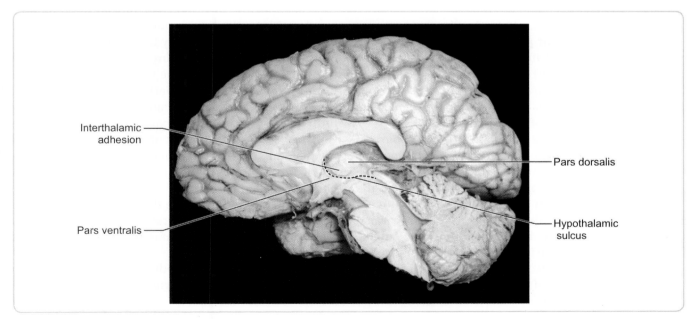

Figure 9.1: Midsagittal section of brain specimen showing parts of diencephalon

TABLE 9.1: Divisions and Important Nuclear Groups of Diencephalon

Divisions	Subdivisions	Important Nuclear Groups
Pars dorsalis diencephali	Thalamus (dorsal thalamus)	Anterior, Medial, Lateral ventral, Lateral dorsal, Non-specific
	Metathalamus	Medial and lateral geniculate bodies
	Epithalamus	Pineal gland, Habenular nucleus
Pars ventralis diencephali	Hypothalamus	Pre-optic, Supraoptic, Tuberal, Mamillary
	Ventral thalamus / Subthalamus	Subthalamic, Zona incerta

Note: The medial and lateral geniculate bodies are distinct from the other regions of the thalamus and are grouped together as the metathalamus and are integral parts of the dorsal thalamus.

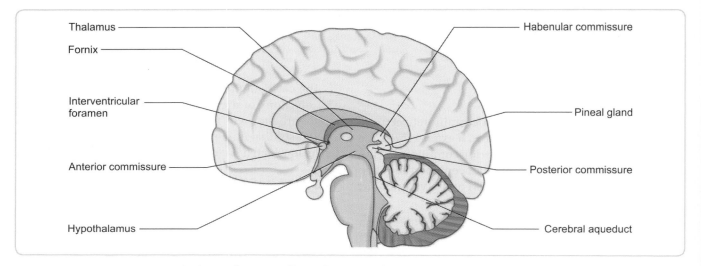

Figure 9.2: Midsagittal section of brain showing thalamus, hypothalamus and epithalamus

ends (or poles), anterior and posterior; and four surfaces, superior, inferior, medial, and lateral.

The **anterior end (or pole)** is narrow and forms the posterior boundary of interventricular foramen. The **posterior end (or pole)** is broader and is called the **pulvinar**. It lies just above and lateral to the superior colliculus. The pulvinar is separated from the geniculate bodies by the **brachium of the superior colliculus**.

The **medial surface** forms the greater part of the lateral wall of the third ventricle and is lined by ependyma. The medial surfaces of the two thalami are usually connected by a mass of grey matter called the **interthalamic adhesion (connexus interthalamicus)** (Figure 9.1). Inferiorly, the medial surface is separated from the hypothalamus by the **hypothalamic sulcus**. This sulcus runs from the interventricular foramen to the cerebral aqueduct (Figure 9.1).

The **lateral surface** of the thalamus is related to the internal capsule, which separates it from the lentiform nucleus (Figure 9.3). This surface itself is separated from internal capsule by the reticular nucleus of thalamus and the external medullary lamina.

The **superior (or dorsal) surface** of the thalamus is related laterally to the body of caudate nucleus, from which it is separated by thalamocaudate groove. A bundle of efferent nerve fibres from amygdala called the **stria terminalis**, and the **thalamostriate vein** lie in this groove. The lateral part of superior surface of thalamus and the body of caudate nucleus together form the floor of the central part of the lateral ventricle (Figure 9.3). The medial part of the superior surface of the thalamus is, however, separated from the ventricle by the fornix and by a fold of pia mater called the **tela choroidea**.

The inferior surface of the thalamus is related to the hypothalamus and the ventral thalamus. The ventral thalamus separates the thalamus from the tegmentum of the midbrain.

At the junction of the medial and superior surfaces of the thalamus, the ependyma of the third ventricle is reflected from the lateral wall to the roof. The line of reflection is marked by a line called the **taenia thalami**. Underlying it there is a narrow bundle of fibres called the **stria medullaris thalami (stria habenularis)**.

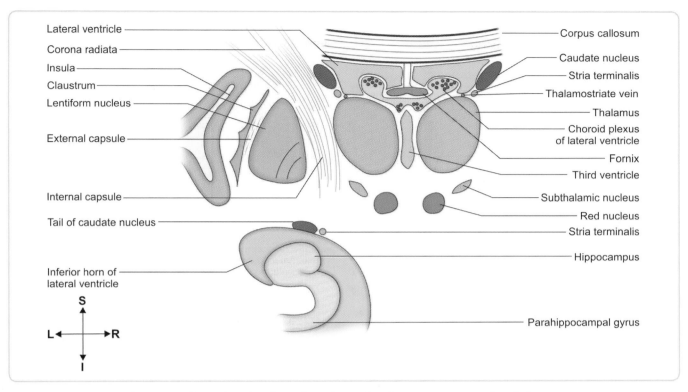

Figure 9.3: Coronal section through cerebrum showing structures related to thalamus

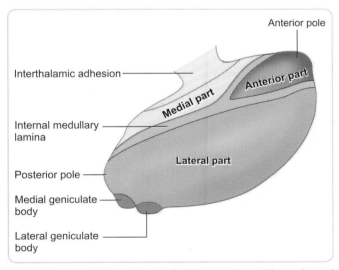

Figure 9.4: Horizontal section of thalamus. Note: The Y-shaped internal medullary lemina divides the thalamus into anterior, lateral, and medial parts

Internal Structure of Thalamus

The thalamus consists mainly of grey matter and a small amount of white matter.

White Matter

The superior surface of thalamus is covered by a thin layer of white matter called the **stratum zonale** and its lateral surface, by a similar layer called the **external medullary lamina.** Internally a 'Y' shaped bundle of white matter called **internal medullary lamina** divides the grey matter of thalamus into three major groups of nuclei: anterior, medial and lateral (Figure 9.4).

Grey Matter

A number of nuclei can be distinguished within each of these parts (Figures 9.5 and 9.6 and Flowchart 9.1). Only the more important of these are listed below:

Nuclei in the Anterior Part
The group of nuclei in this part is collectively referred to as the **anterior nucleus** and is predominantly limbic in function.

Nuclei in the Medial Part
The largest of these is the **medial dorsal nucleus.** It is divisible into a **magnocellular part** (anteromedial) and a **parvocellular part** (posterolateral). This nucleus is also limbic in connections and functions.

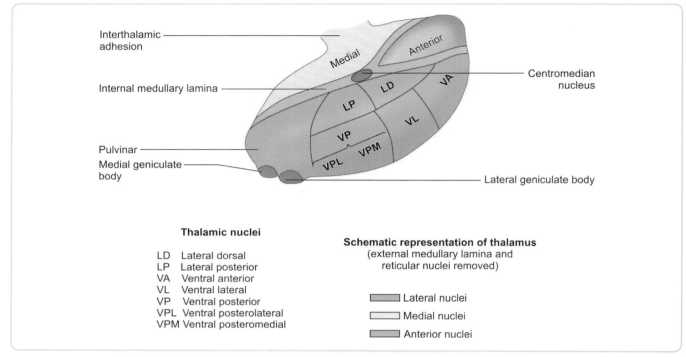

Figure 9.5: Nuclei of thalamus

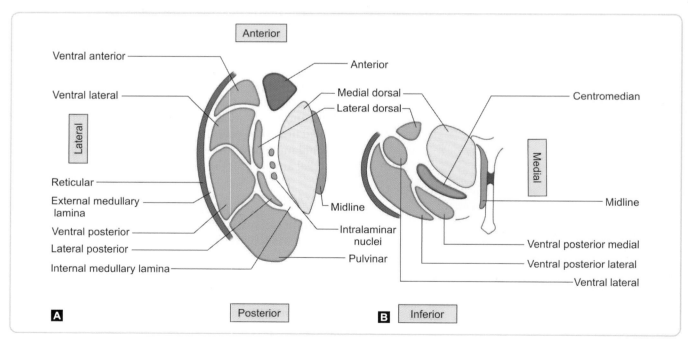

Figures 9.6A and B: Nuclei of thalamus: (A) Superior aspect; (B) Coronal section

Flowchart 9.1: Subdivisions of thalamic nuclei

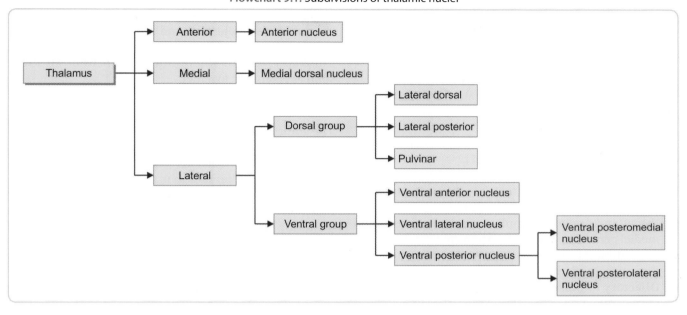

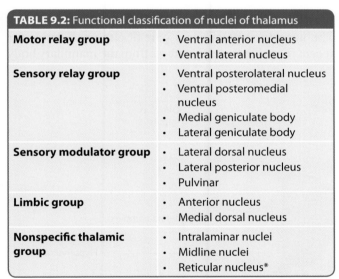

TABLE 9.2: Functional classification of nuclei of thalamus	
Motor relay group	• Ventral anterior nucleus • Ventral lateral nucleus
Sensory relay group	• Ventral posterolateral nucleus • Ventral posteromedial nucleus • Medial geniculate body • Lateral geniculate body
Sensory modulator group	• Lateral dorsal nucleus • Lateral posterior nucleus • Pulvinar
Limbic group	• Anterior nucleus • Medial dorsal nucleus
Nonspecific thalamic group	• Intralaminar nuclei • Midline nuclei • Reticular nucleus*

* The **reticular nucleus** on the lateral aspect of thalamus (Thalamic Reticular Nucleus –TRN) consists of nerve cells which connect with intralaminar nucleus and plays an important role in gating the impulses to and from the cerebral cortex. Recently it has been proposed that this nucleus may have a role in autism. This nucleus is also considered as part of ventral thalalmus because of its proximity to zona incerta.

Nuclei in the Lateral Part

The nuclei in the lateral part are arranged in two tiers as a **ventral group** and a **dorsal group:**

The **nuclei in the ventral group** are as follows (in anteroposterior order):

- **Ventral anterior nucleus**
- **Ventral lateral nucleus** (also called the **ventral intermediate nucleus**)
- **Ventral posterior nucleus**, which is further subdivided into a lateral part, called the **ventral posterolateral nucleus**, and a medial part, called the **ventral posteromedial nucleus** (Figure 9.6 A and B).

While ventral anterior and ventral lateral nuclei are important for motor integration, ventral posteromedial and ventral posterolateral nuclei play an important role in sensory integration.

The **functional classification** of thalamic nuclei is given in Table 9.2

The **nuclei of the dorsal group** are as follows (in anteroposterior order):

- **Lateral dorsal nucleus** (or **dorsolateral nucleus**)
- **Lateral posterior nucleus**
- **Pulvinar**

Other Thalamic Nuclei

In addition to the above, the thalamus contains the following nuclei:

- The **intralaminar nuclei** are embedded within the internal medullary lamina. There are several nuclei in this group. The most important of these is the **centromedian nucleus** .
- The **midline nuclei** consist of scattered cells that lie between the medial part of the thalamus and the

ependyma of the third ventricle. Several nuclei are recognized.

- The **medial and lateral geniculate bodies** (traditionally described under metathalamus) are now included as part of the thalamus.

Connections of Thalamus—An Overview
Afferent

Afferents from a large number of subcortical centres converge on the thalamus (Figure 9.7).

- Exteroceptive and proprioceptive impulses ascend to it through the medial lemniscus, the spinothalamic tracts, and the trigeminothalamic tract.
- Visual and auditory impulses reach the lateral and medial geniculate bodies, respectively.
- Sensations of taste are conveyed to the thalamus through solitariothalamic fibres.
- **Olfactory impulses:** Although the thalamus does not receive direct olfactory impulses they probably reach it through the amygdaloid complex.
- Visceral information is conveyed from the hypothalamus and probably through the reticular formation.

- In addition to these afferents, the thalamus receives profuse connections from all parts of the cerebral cortex, the cerebellum, and the corpus striatum.
  The thalamus is, therefore, regarded as a great integrating centre where information from all these sources is brought together.

Efferent

The information received by thalamus is projected to almost the whole of the cerebral cortex through profuse thalamocortical projections (Figure 9.8). Thalamocortical fibres form large bundles that are described as **thalamic radiations** or as **thalamic peduncles** (Figure 9.9). These radiations are **anterior** (or **frontal**), **superior** (or **dorsal**), **posterior** (or **caudal**), and **inferior (or ventral).** Efferent projections from the thalamus also reach the corpus striatum, the hypothalamus, and the reticular formation.

Connections of Different Parts of Thalamus (Flowcharts 9.2 to 9.8)
Connections of Anterior Group of Thalamic Nuclei

The **anterior nucleus** is a part of circuit of Papez for recent memory. It receives fibres from the mamillary body

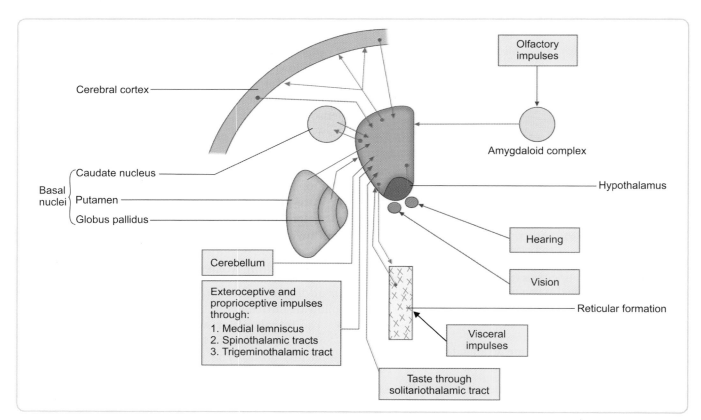

Figure 9.7: Main connections of thalamus (as a whole)

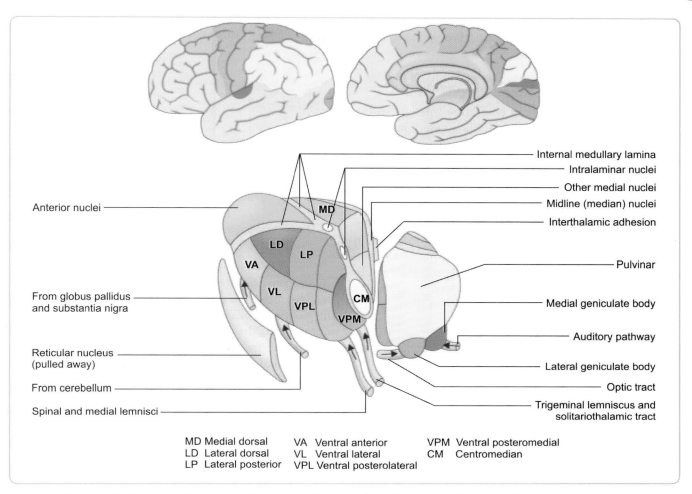

Internal medullary lamina
Intralaminar nuclei
Other medial nuclei
Midline (median) nuclei
Interthalamic adhesion

Pulvinar

Medial geniculate body

Auditory pathway

Lateral geniculate body

Optic tract

Trigeminal lemniscus and solitariothalamic tract

Anterior nuclei

MD

LD
LP
VA
VL
VPL
CM
VPM

From globus pallidus and substantia nigra

Reticular nucleus (pulled away)

From cerebellum

Spinal and medial lemnisci

MD Medial dorsal	VA Ventral anterior	VPM Ventral posteromedial
LD Lateral dorsal	VL Ventral lateral	CM Centromedian
LP Lateral posterior	VPL Ventral posterolateral	

Figure 9.8: Diagram to show areas of superolateral and medial surfaces of cerebral cortex that are connected to individual thalamic nuclei. (The connections are reciprocal.)

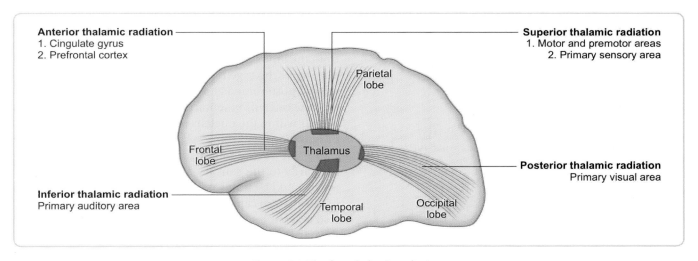

Anterior thalamic radiation
1. Cingulate gyrus
2. Prefrontal cortex

Superior thalamic radiation
1. Motor and premotor areas
2. Primary sensory area

Parietal lobe

Frontal lobe

Thalamus

Posterior thalamic radiation
Primary visual area

Inferior thalamic radiation
Primary auditory area

Temporal lobe

Occipital lobe

Figure 9.9: The four thalamic radiations

through the mamillothalamic tract. Efferent fibres project to the cingulate gyrus (Flowchart 9.5) through the anterior or frontal thalamic radiation.

Connections of Medial Group of Thalamic Nuclei

The **medial dorsal nucleus** (the large nucleus in the medial group) is involved in controlling emotional states and has a role in determining the personality of the individual.

It receives afferent connections from olfactory areas, piriform lobe, amygdala, hypothalamus and corpus striatum. Efferent connections from this nucleus project to prefrontal cortex through anterior or frontal thalamic radiation. This nucleus is concerned with integration of olfactory, visceral and somatic functions and in the mediation of visceral and somatic reflexes. Damage to the nucleus leads to decrease in anxiety, tension and aggression. These functions are similar to those of the prefrontal cortex (Flowchart 9.6).

Connections of the Lateral Part of Thalamus

The lateral part of thalamus is made up of ventral and dorsal tiers of nuclei.

Connections of Ventral Group of Thalamic Nuclei

The **ventral anterior nucleus** receives fibres from the globus pallidus and substantia nigra pars reticularis and sends efferents to the premotor and supplemental motor areas of the cerebral cortex (Flowchart 9.3).

Flowchart 9.2: Connections of the ventral posterior nucleus of thalamus

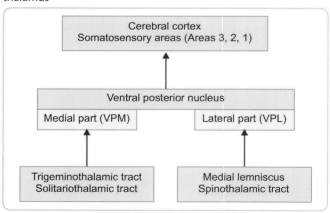

Flowchart 9.3: Connections of the ventral anterior and ventral lateral nucleus of thalamus

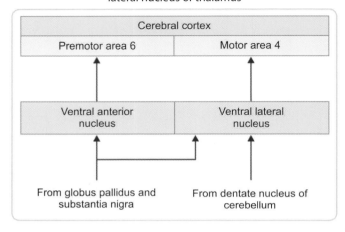

The **ventral lateral nucleus** receives afferents from dentate nucleus of cerebellum. It also receives fibres from the globus pallidus. Efferents from this nucleus project to motor area of the cerebral cortex.

Efferents from these two nuclei pass through superior thalamic radiation.

From a clinical point of view, the most important connections of the thalamus are those of the **ventral posterior nucleus.** This nucleus is divisible into ventral posterolateral and ventral posteromedial parts (that are sometimes mentioned as separate nuclei). This nucleus receives the terminations of the major sensory pathways ascending from the spinal cord and brainstem (Flowchart 9.2). These include the medial lemniscus, the spinothalamic tract, the trigeminal lemniscus, and the solitariothalamic fibres. Within the nucleus, fibres from different parts of the body terminate in a definite sequence. The fibres from the lowest parts of the body end in the most lateral part of the nucleus. The medial lemniscus and spinothalamic tract carrying sensations from the limbs and trunk end in the ventral posterolateral part, while the trigeminal fibres (from the head) end in the ventral posteromedial part, which also receives the fibres for taste carried via solitariothalamic tract. Different layers of cells within the nucleus respond to different modalities of sensation.

All the sensations reaching the nucleus are carried primarily to the sensory area of the cerebral cortex (SI, areas 3,2,1) by fibres passing through the posterior limb of the internal capsule (superior thalamic radiation). They also reach the second somatosensory area (SII) located in the parietal operculum (of the insula).

Flowchart 9.4: Connections of the lateral group of thalamic nuclei

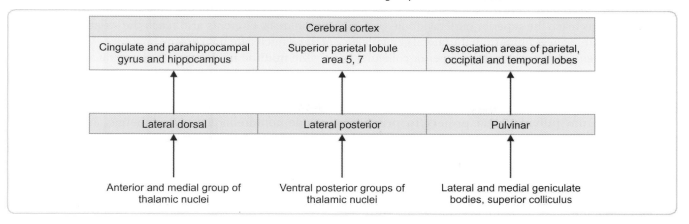

Flowchart 9.5: Connections of the anterior group of thalamic nuclei

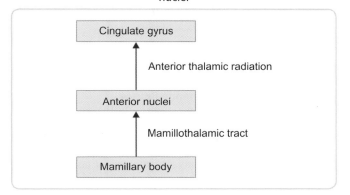

Flowchart 9.6: Connections of the medial dorsal nucleus of thalamus

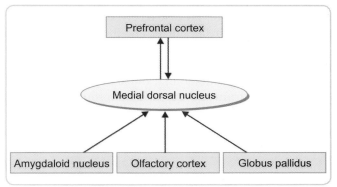

Clinical Anatomy

- In lesions of anterior group of thalamic nuclei, memory for recent events and capacity for new learning are lost as happens in Korsakoff syndrome. The anatomical basis for this is anterior group of thalamic nuclei plays an important role in memory circuit (Papez circuit).
- Ablation of the posterior part of ventral lateral nucleus can reduce tremors in parkinsonism because this nucleus receives inputs from corpus striatum.

Connections of Lateral Group of Nuclei

The **lateral dorsal nucleus** receives impulses from other thalamic nuclei (mainly from the medial and anterior group). Efferent projections reach the limbic lobe—cingulate gyrus, the parahippocampal gyrus, and the hippocampal formation.

Flowchart 9.7: Connections of intralaminar thalamic nuclei

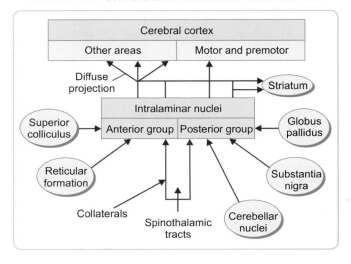

The **lateral posterior nucleus** receives fibres from other thalamic nuclei (mainly from the ventral posterior group). Efferents reach the superior parietal lobule.

The **pulvinar** receives fibres from the lateral geniculate body, medial geniculate body and the superior colliculus. Efferents from the pulvinar project to areas in the occipital and parietal lobes. The pulvinar is described as a lower visual centre.

Efferents from pulvinar also project to primary auditory and auditory association areas in the temporal lobe through inferior thalamic radiation (Flowchart 9.4).

Other Connections

Intralaminar nuclei: There are several nuclei in this group divided into subgroups: anterior and posterior. The posterior subgroup includes the large centromedian nucleus. The nuclei of this group receive inputs from the body through collaterals of spinothalamic tracts (Flowchart 9.7). Fibres are also received from the reticular formation, the cerebellar nuclei, and the substantia nigra. The centromedian nucleus receives many fibres from the globus pallidus.

Efferents from intralaminar nuclei reach the cerebral cortex. Those from the anterior subgroup are diffuse

reaching many parts of the cortex. Those from the posterior group project to the motor, premotor, and supplemental motor areas. Efferents also reach the striatum. Functions of these nuclei are not known.

The **midline nuclei** consist of several small groups of neurons (but there is controversy regarding the groups to be included under this heading). The connections of the nuclei (Flowchart 9.8) are mainly with the limbic system. Afferents include noradrenergic, serotoninergic, and cholinergic bundles ascending from the brainstem. The midline nuclei probably play a role in memory and arousal.

In the past the intralaminar, midline, and reticular nuclei, grouped together as **nonspecific thalamic nuclei** were regarded as part of the ascending reticular activating system, which is responsible for maintaining a state of alertness. They have been described as receiving afferents from the reticular formation (mainly gigantocellular nucleus and ventral reticular nucleus of the medulla; caudal reticular nucleus of pons) and projecting to all parts of the cerebral cortex.

Flowchart 9.8: Connections of the midline nuclei of thalamus

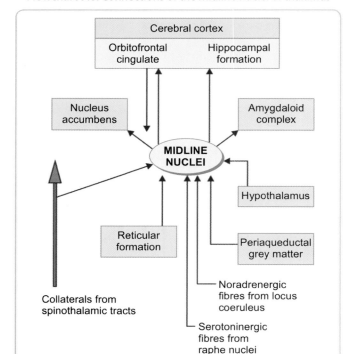

> **Clinical Anatomy**
>
> **Thalamic syndrome of Dejerine-Roussy**
> This occurs due to vascular occlusion of the thalamogeniculate branch of posterior cerebral artery which supplies the posterolateral part of thalamus.
> This condition is characterised by
> - Pansensory loss contralateral to the side of lesion (due to involvement of ventral posterior nuclei)
> - Thalamic pain- severe, persistent, paroxysmal and intolerable pain (Hence this is also known as **painful anaesthesia or anaesthesia dolorosa**) (due to involvement of intralaminar and other non-specific nuclei)
> - Transient hemiparesis (due to involvement of internal capsule)
> - Hemiataxia and choreiform movements (due to involvement of pallidofugal fibres which intersect internal capsule and subthalamus)
> - Homonymous hemianopia (due to involvement of lateral geniculate body)

METATHALAMUS

The metathalamus consists of the medial and lateral geniculate bodies. The medial and lateral geniculate bodies are small oval collections of grey matter situated below the posterior part of the thalamus, lateral to the colliculi of the midbrain (Figure 9.10). Each mass of grey matter is bent on itself, hence the term **"geniculate"**. Traditionally, the geniculate bodies have been grouped

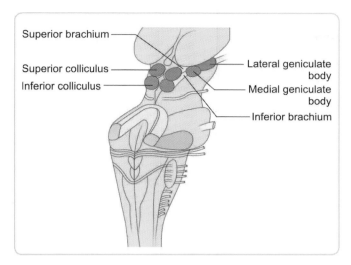

Figure 9.10: Posterolateral view of brainstem showing superior brachium and inferior brachium

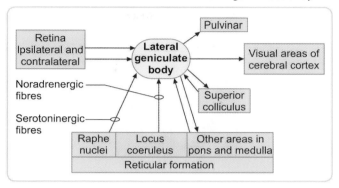

Flowchart 9.9: Connections of the lateral geniculate body

Medial Geniculate Body

The medial geniculate body is a relay station on the auditory pathway. Medial, ventral, and dorsal nuclei are described within it.

Connections

Afferents
The medial geniculate body receives fibres of the lateral lemniscus either directly or after relay in the inferior colliculus (Figure 9.11). These fibres pass through the brachium of the inferior colliculus.

Each medial geniculate body receives impulses from the cochleae of both sides. It also receives fibres from the auditory area of the cerebral cortex. These fibres form part of the **descending auditory pathway.**

Efferents
Fibres arising in the medial geniculate body constitute the auditory radiation. The auditory radiation passes through the sublentiform part of the internal capsule to reach the primary auditory area (Area 41,42) of the cerebral cortex. Different neurons in the ventral nucleus of the medial geniculate body respond to different frequencies of sound (tonotopic organization). The ventral nucleus projects to the primary auditory cortex. The neurons in the dorsal nucleus do not show tonotopic organization. They project to auditory areas around the primary auditory area.

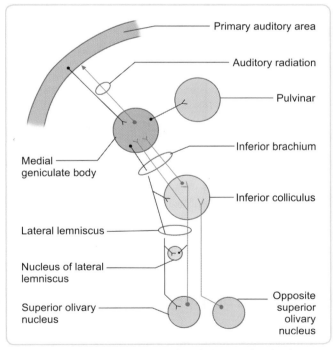

Figure 9.11: Connections of medial geniculate body

together under the heading **metathalamus**, but because of functional relationships, they are now included in the dorsal thalamus.

Lateral Geniculate Body

The lateral geniculate body is a relay station on the visual pathway. It is situated on the inferior aspect of the pulvinar separated from it by the brachium of superior colliculus. It lies anterolateral to the medial geniculate body.

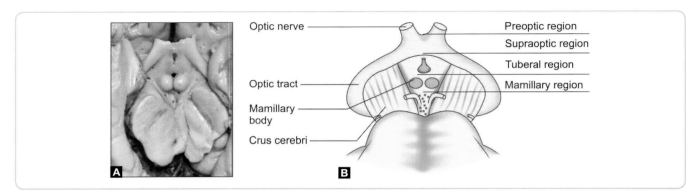

Figures 9.12A and B: Interpeduncular fossa: (A) Specimen; (B) Line diagram

Connections

Afferents

It receives fibres from the retinae of both eyes (Flowchart 9.9).

Apart from retinal fibres, the lateral geniculate body receives fibres from the primary visual cortex and extrastriate visual areas. It also receives fibres from the superior colliculus and the reticular formation of the pons and medulla.

Noradrenergic fibres reach it from the locus coeruleus, and serotoninergic fibres from raphe nuclei (midbrain).

Efferents

Efferents arising in this body constitute the optic radiation, which passes through the retrolentiform part of the internal capsule to reach the primary visual area (Area 17) of the occipital lobe of the cerebral cortex.

HYPOTHALAMUS

The hypothalamus is a part of diencephalon—pars ventralis diencephali. As its name implies, it lies below the thalamus and is separated from it by the hypothalamic sulcus. Most part of hypothalamus is hidden. However, some parts of the hypothalamus can be seen on the external (ventral) surface of the brain. These visible parts of hypothalamus are located in the interpeduncular fossa (Figure 9.12) and they form the floor of third ventricle. On the medial side, it forms the lateral wall of the third ventricle below the level of the hypothalamic sulcus.

Boundaries of Hypothalamus

Laterally, it is in contact with the internal capsule, and (in the posterior part) with the ventral thalamus (subthalamus).

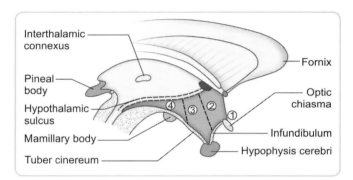

Figure 9.13: Anteroposterior subdivisions of hypothalamus
1. Preoptic 2. Supraoptic 3. Infundibulotuberal 4. Mamillary

Posteriorly, the hypothalamus merges with the ventral thalamus and through it, with the tegmentum of the midbrain.

Anteriorly, it extends up to the lamina terminalis, and merges with certain olfactory structures in the region of the anterior perforated substance.

Inferiorly, the hypothalamus forms structures in the floor of the third ventricle. These are the tuber cinereum, the infundibulum, and the mamillary bodies.

Subdivisions of Hypothalamus

For convenience of description, the hypothalamus may be subdivided, roughly, into a number of regions. Some authorities divide it (from medial to lateral side) into three **zones,** which are as follows:

- **Periventricular**
- **Intermediate**
- **Lateral**

The periventricular and intermediate zones are often described collectively as the **medial zone.** The column of the fornix lies between the medial and lateral zones. The

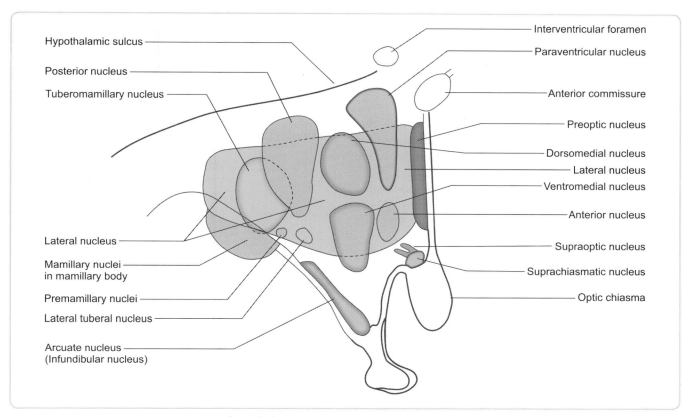

Figure 9.14: Main hypothalamic nuclei as seen from the medial (ventricular) aspect

mamillothalamic tract and the fasciculus retroflexus also lie in this plane.

The hypothalamus is also subdivided anteroposteriorly into four **regions**. These are as follows (Figures 9.12 B and 9.13):

- The **preoptic region** adjoins the lamina terminalis and is anterior to the optic chiasma.
- The **supraoptic (or chiasmatic) region** lies above the optic chiasma.
- The **tuberal (or infundibulotuberal) region** includes the infundibulum, the tuber cinereum, and the region above it.
- The **mamillary (or posterior) region** consists of the mamillary bodies and the region above them.

The preoptic region differs from the rest of the hypothalamus in being a derivative of the telencephalon. The lamina terminalis also belongs to the telencephalon.

Hypothalamic Nuclei

The entire hypothalamus contains scattered neurons within which some aggregations can be recognized. These aggregations, termed the hypothalamic nuclei, are as follows (Figure 9.14):

TABLE 9.3: Hypothalamic regions and nuclei in them	
Region	*Nucleus*
Preoptic region	Preoptic
Supraoptic region	Supraoptic, Paraventricular, Anterior, Suprachiasmatic and Lateral
Tuberal region	Arcuate (infundibular), Ventromedial, Dorsomedial, Lateral tuberal, Premamillary, Tuberomamillary and Lateral
Mamillary region	Posterior, Medial mamillary, Lateral mamillary and Lateral

Nuclei in the Medial Zone

- The **preoptic nucleus lies** in the preoptic region.
- The **paraventricular nucleus**, the **suprachiasmatic nucleus** and the **anterior nucleus** lie in the supraoptic region.
- The **arcuate (infundibular) nucleus** lies in the tuberal region. The tuberal region also contains the **ventromedial nucleus**, the **dorsomedial nucleus** and the **premamillary nuclei**.

- The **posterior nucleus** extends into both the tuberal and mamillary regions.
- The **medial mamillary nucleus** and the **lateral mamillary nucleus** occupy the mamillary region.

Nuclei in the Lateral Zone

The lateral zone contains a diffuse collection of cells that extend through the supraoptic, tuberal, and mamillary regions. These cells constitute the **lateral nucleus.** The lateral zone also contains the following nuclei:

- The **supraoptic nucleus** lies in the supraoptic region (just above the optic tract).
- The **tuberomamillary nucleus** extends into the tuberal and mamillary regions.
- Small aggregations of neurons in the tuberal region constitute the **lateral tuberal nuclei.**

The nuclei present in different regions of hypothalamus are listed in Tables 9.3 and 9.4.

Connections of Hypothalamus

The hypothalamus is concerned with visceral function and is, therefore, connected to other areas having a similar function. These include the various parts of the limbic system, the reticular formation, and autonomic centres in the brainstem and spinal cord (Flowchart 9.10). Apart from its neural connections, the hypothalamus also acts by releasing secretions into the bloodstream and cerebrospinal fluid (CSF).

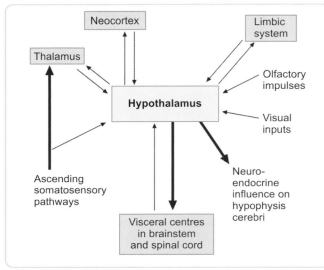

Flowchart 9.10: Connections of hypothalamus

TABLE 9.4: Nuclear groups in the mediolateral zones		
Nuclei in	**Medial zone**	**Lateral zone**
Preoptic region	Preoptic nucleus	Preoptic nucleus
Supraoptic region	Paraventricular Suprachiasmatic Anterior	Supraoptic Lateral
Tuberal region	Arcuate (Infundibular) Ventromedial Dorsomedial Premamillary	Lateral Tuberal Tuberomamillary Lateral
Mamillary region	Medial mamillary Lateral Mamillary Posterior	Lateral

Afferent Connections

The hypothalamus receives visceral afferents (including those of taste) through the spinal cord and brainstem.

Many of these fibres pass through a bundle called the **mamillary peduncle**. Other fibres pass through a bundle called the **dorsal longitudinal fasciculus**. Fibres from the tegmentum of the midbrain also reach the hypothalamus through the **medial forebrain bundle**.

- Afferents from the nucleus of the solitary tract carry taste impulses (and other visceral sensations).
- Somatic afferents reach the hypothalamus through collaterals of major ascending tracts.
- The hypothalamus receives afferents from several centres connected to olfactory pathways and the limbic system.

These are the anterior perforated substance, the septal nuclei, the amygdaloid complex, the hippocampus and the piriform cortex. Many of these fibres reach the hypothalamus through the medial forebrain bundle. Fibres from the hippocampus travel through the fornix.

- **Corticohypothalamic fibres:** In addition to fibres from the piriform cortex (mentioned above), the hypothalamus is believed to receive fibres from the cortex of the frontal lobe. Some of these are direct. Others relay in the thalamus (medial, dorsal, and midline nuclei) and reach the hypothalamus through periventricular fibres (so called because they travel just subjacent to the ependyma). The cingulate gyrus may influence the hypothalamus indirectly through the hippocampal formation. Some fibres from the orbital cortex may reach the hypothalamus through the medial forebrain bundle.

TABLE 9.5: Fibre bundles associated with hypothalamus

A/E	Name of the tract	Connects	Functions
Principally afferents	Fornix	Hippocampal formation	Papez circuit for recent memory
	Stria terminalis	Amygdaloid nucleus	Autonomic effect of aggression
	Ventral amygdalofugal pathway	Amygdaloid nucleus	Autonomic effect of aggression
	Mamillary peduncle	Reticular formation of midbrain	Visceral afferent impulses
	Noradrenergic fibres	Locus coeruleus	Circadian rhythm
	Serotoninergic fibres	Raphe nucleus	Circadian rhythm
	Retinohypothalamic fibres	Retina	Circadian rhythm
Afferent + efferent	Medial forebrain bundle	Anterior olfactory areas, septal areas and tegmentum of the midbrain	Limbic connections to midbrain
Principally efferents	Mamillothalamic tract	Anterior nucleus of the thalamus	Papez circuit for recent memory
	Dorsal longitudinal fasciculus	Central grey matter of brainstem	Projects to parasympathetic nuclei
	Mamillotegmental tract	Tegmental nucleus of the midbrain	Exchange of autonomic information
	Hypothalamospinal tract	Intermediolateral cells of spinal cord	Autonomic connection to T1-L2 and S2-S4
	Paraventriculohypophyseal tract	Neurohypophysis	Release of oxytocin
	Supraopticohypophyseal tract	Neurohypophysis	Release of ADH
	Tuberohypophyseal tract	Adenohypophyseal portal system	Release of GHRH, PIH, TRH, CRH and GnRH

Abbreviations: ADH, antidiuretic hormone; GHRH, growth hormone releasing hormone; PIH, prolactin inhibiting hormone; TRH, thyrotropin releasing hormone; CRH, corticotropin releasing hormone; GnRH, gonadotropin releasing hormone

- The hypothalamus also receives fibres from the subthalamic nucleus and the zona incerta.

Efferent Connections

- The hypothalamus sends fibres to autonomic centres in the brainstem and spinal cord. Centres in the brainstem receiving such fibres include the nucleus of the solitary tract, the dorsal nucleus of the vagus, the nucleus ambiguus, and the parabrachial nucleus. Fibres descending to the spinal cord end in neurons in the intermediolateral grey column. It also sends fibres to the hippocampal formation, the septal nuclei, the amygdaloid complex, and the tegmentum of the midbrain, and autonomic centres in the brainstem and spinal cord. These fibres pass through the same bundles that convey afferent fibres from these centres.
- Fibres from the mamillary body pass through the mamillothalamic tract to reach the anterior nucleus of the thalamus. New fibres arising here project to the cingulate gyrus. Fibres from the mamillary nuclei also reach the subthalamic region and the tegmentum. (through the mamillotegmental tract).

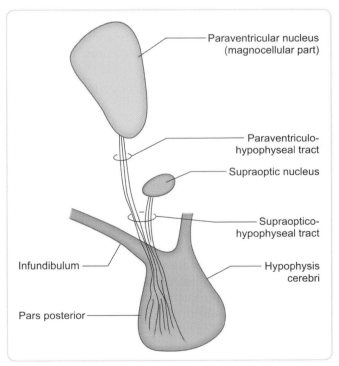

Figure 9.15: Paraventriculohypophyseal and supraopticohypophyseal tracts

- Fibres from the hypothalamus project widely to the neocortex. They play a role in maintaining cortical arousal.

The fibre bundles associated with hypothalamus along with their functions are summarized in Table 9.5.

Control of Hypophysis Cerebri by the Hypothalamus

Neurons in some hypothalamic nuclei produce bioactive peptides that are discharged in the neighbourhood of capillaries or, in some cases, into the cerebrospinal fluid. The process of the production of such bioactive substances by neurons (as distinct from release of neurotransmitters at synapses or efferent nerve endings) is referred to as **neurosecretion**.

Control of Neurohypophysis (Figure 9.15)

Vasopressin (antidiuretic hormone) and **oxytocin**, associated with the neurohypophysis, are really neuro-secretory products synthesized in the supraoptic and paraventricular nuclei of the hypothalamus. Axons of the paraventricular nucleus descend towards the supraoptic nucleus as the **paraventriculohypophyseal tract** (Figure 9.15). They join axons arising from the supraoptic nucleus to form the **supraopticohypophyseal tract**. The axons of the tract pass down into the infundibulum and from there into the neurohypophysis. Here, the axons branch profusely and end in relation to capillaries around which they release their secretion.

Control of the Adenohypophysis by the Hypothalamus

The hypothalamus controls secretion of hormones by the adenohypophysis by producing a number of **releasing factors**. Axons of cells in the infundibular (arcuate) nucleus end in the median eminence and infundibulum, which are closely related to capillaries in the region. The cells of the arcuate (infundibular) nucleus produce releasing factors that travel along their axons and are released into the capillaries. These capillaries carry these factors into the pars anterior of the hypophysis cerebri through the **hypothalamohypophyseal portal system**. In the pars anterior, these factors are responsible for release of appropriate hormones.

Functions of Hypothalamus

The hypothalamus plays an important role in the control of many functions that are vital for the survival of an animal. In exercising such control, the hypothalamus acts in close coordination with higher centres including the limbic system and the prefrontal cortex and with autonomic centres in the brainstem and spinal cord. The main functions attributed to the hypothalamus are as follows:

Regulation of Eating and Drinking Behaviour

The hypothalamus is responsible for feelings of hunger and of satiety. A **feeding centre** has been described in the lateral hypothalamic nucleus and a **satiety centre,** in the ventromedial nucleus.

Regulation of Sexual Activity and Reproduction

The hypothalamus controls sexual activity, both in the male and female. It also exerts an effect on gametogenesis, on ovarian and uterine cycles, and on the development of secondary sexual characters. These effects are produced by influencing the secretion of gonadotropic hormones by the hypophysis cerebri.

Control of Autonomic Activity

The hypothalamus exerts an important influence on the activity of the autonomic nervous system and, thus, has considerable effect on cardiovascular, respiratory, and alimentary functions. Sympathetic activity is said to be controlled predominantly by caudal parts of the hypothalamus and parasympathetic activity, by cranial parts.

Emotional Behaviour

The hypothalamus has an important influence on emotions like fear, anger, and pleasure. Stimulation of lateral areas of the hypothalamus produces sensations of pleasure, while stimulation of medial areas produces pain or other unpleasant effects.

Control of Endocrine Activity

The influence of the hypothalamus in the production of hormones by the pars anterior of the hypophysis cerebri and the elaboration of oxytocin and the antidiuretic hormone by the hypothalamus itself have been described above. Through control of the adenohypophysis, the hypothalamus indirectly influences the thyroid gland, the adrenal cortex, and the gonads.

Response to Stress

Through control over the autonomic nervous system and hormones, the hypothalamus plays a complex role in the way a person responds to stress.

Temperature Regulation

Some neurons in the preoptic nucleus of the hypothalamus act as a thermostat to control body temperature. When body temperature rises or falls, appropriate mechanisms are brought into play to bring the temperature back to normal.

Biological Clock

Several functions of the body show a cyclic variation in activity over the twenty four hours of a day. The most conspicuous of these is the cycle of sleep and waking. Such cycles (called **circadian rhythms**) are believed to be controlled by the hypothalamus, which is said to function as a biological clock. The suprachiasmatic nucleus is believed to play an important role in this regard. Lesions of the hypothalamus disturb the sleep-waking cycle.

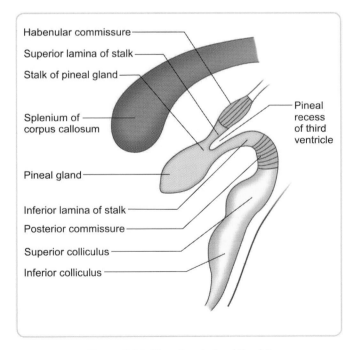

Figure 9.16: The pineal gland (body)

> **Clinical Anatomy**
>
> Effects of lesions of hypothalamic nuclei are seen in Table 9.6

TABLE 9.6: Clinical anatomy of hypothalamic nuclei

Nucleus	Function	Effects of lesion
Preoptic nucleus	Sexually dimorphic	Irregular menstrual cycle and loss of libido
Anterior nucleus	Heat-loss centre	Hyperthermia
Posterior	Heat-rise centre	Hypothermia
Lateral	Hunger centre	Anorexia and emaciation
Medial*	Satiety centre	Obesity
Mamillary body	Recent memory	Wernicke's encephalopathy
Supraoptic nucleus†	ADH secretion	Diabetes insipidus

Abbreviations: ADH, antidiuretic hormone

> **Clinical Anatomy**
>
> * **Kleine-Levin syndrome:** Lesions of medial part of hypothalamus causes problems in satiety resulting in periods of somnolence followed by hyperphagia (Much like the mythological figure 'Kumbhakarna').
> † **Syndrome of Inappropriate ADH secretion (SIADDH):** Lesions of supraoptic nucleus results in improper ADH secretion and diabetes insipidus.

EPITHALAMUS

The epithalamus lies in relation to the posterior part of the roof of the third ventricle and in the adjoining part of its lateral wall. The structures included in the epithalamus are as follows:
- Pineal body
- Habenular nuclei—medial and lateral
- Stria medullaris thalami (stria habenularis) and habenular commissure
- Posterior commissure

Pineal gland (Epiphysis Cerebri)

The pineal gland (or pineal body) is a small piriform structure present in relation to the posterior wall of the third ventricle of the brain (Figure 9.16). It has for long been regarded as a vestigeal structure of no functional importance. However, it is now known to be an endocrine gland of considerable significance. The pineal body is made up of cells called **pinealocytes.** Pinealocytes are separated from one another by neuroglial cells that resemble astrocytes in structure.

The attachment of the pineal body to the posterior wall of the third ventricle is through a stalk that has two laminae: superior and inferior. The superior lamina is traversed by fibres of the **habenular commissure** and the inferior lamina, by fibres of the **posterior commissure.**

The pineal body is innervated by postganglionic sympathetic neurons located in the superior cervical sympathetic ganglia. The fibres travel through the **nervus conarii.** The fibres of this nerve end in the habenular nuclei. Fibres arising in these nuclei form the **habenulopineal tract.** A ganglion (**ganglion conarii)** has been described at the apex of the pineal body.

Function

The pineal body produces a number of hormones (chemically indolamines or polypeptides). These hormones have an important regulatory influence on many endocrine organs, including the hypophysis cerebri, the thyroid, the parathyroids, the adrenals, and the gonads. The hormones of the pineal body reach the hypophysis cerebri both through blood and through the cerebrospinal fluid.

Some activities of the pineal body (for example, the secretion of the hormone **melatonin**) show a marked circadian rythm, which appears to be strongly influenced by exposure of the animal to light.

Clinical Anatomy

A tumour of the pineal body can produce precocious puberty. Melatonin is believed to regulate the onset of puberty.

Habenular Nuclei

The habenular nuclei (medial and lateral) are situated in relation to a triangular depression in the wall of the third ventricle called the **habenular trigone.** The trigone lies in relation to the dorsomedial part of the thalamus. It is medial to the pulvinar, separated from it by the sulcus habenulae. The superior colliculus lies just behind and below the trigone. The habenular nuclei of the two sides are connected by fibres that form the habenular commissure. The habenular nuclei influence neurons concerned with various visceral and endocrine functions. They may be involved in control of sleep and in temperature regulation.

Stria Medullaris Thalami (Stria Habenularis) and Habenular Commissure

The **stria medullaris thalami** is a bundle of fibres lying deep to the taenia thalami (along the junction of the medial and superior surfaces of the thalamus). It begins near the anterior pole of the thalamus and runs backwards to reach the habenular region. Many afferents to the habenular nuclei are from the septal nuclei and pass through the stria medullaris thalami.

Some fibres of the stria medullaris thalami cross in the superior (or anterior) lamina of the pineal stalk to reach the habenular nuclei of the opposite side. These fibres constitute the **habenular commissure.**

Several neuromediators have been demonstrated in the fibres of the stria medullaris. These include acetylcholine, noradrenaline, serotonin, and gamma-aminobutyric acid (GABA).

Posterior Commissure

The posterior commissure lies in the inferior lamina of the stalk of the pineal body. A number of small nuclei are present in relation to the commissure. These include the interstitial and dorsal nuclei of the posterior commissure, the nucleus of Darkschewitsch, and the interstitial nucleus of Cajal. Some fibres arising from these nuclei pass through the posterior commissure. Other fibres continue into it from the medial longitudinal bundle. Some fibres arising

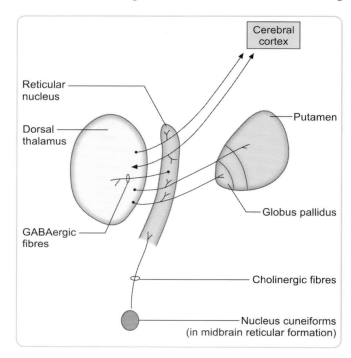

Figure 9.17: Connections of reticular nucleus of the thalamus

in the thalamus, the tectum, and the pretectal nuclei also pass through the posterior commissure.

VENTRAL THALAMUS

The part of the diencephalon that is called the ventral thalamus lies below the posterior part of the thalamus, behind and lateral to the hypothalamus.

Inferiorly, the ventral thalamus is continuous with the tegmentum of the midbrain. Laterally, it is related to the lowest part of the internal capsule.

The main masses of grey matter that are included in the ventral thalamus are the reticular nucleus (previously described as part of the dorsal thalamus) and the zona incerta.

Reticular Nucleus

The reticular nucleus is made up of a thin layer of neurons covering the lateral aspect of the (dorsal) thalamus, separated from the latter by the external medullary lamina. Laterally, the nucleus is related to the internal capsule. Inferiorly, it becomes partially continuous with the zona incerta.

Most fibres emerging from the dorsal thalamus have to traverse the reticular nucleus (The fibres crossing through it give the nucleus a reticulated appearance, and hence, the name). As they pass through it, the fibres give collaterals to the reticular nucleus.

In this way, the nucleus receives somatic, visceral, and auditory impulses. The main efferents of the reticular nucleus pass back into the dorsal thalamus. These fibres are GABAergic. They may influence conduction through the dorsal thalamus (Figure 9.17). The reticular nucleus also receives fibres from the nucleus cuneiformis (in the reticular formation of the midbrain).

Zona Incerta

The zona incerta is a thin lamina of grey matter continuous with the reticular nucleus of the thalamus. It intervenes between the subthalamic nucleus and the thalamus (Figure 9.18). Its functions are not known.

- Some neurons lie along the lower edge of the zona incerta (near the upper end of the red nucleus). These are termed the nuclei of the prerubral field.

Fibre Bundles Passing Through Subthalamic Region

In addition to its grey matter, the subthalamic region contains a number of fibre bundles (Figure 9.18).

Ascending tracts (medial lemniscus, spinal lemniscus, trigeminal lemniscus) pass through it on their way from the midbrain to the thalamus. They are accompanied by dentatothalamic and rubrothalamic fibres.

The subthalamic region also contains two bundles of fibres that connect the globus pallidus to the thalamus. These are the **ansa lenticularis** and the **fasciculus lenticularis**. Associated with these bundles, there are certain regions called the fields of Forel (H, H1, and H2) as shown in Figure 9.18.

Starting from the globus pallidus, the **ansa lenticularis** winds round the ventral and posterior border of the internal capsule to reach the subthalamic region, where it lies ventral and medial to the subthalamic nucleus. Fibres of the **fasciculus lenticularis** intersect those of the internal capsule to reach the subthalamic region. Here, they pass medially above the subthalamic nucleus and below the zona incerta. This region is field H2 of Forel.

The **subthalamic fasciculus** (connecting the globus pallidus to the subthalamic nucleus) occupies a position intermediate between the ansa lenticularis and the fasciculus lenticularis. The fibres of the ansa lenticularis and of the fasciculus lenticularis join together medial to the subthalamic nucleus (in field H of Forel) to form the **thalamic fasciculus** (which is also joined by dentatothalamic and rubrothalamic fibres). The thalamic fasciculus passes above the zona incerta (field H1 of Forel) to reach the thalamus.

Subthalamic Nucleus (of Luys)

As explained above the subthalamic nucleus, which has traditionally been described as a part of the subthalamic region is now grouped functionally with the basal nuclei/ganglia.

ARTERIAL SUPPLY OF DIENCEPHALON

The thalamus is supplied mainly by perforating branches of the posterior cerebral artery. The posteromedial group of branches (also called thalamogeniculate arteries) supply the medial and anterior part. The posterolateral group (also called thalamogeniculate branches) supply the posterior and lateral parts of the thalamus. The thalamus also receives some branches from the posterior communicating, anterior choroidal, posterior choroidal, and middle cerebral arteries (Figure 9.19).

The anterior part of **the hypothalamus** is supplied by central branches of the anteromedial group (arising from the anterior cerebral artery). The posterior part is supplied by central branches of the posteromedial group (arising from the posterior cerebral and posterior communicating arteries).

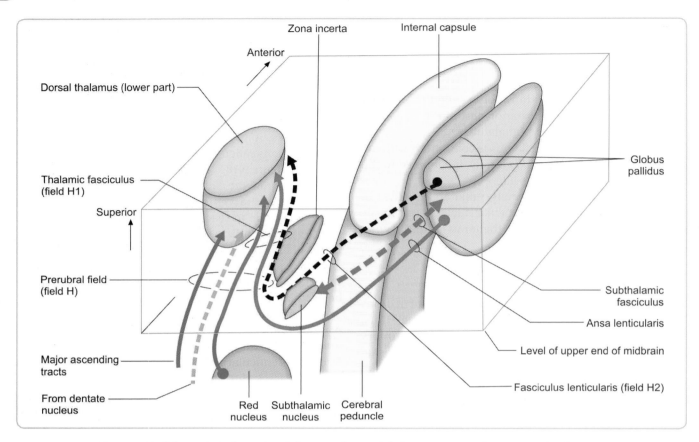

Figure 9.18: Schematic 3-dimensional diagram of ventral thalamic region to show some of its features

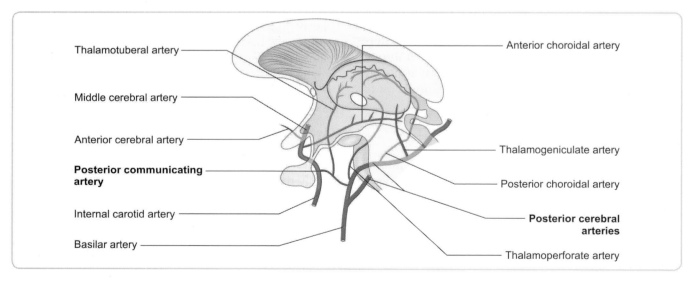

Figure 9.19: Arterial supply of diencephalon

MULTIPLE CHOICE QUESTIONS

Q1. Which of the following nuclei is functionally a part of basal nuclei?
A. Dorsal thalamus
B. Epithalamus
C. Metathalamus
D. Subthalamus

Q2. The lateral surface of the thalamus is related to:
A. Globus pallidus
B. Head of the caudate nucleus
C. Posterior limb of internal capsule
D. Third ventricle

Q3. The sheet of white matter that divides the thalamus into different groups of nuclei is known as:
A. Internal medullary lamina
B. Lamina terminalis
C. Stratum zonale
D. Stria medullaris thalami

Q4. The medial group of thalamic nuclei is concerned with:
A. Emotional aspect of the behaviour
B. Receiving somatosensory impulses
C. Recent memory
D. Relay station from corpus striatum

Q5. Which of the following thalamic peduncles passes through the posterior limb of the internal capsule?
A. Anterior
B. Inferior
C. Posterior
D. Superior

Q6. Which of the following is the most posterior part of the hypothalamus?
A. Infundibulum
B. Lamina terminalis
C. Mamillary bodies
D. Tuber cinereum

Q7. Which of the following group of nuclei of the hypothalamus secretes the hormones of neurohypophysis?
A. Arcuate and tuberomamillary
B. Mamillary and suprachiasmatic
C. Preoptic and infundibular
D. Supraoptic and paraventricular

Q8. The centre located at the lateral part of hypothalamus regulates:
A. Autonomic activity
B. Hunger and thirst
C. Sexual activity
D. Temperature

Q9. Which sensory pathway reaches cerebral cortex bypassing thalamus?
A. Auditory
B. Gustatory
C. Olfactory
D. Visual

Q10. Nervus conarii supplying pineal gland arises from:
A. Nucleus of reticular formation
B. Preganglionic fibres from vagus nerve
C. Superior cervical sympathetic ganglion
D. Suprachiasmatic nucleus

ANSWERS

1. D   2. C   3. A   4. A   5. D   6. C   7. D   8. B   9. C   10. C

SHORT NOTES

1. Lateral geniculate body
2. Metathalamus
3. Intralaminar nuclei of thalamus
4. Hypothalamus
5. Subdivisions of diencephalon

LONG QUESTION

Describe the dorsal thalamus under the following headings: Morphology, connections, blood supply and clinical anatomy.

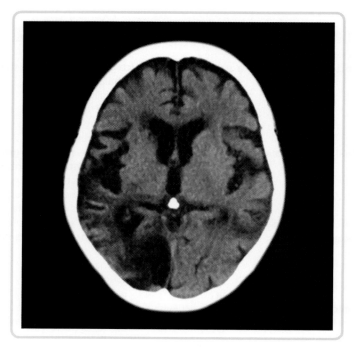

Figure 9.20: CT scan of brain showing calcified pineal gland (*Courtesy:* Dr HD Deshmukh, Professor & Head, Department of Radiology, Seth GS Medical College & KEM Hospital, Mumbai.)

Clinical Cases

9.1: A CT scan of an eighteen year old boy showed a calcified mass located in the groove between the two thalamic bodies. A diagnosis of calcified pineal gland (Figure 9.20) was made .
Explain how the knowledge of location of pineal gland is important clinically.

9.2: Thalamus is an integrating centre and relay station for all types of sensations.
Which sensation is not relayed in thalamus? Why?

9.3: In thalamic syndrome (Dejerine-Roussy) there is increased response to tactile stimuli, abnormal voluntary movements. Which artery is affected?

INTRODUCTION

The cerebrum is the largest part of the brain. It has an ovoid shape. It consists of two incompletely separated cerebral hemispheres (Figure 10.1). The outer surface of the cerebral hemisphere is covered with a shell of grey matter called cortex, which is highly folded due to the presence of convolutions called as gyri which are separated by grooves called as sulci. The core of the hemisphere consists of white matter and a group of nuclei called basal nuclei (basal ganglia) deeper to that. The cavity inside each hemisphere is called the lateral ventricle (Figure 10.2).

The **longitudinal fissure** of cerebrum intervenes between the medial surfaces of the right and left hemispheres. At the bottom of the fissure lies the corpus callosum, which connects the two hemispheres. The contents of the longitudinal fissure are:
• Falx cerebri and the accompanying arachnoid mater
• Pia mater covering the medial surfaces of the hemispheres

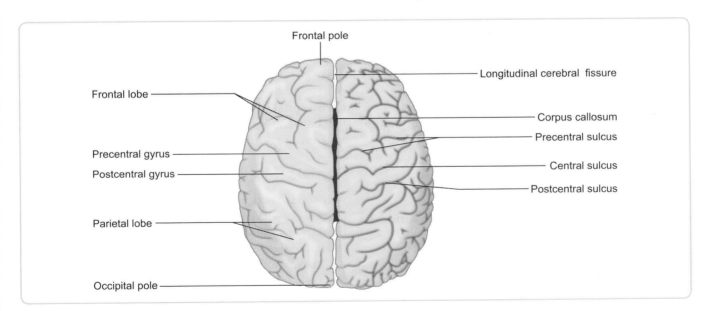

Figure 10.1: Superior view of the cerebrum

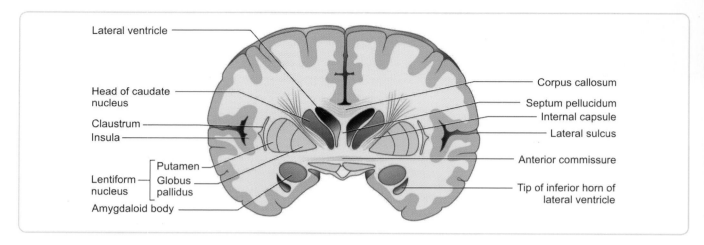

Figure 10.2: Coronal section of cerebrum showing cerebral cortex, white matter and basal nuclei

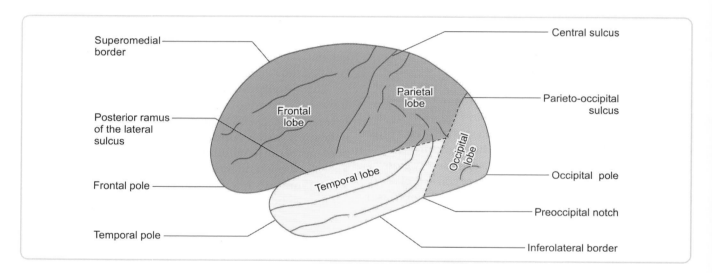

Figure 10.3: Lateral aspect of the cerebral hemisphere to show borders, poles, and lobes

- Anterior cerebral vessels
- Indusium griseum, a thin layer of grey matter on the superior surface of the corpus callosum.

EXTERNAL FEATURES OF CEREBRAL HEMISPHERES

Each cerebral hemisphere has **three poles, three surfaces, and three borders.**

Poles

Three somewhat pointed ends or poles can be recognized when the cerebral hemisphere is viewed from the lateral aspect (Figure 10.3). These are the **frontal pole** anteriorly, the **occipital pole** posteriorly, and the **temporal pole** that lies between the frontal and occipital poles and points forward and downward.

Borders

A coronal section through the cerebral hemispheres (Figure 10.4) shows that each hemisphere has three borders: (1) **superomedial,** (2) **inferolateral,** and (3) **inferomedial.**

The inferomedial border is divided into an anterior part called the **medial orbital border** and a posterior part called the **medial occipital border**. The orbital part of the inferolateral border is called the **superciliary border** (as it lies just above the level of the eyebrows) (Figure 10.5).

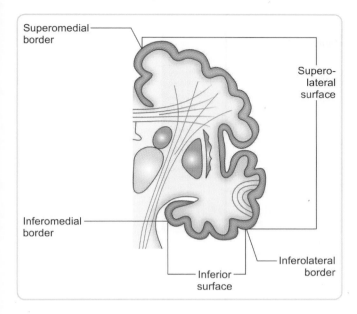

Figure 10.4: Coronal section through cerebral hemisphere to show its borders and surfaces

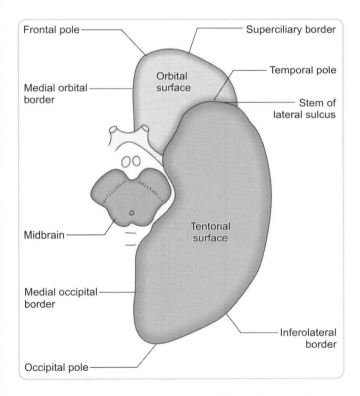

Figure 10.5: Inferior aspect of a cerebral hemisphere to show its borders, poles, and surfaces

Surfaces

Each cerebral hemisphere has three surfaces:
1. **Superolateral surface** between the superomedial border and the inferolateral border (Figure 10.3).
2. **Medial surface** between the superomedial border and the inferomedial border.
3. **Inferior surface** between the inferolateral and inferomedial borders (Figure 10.4).

The **inferior surface** is subdivided into **orbital** and **tentorial surfaces** by the stem of the lateral sulcus (Figure 10.5).

A little anterior to the occipital pole, the inferolateral border shows a slight indentation called the **preoccipital notch (or preoccipital incisure).**

Sulci and Gyri

The surfaces of the cerebral hemisphere are not smooth. They show a series of grooves or **sulci** (Figure 10.6), which are separated by intervening areas that are called **gyri.** There are four different types of sulci described:
1. **Limiting sulcus:** Such a sulcus separates two functionally different areas, e.g. central sulcus.
2. **Axial sulcus:** A sulcus growing in the long axis of a rapidly growing homogeneous area is called an axial sulcus, e.g. posterior part of calcarine sulcus.
3. **Operculated sulcus:** A sulcus, which has one particular type of functional area on the surface and has another functional area in its depth, which is concealed, is called an operculated sulcus, e.g. posterior part of calcarine sulcus which has primary visual area in its depth and has peristriate and parastriate areas which are secondary visual areas on the surface.
4. **Complete sulcus:** A sulcus, which is deep enough to produce an elevation on the ventricular wall is a complete sulcus, e.g. collateral sulcus which produces collateral eminence in the floor of the inferior horn of lateral ventricle.

Lobes

There are four major lobes in the cerebrum namely, frontal, parietal, occipital, and temporal, which subserve different functions. These are well-demarcated on the superolateral surface (Figure 10.3) separated by prominent sulci. Apart from these four lobes, two more lobes are described namely, insular lobe and limbic lobe.

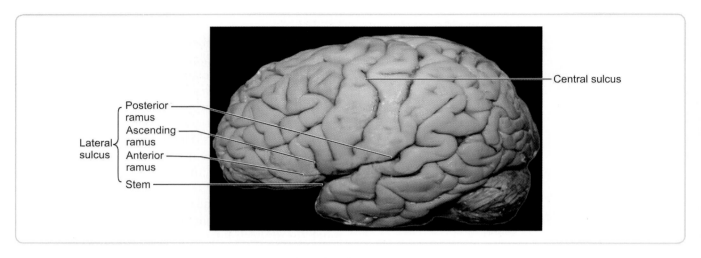

Figure 10.6: Superolateral surface as seen in a brain specimen

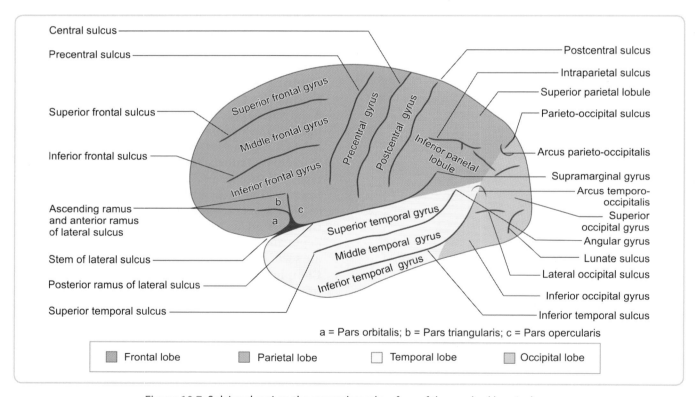

a = Pars orbitalis; b = Pars triangularis; c = Pars opercularis

| Frontal lobe | Parietal lobe | Temporal lobe | Occipital lobe |

Figure 10.7: Sulci and gyri on the superolateral surface of the cerebral hemisphere

On the superolateral surface of the hemisphere, there are two prominent sulci (Figure 10.6). One of these is the **posterior ramus of the lateral sulcus,** which begins near the temporal pole and runs backward and slightly upward. Its posterior most part curves sharply upward. The second sulcus that is used to delimit the lobes is the **central sulcus.** It begins on the superomedial margin, a little behind the midpoint between the frontal and occipital poles and runs downward and forward to end a little above the posterior ramus of the lateral sulcus.

On the medial surface of the hemisphere, there is a "Y" shaped sulcus posteriorly. The upper limb of the "Y" shaped sulcus is called the **parieto-occipital sulcus** (Figure 10.8). The upper end of this sulcus crosses the superomedial border and a small part of it can be seen on the superolateral surface (Figure 10.7).

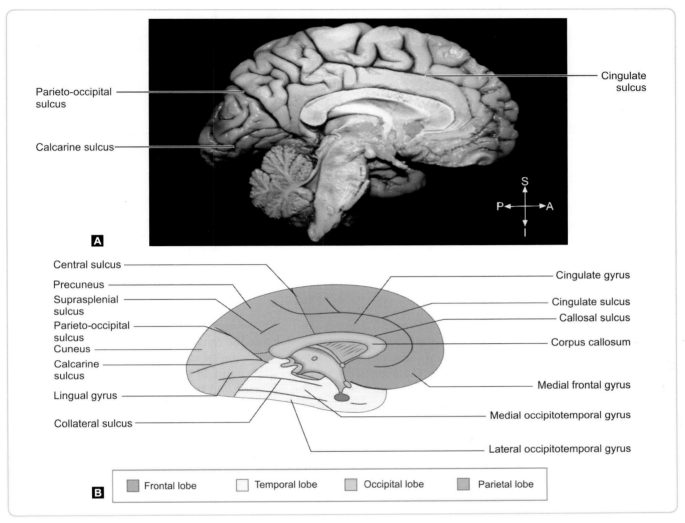

Figures 10.8A and B: (A) Medial surface of the cerebrum as seen in a specimen of brain; (B) The medial surface of the cerebral hemisphere showing gyri and sulci

To define the limits of various lobes, central sulcus and the posterior ramus of lateral sulcus are taken into consideration. Two imaginary lines are also drawn on the superolateral surface to make the divisions complete. The first imaginary line connects the upper end of the parieto-occipital sulcus to the preoccipital notch. The second imaginary line is a backward continuation of the posterior ramus of the lateral sulcus (excluding the posterior upturned part) to meet the first line. The limits of the various lobes are as follows (Figure 10.7):

- The **frontal lobe** lies anterior to the central sulcus and above the posterior ramus of the lateral sulcus
- The **parietal lobe** lies behind the central sulcus. It is bounded below by the posterior ramus of the lateral sulcus and by the second imaginary line and behind by the upper part of the first imaginary line

- The **occipital lobe** is the area lying behind the first imaginary line
- The **temporal lobe** lies below the posterior ramus of the lateral sulcus and the second imaginary line. It is separated from the occipital lobe by the lower part of the first imaginary line
- The **insula or insular lobe (island of Reil)** is an area of the cortex that lies in the depth of the lateral sulcus and hence hidden from the surface view (Figure 10.9)
- The **limbic lobe** is a part of limbic system, forming a border (Limbus = Border) between telencephalic and diencephalic structures and comprising of cingulate, subcallosal and parahippocampal gyri. The limbic lobe is seen on the medial and inferior surfaces of the cerebral hemisphere

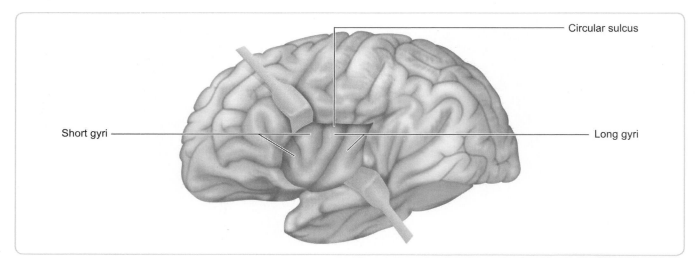

Figure 10.9: The insula of the cerebrum exposed

- The upper end of the central sulcus winds round the superomedial border to reach the medial surface. Here its end is surrounded by a gyrus called the **paracentral lobule** (Figure 10.8B). The lower end of the central sulcus is always separated by a small interval from the posterior ramus of the lateral sulcus (Figure 10.7)
- The lateral sulcus begins on the inferior aspect of the cerebral hemisphere, where it lies between the orbital surface and the anterior part of the temporal lobe (Figures 10.6 and 10.11). It runs laterally to reach the superolateral surface. On reaching this surface, it divides into three rami (branches). These rami are **anterior (or anterior horizontal), ascending (or anterior ascending),** and **posterior** (Figures 10.6 and 10.7). The anterior and ascending rami are short and run into the frontal lobe in the directions indicated by their names. The posterior ramus has already been considered. Unlike most other sulci, the lateral sulcus is very deep. Its walls cover a fairly large area of the surface of the hemisphere called the **insula** (Figure 10.9).

SUPEROLATERAL SURFACE OF CEREBRAL HEMISPHERE

The subdivisions of the superolateral surface are described here and are shown in Figure 10.7.

Frontal Lobe

The frontal lobe is further subdivided as follows. The **precentral sulcus** runs downward and forward parallel

to and a little anterior to the central sulcus. The area between it and the central sulcus is the **precentral gyrus.** In the region anterior to the precentral gyrus there are two sulci that run in an anteroposterior direction. These are the **superior** and **inferior frontal sulci.** They divide this region into **superior, middle,** and **inferior frontal gyri.** The anterior and ascending rami of the lateral sulcus extend into the inferior frontal gyrus, dividing it into three parts: (1) the part below the anterior ramus is the **pars orbitalis;** (2) that between the anterior and ascending rami is the **pars triangularis;** and (3) the part posterior to the ascending ramus is the **pars opercularis.**

Temporal Lobe

The temporal lobe has two sulci that run parallel to the posterior ramus of the lateral sulcus. They are termed the **superior** and **inferior temporal sulci.** They divide the superolateral surface of this lobe into **superior, middle,** and **inferior temporal gyri.**

Parietal Lobe

The parietal lobe shows the following subdivisions. The **postcentral sulcus** runs downward and forward parallel to and a little behind the central sulcus. The area between these two sulci is the **postcentral gyrus.** The rest of the parietal lobe is divided into a **superior parietal lobule** and an **inferior parietal lobule** by the **intraparietal sulcus.** The upturned posterior end of the posterior ramus of the lateral sulcus extends into the inferior parietal lobule. The posterior end of the superior temporal sulcus also turns upward to enter this lobule. The part that arches over the upturned posterior end of the posterior ramus of the lateral sulcus is called the **supramarginal gyrus.** The part that arches over the superior temporal sulcus is called the **angular gyrus.**

Occipital Lobe

The occipital lobe shows three rather short sulci. One of these, the **lateral occipital sulcus** lies horizontally and divides the lobe into **superior and inferior occipital gyri.** The **lunate sulcus** runs downward and slightly forward just in front of the occipital pole. The **transverse occipital sulcus** is located in the uppermost part of the occipital lobe. The upper end of the parieto-occipital sulcus (which just reaches the superolateral surface from the medial surface) is surrounded by the **arcus parieto-occipitalis.** As its name suggests, it belongs partly to the parietal lobe and partly to the occipital lobe.

Insula

In the depth of the stem and posterior ramus of the lateral sulcus, there is a part of the cerebral hemisphere called the **insula** (insula = hidden) (Figure 10.9). It is surrounded by a **circular sulcus.** During development of the cerebral hemisphere, this area grows less than surrounding areas, which therefore, come to overlap it and occlude it from surface view. These surrounding areas are called **opercula** (= lids). The **frontal operculum** lies between the anterior and ascending rami of the lateral sulcus. The **frontoparietal operculum** lies above the posterior ramus of the lateral sulcus. The **temporal operculum** lies below this sulcus. The temporal operculum has a superior surface hidden in the depth of the lateral sulcus. On this surface are located two gyri called the **anterior and posterior transverse temporal gyri.** The surface of the insula itself is divided into a number of gyri.

MEDIAL SURFACE OF CEREBRAL HEMISPHERE

The features of the medial surface include the sulci and gyri, as well as the corpus callosum and the midline structures below it (Figures 10.8 and 10.10).

The **corpus callosum** is a prominent arched structure consisting of commissural fibres passing from one hemisphere to the other.

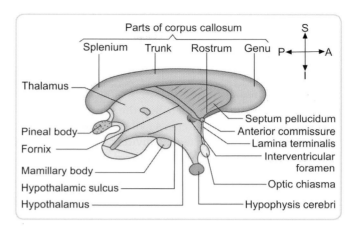

Figure 10.10: Structures seen below corpus callosum

Frontal Lobe

The **lamina terminalis** is a thin lamina of nervous tissue between the anterior commissure and the optic chiasma. Just in front of the lamina terminalis, there are the **paraterminal gyrus** and the **parolfactory gyrus.**

Above the corpus callosum (and also in front of and behind it), are the sulci and gyri of the medial surface of the hemisphere (Figure 10.8). Just above the corpus callosum is callosal sulcus. Parallel to this is cingulate sulcus. Between the two is **cingulate gyrus.** The gyrus above cingulate gyrus (in frontal lobe) is **medial frontal gyrus**. The cingulate sulcus splits to enclose the **paracentral lobule.**

Parietal Lobe

The cingulate gyrus (in parietal lobe) is limited by suprasplenial sulcus. Above the sulcus is **precuneus.**

Occipital Lobe

In the occipital lobe, the region between parieto-occipital sulcus and calcarine sulcus is **cuneus.** Below the calcarine sulcus is **lingual gyrus.** Cingulate gyrus is continuous with parahippocampal gyrus through **isthmus.**

INFERIOR SURFACE OF CEREBRAL HEMISPHERE

When the cerebrum is separated from the hindbrain by cutting across the midbrain and is viewed from below, the structures seen are shown in Figure 10.11. The stem of lateral sulcus divides the inferior surface into orbital surface (of frontal lobe) and tentorial surface (of occipitotemporal lobe).

Orbital Surface

Close to the medial border of the orbital surface, there is an anteroposterior sulcus called the **olfactory sulcus.** The area medial to this sulcus is called the **gyrus rectus**. The rest of the orbital surface is divided by an H-shaped **orbital sulcus** into **anterior, posterior, medial,** and **lateral orbital gyri.**

Tentorial Surface

The tentorial surface is marked by two major sulci that run in an anteroposterior direction. These are the **collateral sulcus,** medially and the **occipitotemporal sulcus,** laterally. Medial to collateral sulcus is the **parahippocampal gyrus.** The anterior end of the parahippocampal gyrus is cut off from the curved temporal pole of the hemisphere by a curved **rhinal sulcus.** This part of the parahippocampal gyrus forms a hook-like structure called the **uncus.** Posteriorly, the parahippocampal gyrus becomes continuous with the gyrus cinguli through the isthmus (Figures 10.8 and 10.11).

The area on either sides of the occipitotemporal sulcus is the **medial occipitotemporal gyrus** and **lateral occipitotemporal gyrus.**

FUNCTIONAL AREAS OF CEREBRAL CORTEX

Various authors have worked out "maps" of the cerebral cortex indicating areas of differing structure and functions. The best known scheme is that of Brodmann, who represented different areas by numbers. Areas of the cortex are very frequently referred to by Brodmann numbers. The numbers most commonly referred to are indicated in Figure 10.12.

Primary Motor Area (Area 4 of Brodmann)

The **primary motor area (MI)** is located in the precentral gyrus on the superolateral surface of the hemisphere (Figures 10.12A and 10.13A) and in the anterior part of the paracentral lobule on the medial surface (Figure 10.13B). When these areas are stimulated electrically, movements occur in various parts of the body. Anatomically, these areas give origin to projection fibres that form the corticospinal and corticonuclear tracts.

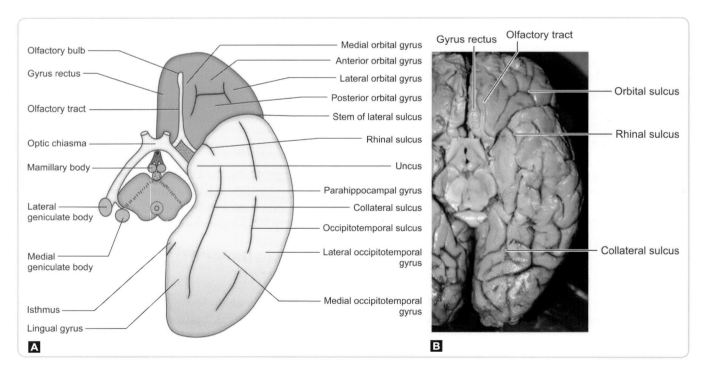

Figures 10.11A and B: (A) Structures seen on the inferior aspect of the cerebrum; (B) Inferior surface seen in a brain specimen

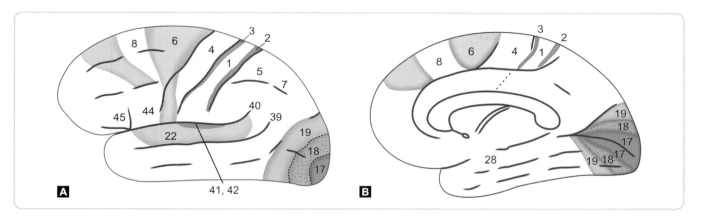

Figures 10.12A and B: (A) Location of some of the areas of Brodmann on the superolateral aspect; and (B) On the medial aspect of the cerebral hemisphere

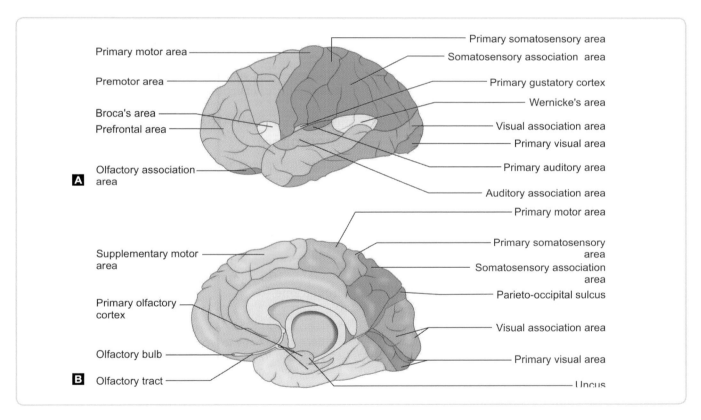

Figures 10.13A and B: (A) Functional areas on the superolateral aspect of the cerebral hemisphere; (B) Functional areas on the medial aspect of the cerebral hemisphere

Specific regions within the area are responsible for movements in specific parts of the body. The body representation is upside down (inverted homunculus) (Figure 10.14).

The area of cortex representing a part of the body is not proportional to the size of the part, but rather to intricacy of movements in the region. Thus, relatively large areas of cortex represent the hands and lips.

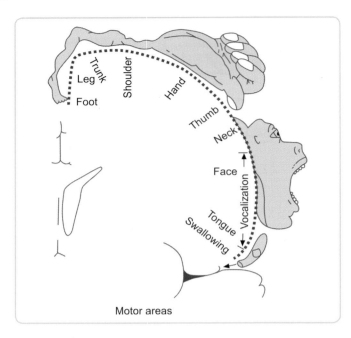

Figure 10.14: The motor homunculus

Premotor Area (Areas 6 and 8 of Brodmann)

The premotor area is located just anterior to the motor area. It occupies the posterior parts of the superior, middle, and inferior frontal gyri (Figures 10.12 A and 10.13 A).

Stimulation of the premotor area results in movements, but these are more intricate than those produced by stimulation of the motor area.

The premotor area is responsible for programming the intended movements and control of movements in progress.

Apart from its corticospinal output, the motor area is connected (in a point-to-point manner) with the main sensory cortex (SI). This explains why neurons in area 4 are responsive to peripheral stimulation. Area 4 receives afferents from the posterior part of the ventral lateral nucleus of the thalamus. This nucleus receives fibres from cerebellar nuclei. In this way, the cerebellum projects to area 4. Area 4 also receives fibres from some other parts of the thalamus, the hypothalamus, and some other parts of the cerebral cortex (including the primary sensory area SI).

Supplementary Motor Area

Supplementary motor area (MII) lies on the medial surface of the cerebral hemisphere on the medial frontal gyrus (Figure 10.12B). It has extensions of Brodmann's areas 4, 6 and 8 on to the medial surface.

Frontal Eye Field (Area 8 of Brodmann)

The frontal eye field lies in the middle frontal gyrus (Figure 10.12A). Stimulation of this area causes both eyes to move to the opposite side. These are called **conjugate movements.**

Prefrontal Area

The part of the frontal lobe excluding the motor and premotor areas is referred to as the prefrontal area (Figure 10.13A). It includes the parts of the frontal gyri anterior to the premotor area, the orbital gyri, most of the medial frontal gyrus.

The prefrontal area is concerned with normal expression of emotions and the ability to predict consequences of actions.

Motor Speech Area (Areas 44 and 45 of Brodmann)

The motor speech area of Broca lies in the inferior frontal gyrus (Figures 10.12A and 10.13A) of the dominant hemisphere. Injury to this region results in inability to speak **(aphasia),** even though the muscles concerned are not paralyzed. These effects occur only if damage occurs in the left hemisphere in right-handed persons and also in many left-handed persons.

Table 10.1 summarizes the functional areas of the frontal lobe.

> ### Clinical Anatomy
>
> **Effects of Damage to Frontal Lobe**
> - A localized lesion of the primary motor area normally produces contralateral monoplegia. An extensive lesion can cause hemiplegia.
> - Lesions of the premotor area have an adverse effect on skilled movements.
> - Lesions of the frontal eye field result in deviation of both eyes to the side of lesion.
> - Lesions of the motor speech area destroy the ability to speak.
> - Lesions of the prefrontal area lead to personality changes such as making the person not only more docile but also negligent and lacking in concentration and willpower.

TABLE 10.1: Functional areas of frontal lobe

Surface	Names of gyri	Functional areas	Brodmann's numbers	Blood supply
Superolateral surface	Precentral gyrus	Motor area	4	MCA, ACA
	Superior frontal gyrus	Premotor area, Frontal eye field	6, 8	MCA, ACA
	Middle frontal gyrus		8	
	Inferior frontal gyrus	Broca's motor speech area	44, 45	MCA
Medial surface	Medial frontal gyrus	Supplementary motor area	4, 6, 8	ACA
	Cingulate gyrus, septal area	Limbic lobe	24, 32	ACA
	Paracentral lobule	Motor area	4	ACA
Inferior surface	Gyrus rectus	Prefrontal area	9, 10, 11, 12	MCA, ACA
	Orbital gyri: Medial, posterior, lateral and anterior			
Around frontal pole				

Abbreviations: ACA, anterior cerebral artery; MCA, middle cerebral artery

Primary Somatosensory Area (Areas 3, 1 and 2 of Brodmann)

The sensory area located in the postcentral gyrus is called the **primary somatosensory area (SI)** (Figure 10.13A). It also extends onto the medial surface of the hemisphere where it lies in the posterior part of the paracentral lobule. Responses can be recorded from the sensory area when individual parts of the body are stimulated. Like the motor area, the body representation is upside down (inverted homunculus).

It receives projections from the ventral posteromedial and ventral posterolateral nuclei of the thalamus, conveying impulses received through the medial, spinal, and trigeminal lemnisci.

The area of cortex that receives sensations from a particular part of the body is not proportional to the size of that part but rather to the complexity of sensations received from it. Thus, the digits, the lips, and the tongue have a disproportionately large representation (Figure 10.15).

A second area predominantly somatosensory in function (**second somatosensory area or SII**) has been described in relation to the superior lip of the posterior ramus of the lateral sulcus.

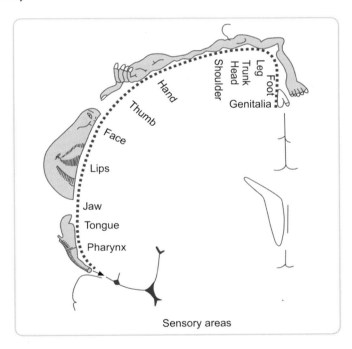

Figure 10.15: The sensory homunculus

Somatosensory Association Area (Areas 5 and 7 of Brodmann)

Parts of the superior parietal lobule help us recognize shape, size, and texture of objects.

Sensory Speech Area (Areas 22, 39 and 40 of Brodmann)

The sensory speech area of Wernicke lies in the posterior part of the superior and middle temporal gyri of the

TABLE 10.2: Functional areas of parietal lobe

Surface	Names of gyri	Functional areas	Brodmann's numbers	Blood supply
Superolateral surface	Postcentral gyrus	Primary somatosensory area	3, 1, 2	MCA, ACA
	Superior parietal lobule	Somatosensory association area	5, 7	MCA, ACA
	Inferior parietal lobule	Secondary somatosensory area, Part of Wernicke's sensory speech area	39, 40	MCA
Medial surface	Paracentral lobule	Primary somatosensory area	3, 1, 2	ACA
	Precuneus	Somatosensory association area	7	ACA

Abbreviations: ACA, anterior cerebral artery; MCA, middle cerebral artery

language dominant hemisphere. It extends into **areas 39 and 40** of the parietal lobe. This area is responsible for interpretation of speech.

Table 10.2 summarizes the functional areas of parietal lobe.

> **Clinical Anatomy**
>
> **Effects of Damage to Sensory Areas**
> - Damage to the first somatosensory area causes loss of sensation (both exteroceptive and proprioceptive) from the opposite side of the body.
> - Damage to superior parietal lobule interferes with ability to identify objects by feeling them (Astereognosis).
> - Damage to the area of Wernicke leads to failure to understand spoken as well as written speech.

Visual Areas (Areas 17, 18 and 19 of Brodmann)

The primary visual area is located in the occipital lobe, mainly on the medial surface, both above and below the calcarine sulcus (Brodmann's area 17). Area 17 extends into the cuneus and into the lingual gyrus (Figure 10.13B). Posteriorly, it may extend onto the superolateral surface, where it is limited (anteriorly) by the lunate sulcus.

It receives fibres of the optic radiation. It is also called the **striate cortex.**

Area 18 **(parastriate area)** and area 19 **(peristriate area)** are responsible mainly for interpretation of visual impulses reaching area 17, and they often described as **visual association area.**

The visual areas give off efferent fibres also. These reach various parts of the cerebral cortex in both hemispheres. In particular, they reach the frontal eye field, which is concerned with eye movements. Like other "sensory" areas, the visual areas also connect with functionally related motor areas. This is substantiated by the fact that movements of the eyeballs and head can be produced by stimulation of areas 17 and 18, which constitute the **occipital eye field.** Efferents from the visual areas also reach the superior colliculus, the pretectal region, and the nuclei of cranial nerves supplying muscles that move the eyeballs.

Table 10.3 summarizes the functional areas of occipital lobe.

TABLE 10.3: Functional areas of occipital lobe

Surface	Names of gyri	Functional areas	Brodmann's numbers	Blood supply
Medial surface	Cuneus, lingual gyrus	Primary visual area Visual association area	17 18, 19	PCA
Superolateral surface	Superior occipital gyrus	Visual association area	18	PCA
	Inferior occipital gyrus	Visual association area	18	PCA
Around occipital pole	-	Primary visual area for macular vision	17	MCA and PCA

Abbreviations: MCA, middle cerebral artery; PCA, posterior cerebral artery

Auditory (Acoustic) Areas (Areas 41, 42 and 22 of Brodmann)

The primary auditory area or the area for hearing is situated in the temporal lobe. It lies in that part of the superior temporal gyrus, which forms the inferior wall of the posterior ramus of the lateral sulcus (Figure 10.16). In this location, there are two short oblique gyri called the anterior and posterior **transverse temporal gyri.** The auditory area lies in the anterior transverse temporal gyrus and extends to a small extent onto the surface of the hemisphere in the superior temporal gyrus (area 41, 42).

It receives the auditory radiation. Auditory association area lies in the superior temporal gyrus (Brodmann's area 22) anterior to primary auditory area.

Essentially, the fibres of each lateral lemniscus are bilateral. Hence, the auditory areas in each cerebral cortex receive fibres from both the right and left cochleae. The close relationship of the auditory areas to Wernicke's speech area is to be noted. The association is significant in view of the obvious relationship between hearing and speech.

Table 10.4 summarizes the functional areas of temporal lobe.

STRUCTURE OF CEREBRAL CORTEX

Due to the presence of a large number of sulci, only about one-third of the total area of cerebral cortex is seen on the surface of the brain. The total area of the cerebral cortex is estimated to be about 2500 cm².

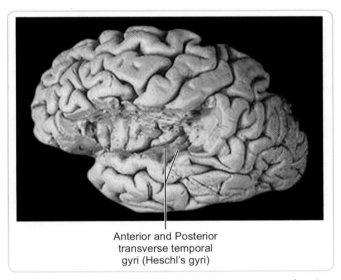

Anterior and Posterior transverse temporal gyri (Heschl's gyri)

Figure 10.16: Anterior and posterior transverse temporal gyri--auditory area

Surface	Names of gyri	Functional areas	Brodmann's numbers	Blood supply
Superolateral surface	Superior temporal gyrus	Part of Wernicke's sensory speech area, auditory association area	22	MCA
	Middle temporal gyrus	-	-	MCA
	Inferior temporal gyrus	-	-	MCA, PCA
	Anterior and posterior transverse temporal gyri	Primary auditory area	41, 42	MCA
Inferior surface	Parahippocampal gyrus	Entorhinal area	28	PCA
	Medial occipitotemporal gyrus	-	-	PCA
	Lateral occipitotemporal gyrus	-	-	PCA

TABLE 10.4: Functional areas of temporal lobe

Abbreviations: MCA, middle cerebral artery; PCA, posterior cerebral artery

Like other masses of grey matter, the cerebral cortex contains the cell bodies of an innumerable number of neurons along with their processes, neuroglia, and blood vessels. The neurons are of various sizes and shapes. They establish extremely intricate connections with each other and with axons reaching the cortex from other masses of grey matter.

NEURONS IN CEREBRAL CORTEX

Cortical neurons vary in size, shape of their cell bodies, and lengths, branching patterns, and orientation of their processes. The cerebral cortex consists of many types of nerve cells but two principal nerve cells are the pyramidal cells and stellate cells (Table 10.5 and Figure 10.17).

Pyramidal Cells

They are the most abundant type of cortical neurons. In contrast, all other neurons in the cortex are referred to as nonpyramidal neurons. About two-thirds of all cortical

TABLE 10.5: Important nerve cells of cerebral cortex

Pyramidal cells (P) (almost two-thirds of cortical neurons)	Cells of Martinotti (M)
Stellate cells (S) (almost one-third of cortical neurons)	Fusiform cells (F)
	Horizontal cells of Cajal (H)

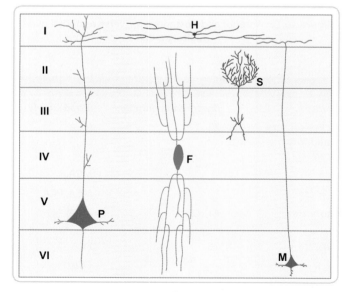

Figure 10.17: Important types of cells seen in the cerebral cortex. P, pyramidal cell; S, stellate cell; F, fusiform cell; H, horizontal cell of Cajal; M, Martinotti cell

neurons are pyramidal, with the apex generally directed towards the surface of the cortex. A large dendrite arises from the apex. Other dendrites arise from basal angles. The axon arises from the base of the pyramid. The processes of pyramidal cells extend vertically through the entire thickness of cortex and establish numerous synapses. The axon of a pyramidal cell may terminate in one of the following ways:
- It may travel to noncortical regions such as the basal ganglia, the brainstem, or the spinal cord.
- It may cross to the opposite side (through a commissure) and reach the corresponding region of the opposite hemisphere.
- It may enter the white matter to travel to another part of the cortex.
- It may be short and may terminate within the same area of the cortex.

Stellate Cells

The **stellate neurons** are relatively small and multipolar. They form about one-third of the total neuronal population of the cortex. Under low magnifications (and in preparations in which their processes are not demonstrated), these neurons look like granules. They have, therefore, been termed **granular neurons**. Their axons are short and end within the cortex. Their processes extend chiefly in a vertical direction within the cortex. In addition to the stellate and pyramidal neurons, the cortex contains numerous other cell types such as the fusiform cells, the horizontal cells of Cajal, and the cells of Martinotti.

LAMINAE OF CEREBRAL CORTEX

On the basis of light microscopy (cell bodies displayed by Nissl method and the myelinated fibres stained by Weigert method), the cerebral cortex is described as having six layers or laminae (Figure 10.18). From superficial to deep, these laminae are:
- Plexiform or molecular layer
- External granular layer
- Pyramidal cell layer
- Internal granular layer
- Ganglionic layer
- Pleomorphic or multiform layer

The plexiform layer is predominantly made up of fibres, although a few cells are present. All the remaining layers contain both stellate and pyramidal neurons, as well as other types of neurons. The external and internal granular layers have predominance of stellate (granular) cells. The prominent neurons in the pyramidal layer and the ganglionic layer are pyramidal neurons. The largest pyramidal cells (giant pyramidal cells of Betz) are found in

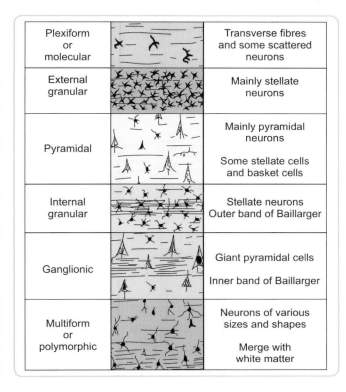

Plexiform or molecular		Transverse fibres and some scattered neurons
External granular		Mainly stellate neurons
Pyramidal		Mainly pyramidal neurons Some stellate cells and basket cells
Internal granular		Stellate neurons Outer band of Baillarger
Ganglionic		Giant pyramidal cells Inner band of Baillarger
Multiform or polymorphic		Neurons of various sizes and shapes Merge with white matter

Figure 10.18: Laminae of cerebral cortex

the ganglionic layer. The multiform layer contains cells of various sizes and shapes.

In addition to the cell bodies of neurons, the cortex contains abundant nerve fibres. Many of these are vertically oriented. Some of these fibres represent afferents entering the cortex. In addition to the vertical fibres, the cortex contains transversely running fibres that form prominent aggregations in certain situations. One such aggregation, present in the internal granular layer is called the **external band of Baillarger**. Another, present in the ganglionic layer is called the **internal band of Baillarger**. The space between the cell bodies of neurons is permeated by a dense plexus formed by their processes. This plexus is referred to as the **neuropil.**

VARIATIONS IN CORTICAL STRUCTURE

The structure of the cerebral cortex shows considerable variation from region to region, both in terms of thickness and the prominence of the various laminae described earlier. As already mentioned, finer variations form the basis of the subdivisions into Brodmann areas. Other workers divide the cortex into five broad varieties. These are as follows:

- In the **agranular cortex,** the external and internal granular laminae are inconspicuous. This type of cortex

is seen most typically in the precentral gyrus (area 4) and is, therefore, typical of "motor" areas. It is also seen in areas 6 and 8, and in parts of the limbic system.
- In the **granular cortex,** the granular layers are highly developed, while the pyramidal and ganglionic layers are poorly developed or absent. This type of cortex is seen most typically in "sensory" areas, including the postcentral gyrus, the visual cortex, and the auditory areas. In the visual area, the external band of Baillarger is prominent and forms a white line that can be seen with the naked eye when the region is freshly cut across. This **stria of Gennari** gives the name **striate cortex** to the visual cortex.

Between these two extremes represented by the agranular and granular varieties of cortex, three intermediate types are described as follows:
- **Frontal cortex**
- **Parietal cortex**
- **Polar cortex**

The frontal type is nearest to the agranular cortex, the pyramidal cells being most prominent, while the polar type is nearest to the granular cortex.

Phylogenetically, cerebral cortex is of three types:
1. **Archipallium (Ancient cortex):** Only three laminae are seen, e.g. hippocampal gyrus.
2. **Paleopallium (Primal cortex):** Four to five laminae are seen, e.g. subiculum and olfactory cortex.
3. **Neopallium (New cortex):** Six laminae are seen, e.g. precentral gyrus and postcentral gyrus.

ARTERIAL SUPPLY OF CEREBRAL CORTEX

The cerebral cortex is supplied by cortical branches of the anterior, middle, and posterior cerebral arteries.

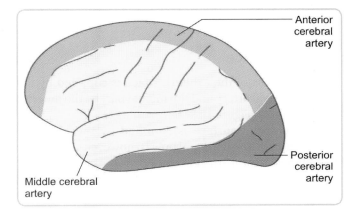

Figure 10.19: Distribution of the anterior, posterior and middle cerebral arteries on the superolateral surface of the cerebral hemisphere

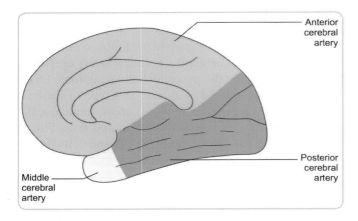

Figure 10.20: Arteries supplying the medial surface of the cerebral hemisphere

Superolateral Surface

The greater part of the superolateral surface is supplied by the middle cerebral artery (Figure 10.19). The areas not supplied by this artery are as follows:

- A strip half to one inch wide along the superomedial border, extending from the frontal pole to the parieto-occipital sulcus is supplied by the anterior cerebral artery.
- The area belonging to the occipital lobe is supplied by the posterior cerebral artery.
- The inferior temporal gyrus (excluding the part adjoining the temporal pole) is also supplied by the posterior cerebral artery.

Medial Surface

The main artery supplying the medial surface is the anterior cerebral artery (Figure 10.20). The area of this surface belonging to the occipital lobe is supplied by the posterior cerebral artery.

Inferior Surface

The lateral part of the orbital surface is supplied by the middle cerebral artery and the medial part by the anterior cerebral artery (Figure 10.21).

The tentorial surface is supplied by the posterior cerebral artery. The temporal pole is, however, supplied by the middle cerebral artery (Figure 10.21).

How does the (left) cerebral hemisphere use and interpret "words" as symbols of communication (language) and how do cortical disorders result in various types of "speech" disturbances (aphasias) is seen in Figure 10.22. Such lesions of the cerebral cortex could be caused by

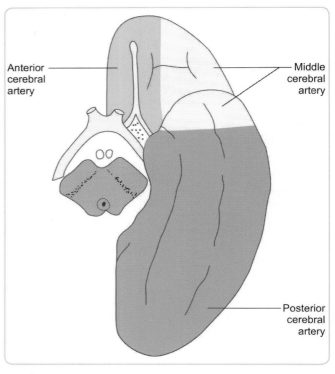

Figure 10.21: Arteries supplying the orbital and tentorial surfaces of the cerebral hemisphere

vascular accidents, tumours, and injuries. A summary of lesion of various areas in the cerebral cortex are tabulated in Table 10.6.

LATERALIZATION OF CEREBRAL HEMISPHERES

The two hemispheres show bilateral asymmetry, both in structure and in function. Structurally, the posterior ramus of lateral sulcus generally is longer in the left hemisphere (planum temporale) than in the right hemisphere. Functionally, Broca's area and Wernicke's area are located in the left cerebral hemisphere in almost all right-handed individuals and most left-handed as well.

Functional specialization has been studied in split-brain patients (who had corpus callosotomy due to severe epilepsy). New methods that allow in vivo comparison of the two hemispheres in normal individuals include positron emission tomography (PET) and functional magnetic resonance imaging (fMRI). These led to a better understanding of functional laterality of the cerebral hemispheres (Figure 10.23).

Clinical Anatomy

Effects of Occlusion of Unilateral Anterior Cerebral Artery
- Contralateral monoplegia of lower limb—involvement of the upper part of the motor area
- Contralateral anaesthesia of lower limb—involvement of the upper part of the sensory area
- Astereognosis—involvement of superior parietal lobule

Effects of Occlusion of One Anterior Cerebral Artery (ACA) When Only One ACA is Present (Unpaired ACA)
- Personality changes, i.e. attention deficit, difficulty in planning, emotional lability, (excessive emotional reactions and frequent mood changes), inappropriate social behaviour, apathy, abulia (loss of willpower)—involvement of prefrontal cortex
- Uninhibited bladder—involvement of medial frontal cortex
- Cortical paraplegia—involvement of paracentral lobule

Effects of Occlusion of Middle Cerebral Artery
- Contralateral hemiplegia and loss of sensations (the face and arms are most affected while lower limb shows slight weakness due to cerebral oedema that is associated with a large infarct)—involvement of primary motor and somatosensory cortex
- Astereognosis or tactile agnosia—involvement of somatosensory association area
- Hearing may be slightly affected in both ears—involvement of primary auditory area
- Aphasia, if the thrombosis is in the left hemisphere—involvement of Broca's, Wernicke's areas and/or involvement of arcuate fasciculus connecting the two areas
- Aprosodia (prosody means rhythm, pitch, stress, intonation of speech), if the thrombosis is in the right hemisphere—involvement of similar areas of right hemisphere
- Word deafness/auditory verbal agnosia—involvement of auditory association area of left side
- Acalculia, anomia, finger agnosia, left-right confusion—involvement of left inferior parietal lobule
- Left hemineglect, construction apraxia, dressing apraxia, anosognosia (unaware of the existence of the disability)—involvement of right inferior parietal lobule

Effects of Occlusion of Posterior Cerebral Artery
- Contralateral homonymous hemianopia with macular sparing—involvement of primary visual area
- Visual hallucinations, distortion of colour vision—involvement of visual association area
- Pure word blindness/alexia—involvement of visual association area of left hemisphere
- Peripheral visual loss with macular sparing/Gun-barrel vision—bilateral involvement of primary visual area

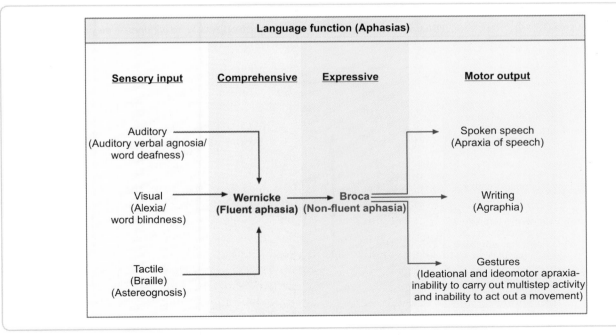

Figure 10.22: A comprehensive look at using words as symbol of communication (Language function)

TABLE 10.6: Lesions of various areas in the cerebral cortex (Brodmann number in brackets) and their effects

Site of lesion		Result of lesion
Primary motor area (4)		*Epileptic seizures:* Due to irritative lesion *Hemiplegia* (contralateral flaccid paralysis)
Premotor area (6)		*Apraxia* (difficulty in performing skilled movements)
Frontal eye field (8)		Contralateral voluntary *conjugate movements of the eye are lost* and the eye deviates to the side of lesion. However, pursuit movements on both sides are normal (controlled by occipital lobe)
Broca's motor speech area (44, 45)		*Expressive/motor aphasia:* Difficulty in spoken speech or writing *(agraphia).* Nonfluent speech and telegraphic language. Key words spoken are normal
Supplementary motor area M II		No permanent loss of movement, bilateral *flexor hypotonia* is present
Sensory speech area of Wernicke (posterior 22, inferior 39, 40)		*Receptive aphasia:* Loss of ability to understand spoken and written speech. Spoken speech is fluent but contains paraphasias (substitution of a word with a nonword, out of context word, and neologism)
Prefrontal area (9, 10, 11, 12)		*Personality changes:* Attention deficit, difficulty in planning, emotional lability, inappropriate social behaviour, apathy, abulia
Primary somatosensory area (3, 1, 2)		*Contralateral sensory loss*
Somatosensory association area (5, 7)		*Astereognosis or tactile agnosia:* Inability to perceive the shape, size, roughness and texture of the objects by touch alone
Left inferior parietal lobule (39, 40)		Acalculia, anomia, finger agnosia, left-right confusion
Right inferior parietal lobule (39, 40)		Left hemineglect, construction apraxia, dressing apraxia, anosognosia (unaware of the existence of the disability)
Left perisylvian area		*Global aphasia:* Involvement of Broca's and Wernicke's area
Right perisylvian area		*Aprosodia:* Inability of a person to properly convey or interpret emotional prosody (prosody in language refers to the ranges of rhythm, pitch, stress, intonation, etc.)
Primary auditory area (41, 42)		Slight bilateral loss of hearing if one side is affected. Bilateral involvement of auditory area will result in *deafness*
Auditory association area (22)		*Word deafness (auditory verbal agnosia):* Inability to interpret meaning of the sounds heard
Primary visual area (17)		*Contralateral homonymous hemianopia with macular sparing* in vascular lesions (no macular sparing in trauma or tumours)
Visual association area (18, 19)		*Visual agnosia:* Loss of ability to recognize objects, *word blindness—alexia*

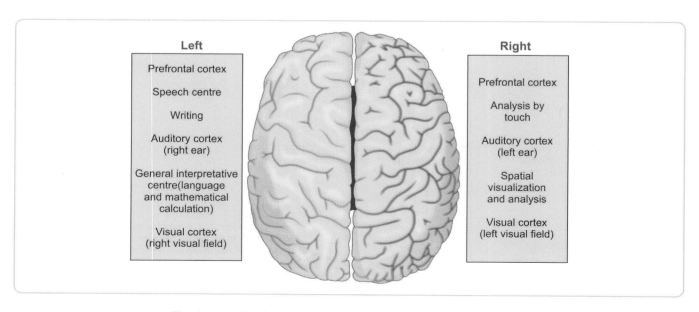

Figure 10.23: Cerebral dominance—Lateralization of cerebral functions

Language functions such as grammar, vocabulary, and literal meaning are typically lateralized to the left hemisphere. The rhythm, stress, intonation of speech, the emotional state of the speaker, the presence of irony or sarcasm, emphasis, contrast and focus (all together called prosody), are comprehended and expressed by the right hemisphere. Arithmetic ability (numerical calculation) and fact retrieval are associated with left hemisphere while geometric understanding, facial perception, and artistic ability (including music) are predominantly right-sided. Analytical, sequential, and logical thinking are by left hemisphere while synthetic, spatial and creative thinking (lateral thinking/thinking out-of-the-box) are predominantly by the right hemisphere.

The functional advantage of lateralization allows each hemisphere to hone its specialization rather than be a jack-of-all-and-master-of-none. The evolutionary advantage of lateralization comes from the ability to perform separate parallel tasks, simultaneously, in each hemisphere of the brain. (Put all the eggs in one basket and watch that basket!)

MULTIPLE CHOICE QUESTIONS

Q1. The cingulate gyrus is related inferiorly to:
A. Corpus callosum
B. Uncus
C. Hippocampus
D. Pineal body

Q2. The collateral sulcus is seen on which surface of the cerebral hemisphere?
A. Superolateral
B. Medial
C. Orbital
D. Tentorial

Q3. The paracentral lobule is located on which surface of cerebral hemisphere?
A. Medial
B. Tentorial
C. Superolateral
D. Orbital

Q4. Which structure lies posterior to the parieto-occipital sulcus on the medial surface of cerebral hemisphere?
A. Cuneus
B. Precuneus
C. Inferior parietal lobule
D. Paracentral lobule

Q5. The artery related to the trunk of the corpus callosum is:
A. Middle cerebral
B. Anterior cerebral
C. Posterior cerebral
D. Anterior choroidal

Q6. Which of the following parts of the body has maximum representation in the cerebral cortex?
A. Thigh
B. Trunk
C. Hand
D. Neck

Q7. Which of the following sulci is related to the primary visual area (17)?
A. Calcarine
B. Parieto-occipital
C. Occipito-temporal
D. Lateral occipital sulcus

Q8. On the superolateral surface of the cerebrum, which sulcus limits the primary visual area?
A. Calcarine
B. Parieto-occipital
C. Lunate
D. Lateral occipital

Q9. Lesion of Brodmann's area results in:
A. Auditory agnosia
B. Astereognosis
C. Visual agnosia
D. Alexia

Q10. Broca's area is located in:
A. Superior temporal gyrus
B. Inferior parietal lobule
C. Inferior frontal gyrus
D. Angular gyrus

ANSWERS

| 1. A | 2. D | 3. A | 4. A | 5. B | 6. C | 7. A | 8. C | 9. A | 10. C |

SHORT NOTES

1. Write a short note on Broca's motor speech area
2. Specify the functional areas of frontal lobe
3. Write a short note on visual cortex
4. Specify the layers of cerebral cortex

LONG QUESTIONS

1. Describe the frontal lobe under the following headings: sulci, gyri, functional areas, blood supply and applied anatomy.
2. Describe the parietal lobe under the following headings: sulci, gyri, functional areas, blood supply and applied anatomy.
3. Draw and label the sulci and gyri on the superolateral surface of the cerebral hemisphere.
4. Draw and label the structures seen on the medial surface of the cerebral hemisphere.
5. Describe the occipital lobe under the following headings: sulci, gyri, functional areas, blood supply and applied anatomy.
6. Describe the temporal lobe under the following headings: sulci, gyri, functional areas, blood supply and applied anatomy.

Clinical Cases

10.1: A 20-year-old man complained of headache, progressive weakness of both lower limbs and incontinence of urine. On investigation, the MRI showed a parasagittal meningioma pressing on the superomedial border.
   A. Based on the signs and symptoms, which area of the brain is affected in this patient?
   B. Which artery supplies that area?

10.2: A patient with middle cerebral artery occlusion was finding it difficult to identify the object placed in his hand, with eyes closed.
   A. What is this condition called as?
   B. Which functional area is affected?

Chapter 11

White Matter of Cerebral Hemispheres

Specific Learning Objectives

At the end of learning, the student shall be able to:
➢ Classify the white fibres of cerebrum into association, commissural and projection fibres
➢ Describe the corpus callosum
➢ Describe the internal capsule
➢ Explain the anatomical basis of stroke

INTRODUCTION

The interior of each cerebral hemisphere consists of a core of white matter, which is composed of myelinated nerve fibres. The fibres of white matter are classified into three types (Figure 11.1):
1. Association fibres
2. Commissural fibres
3. Projection fibres

ASSOCIATION FIBRES

The association fibres connect different parts of the cerebral cortex of the same hemisphere to each other. These are of two types (Figure 11.2):

1. **Short-association fibres**, which connect the adjacent gyri to each other
2. **Long-association fibres**, which connect the gyri located at a distance from each other

Long-association Bundles

- The **cingulum** (girdle-shaped) is located within the cingulate gyrus. It extends from the paraterminal gyrus to the uncus. The cingulum is part of the Papez circuit of the limbic system.
- The **uncinate fasciculus** is a curved fibre bundle. It connects the inferior frontal gyrus and the orbital gyri of the frontal lobe to the hippocampus and amygdaloid

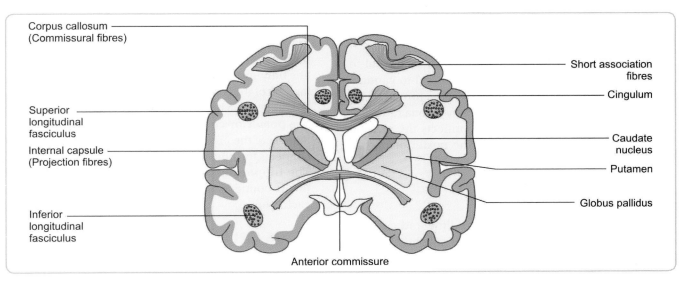

Corpus callosum (Commissural fibres)

Superior longitudinal fasciculus

Internal capsule (Projection fibres)

Inferior longitudinal fasciculus

Short association fibres

Cingulum

Caudate nucleus

Putamen

Globus pallidus

Anterior commissure

Figure 11.1: Coronal section of the brain showing association, commissural and projection fibres

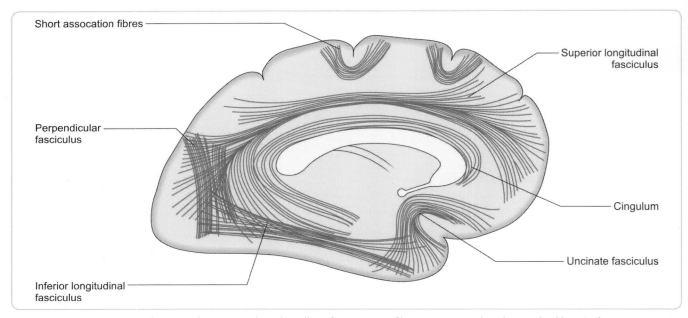

Figure 11.2: Schematic diagram to show bundles of association fibres present within the cerebral hemisphere

nucleus of the temporal lobe. Thus, it connects the limbic areas of the cerebral hemispheres.

- The **superior longitudinal fasciculus** is a long bundle that begins in the frontal lobe and arches back via the parietal lobe to the occipital lobe, from where it turns into the temporal lobe. Thus, it connects the occipital lobe to the frontal eye field. (The **arcuate fasciculus** is a bundle of axons that forms part of the superior longitudinal fasciculus that connects temporal lobe and the frontal lobe. Thus, it connects the sensory and motor speech areas to each other in the dominant hemisphere).
- The **inferior longitudinal fasciculus** connects the occipital lobe to the temporal lobe.
- The **fronto-occipital fasciculus** connects frontal to occipital and temporal lobes. It is lateral to caudate nucleus, lies medial to the superior longitudinal fasciculus and is separated from it by corona radiata.
- The **perpendicular fasciculus** connects the parietal lobe to the occipital lobe and the posterior part of temporal lobe.

COMMISSURAL FIBRES

The commissural fibres cross the midline and connect functionally identical parts of the two hemispheres.

Note: All fibres crossing from one side of the brain or spinal cord to the opposite side are not commissural fibres. When fibres originating in a mass of grey matter in one-half of the central nervous system (CNS) end in some other mass of grey matter in the opposite half, they are referred to as **decussating fibres**, and the sites where such crossings take place are referred to as decussations.

Important Commissures

- The **corpus callosum** is the largest commissure of the brain connecting various parts of neocortex of both the hemispheres.
- The **anterior commissure** connects the right and left temporal lobes. It is in the shape of a cupid's bow. It crosses the midline in the upper part of the lamina terminalis anterior to the columns of fornix.
- The **habenular commissure** is located in the superior lamella of the pineal stalk and is a part of epithalamus. It connects the habenular nuclei of both sides.
- The **posterior commissure** is located in the inferior lamella of the pineal stalk and is a part of brainstem. It connects the nuclei of III, IV, VI and VIII cranial nerves.
- The **hippocampal commissure** or **commissure of fornix** connects the hippocampus of the two sides to each other.

CORPUS CALLOSUM

This is located in the floor of the median longitudinal fissure (Figure 11.3).

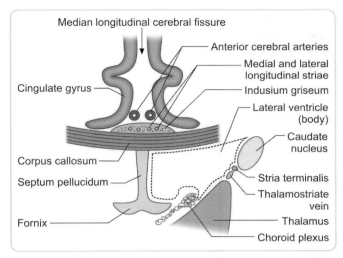

Figure 11.3: Schematic diagram to show relations of the corpus callosum

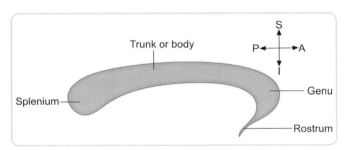

Figure 11.4: Parts of corpus callosum

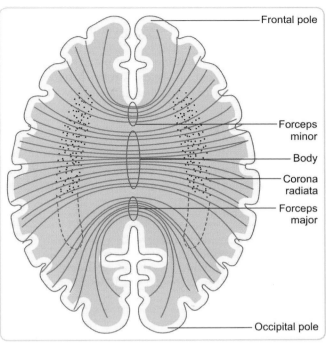

Figure 11.5: Cerebrum viewed from above, showing the different fibre systems of corpus callosum

Parts

The corpus callosum consists of four parts. Its anterior part is called the **genu**, the central part is the **trunk** and the posterior bulbous part forms the **splenium**. The prolongation from the genu to the upper end of lamina terminalis is called rostrum (Figure 11.4).

Relations

- The superior aspect of the corpus callosum is covered with **indusium griseum**, in which medial and lateral longitudinal striae are embedded. The indusium griseum is the rudimentary grey matter of dorsal hippocampus.
- Transverse fissure separates the splenium from the superior colliculi and pineal gland. It gives passage to the tela choroidea of third and lateral ventricles. The posterior choroidal arteries enter the fissure and the internal cerebral veins leave it and unite to form the great cerebral vein beneath the splenium.

- The anterior and superior aspects of the corpus callosum are in close relation to the anterior cerebral vessels.
- The inferior aspect of the corpus callosum gives attachment to the septum pellucidum, anteriorly and the fornix, posteriorly.
- The rostrum and genu form the boundaries of the anterior horn, and the trunk forms the roof of the central part of the lateral ventricle.

Connections of Corpus Callosum

The fibres of the corpus callosum interconnect the corresponding parts of the right and left hemispheres.
- The fibres passing through the rostrum connect the orbital surfaces of the frontal lobes.
- The fibres passing through the genu interconnect the two frontal lobes by means of a fork-like bundle of fibres called **forceps minor** (Figures 11.5 and 11.6).
- The fibres passing through the splenium interconnect the occipital lobes by means of a fork-like bundle of fibres called **forceps major**. The forceps major bulges into the medial wall of the posterior horn of lateral ventricle to give rise to an elevation called the **bulb** of the posterior horn.

- A large number of fibres from the trunk run transversely to intersect with the fibres of the corona radiata. Some fibres of the trunk and adjacent splenium, which do not intersect with corona radiata, are known as the **tapetum**. The tapetum is closely related to the inferior horn and posterior horn of lateral ventricle.

Arterial Supply

The rostrum, genu and body of corpus callosum receive branches from the anterior cerebral arteries. The splenium receives branches from the posterior cerebral arteries.

> ### Clinical Anatomy
>
> - Corpus callosum may be congenitally absent, which results in the two hemispheres being disconnected. This results in **split brain syndrome** or **callosal syndrome**. The skills learnt using one hand cannot be replicated using the other hand.
> - Corpus callosum may be surgically divided in cases of **intractable epilepsy**. The anatomical basis for such a surgery is to disconnect the transfer of impulses from an irritable focus of one cerebral hemisphere to another.
> - **Callosal syndrome** shows the following symptoms:
>   - **Hemialexia**: Patients with callosal disconnection will not be able to read matter presented to them in the left hemivisual field.
>   - **Left ideomotor apraxia**: These patients will not be able to carry out work with their left hand in response to verbal command.
>   - **Left agraphia**: They will not be able to write with their left hand.
>   - **Left tactile anomia**: They will not be able to name an object held in their left hand with eyes closed.
>
> The anatomical basis of these symptoms is the inability of the senses perceived by the left hemisphere to go to right hemisphere through corpus callosum.

PROJECTION FIBRES

The projection fibres connect the cerebral cortex to other regions of CNS below it by corticopetal or **ascending** and corticofugal or **descending** fibres.

Projection Fibre Bundles

- The **corona radiata** (Figure 11.7) is a mass of white matter composed of the projection fibres, which converge from the cerebral cortex to the internal capsule and fan out from the internal capsule toward the cortex.
- The **internal capsule** (Figures 11.6 and 11.7) transmits the corticofugal projection fibres like corticospinal, corticonuclear and corticopontine fibres. These fibres

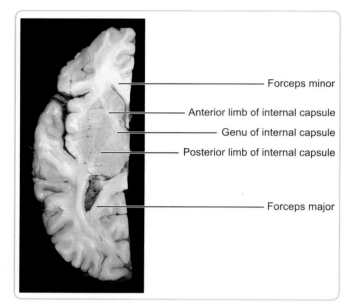

Figure 11.6: Horizontal section of cerebrum to show fibres of corpus callosum and parts of internal capsule

— Forceps minor
— Anterior limb of internal capsule
— Genu of internal capsule
— Posterior limb of internal capsule
— Forceps major

arise in the cerebral cortex and terminate on the lower neurons (like anterior horn cells, cranial nerve nuclei in brainstem and pontine nuclei). The internal capsule also gives passage to corticopetal thalamic radiations (comprising of connections between cerebral cortex and thalamic nuclei).

- The **external capsule** is a bundle of fibres, which lies lateral to putamen of lentiform nucleus and contains corticostriate fibres.

The **fornix** is composed of **projection fibres, commissural fibres** and **association fibres**, which take origin from the hippocampus. The projection fibres in the fornix are connected to the neurons of the mamillary body of hypothalamus. The commissural fibres of fornix cross beneath the splenium to the opposite side fornix and end in the hippocampus of opposite side. The association fibres in the fornix connect the hippocampus with the neighboring parahippocampal gyrus and septal areas.

INTERNAL CAPSULE

A large number of nerve fibres project from the cerebral cortex to interconnect with subcortical centres in the brainstem and spinal cord. This compact bundle of fibres is collectively called the **internal capsule** (Figure 11.6).

Relations

These fibres fan-out cranially to form corona radiata and condense caudally to form the crus cerebri of the

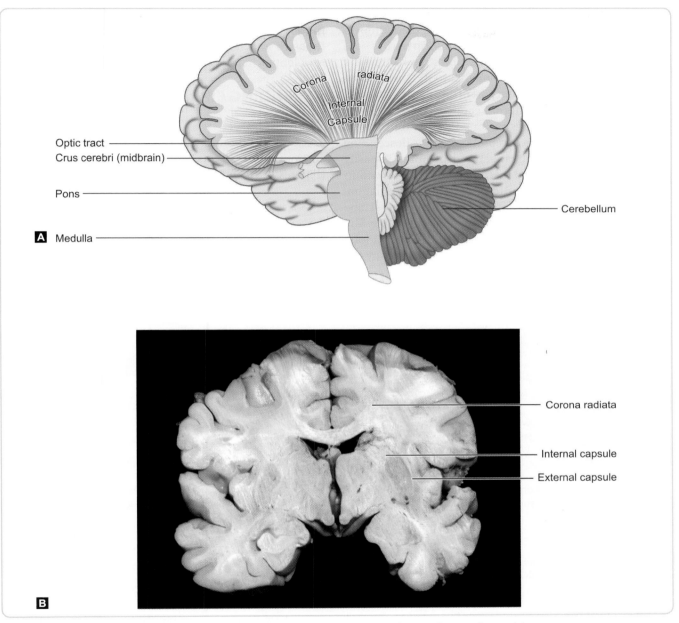

Figures 11.7A and B: Projection fibres (corona radiata and internal capsule)

midbrain (Figure 11.7). Most of these fibres pass through the interval between the thalamus and caudate nucleus medially and the lentiform nucleus laterally (Figure 11.8) to form a thick sheet of fibres called the **internal capsule.**

Parts

The internal capsule shows the following parts (Figure 11.9):

- **Anterior limb**: The anterior limb lies between the caudate nucleus medially and the anterior part of the lentiform nucleus laterally.
- **Posterior limb**: The posterior limb lies between the thalamus medially and the posterior part of the lentiform nucleus laterally.
- **Genu**: In transverse section through the cerebral hemisphere, the anterior and posterior limbs of the internal capsule meet at an angle open outwards. This angle is called the **genu** (**genu = bend**).

- **Retrolentiform part**: Some fibres of the internal capsule lie behind the posterior end of the lentiform nucleus. They constitute its retrolentiform part.
- **Sublentiform part**: Some other fibres pass below the lentiform nucleus (and not medial to it). These fibres constitute the sublentiform part of the internal capsule.

Various parts of the internal capsule consist of large number of fibres. The fibres passing through the capsule may be ascending (to the cerebral cortex) or descending (from the cortex). The arrangement of fibres is easily remembered, if it is realized that any group of fibres within the capsule **takes the most direct path** to its destination. Thus, fibres to and from the anterior part of the frontal lobe pass through the anterior limb of the internal capsule. The fibres to and from the posterior part of the frontal lobe and from the greater part of the parietal lobe occupy the genu and posterior limb of the capsule. Fibres to and from the temporal lobe occupy the sublentiform part, while those to and from the occipital lobe pass through the retrolentiform part.

ASCENDING FIBRES (CORTICOPETAL FIBRES)

These are **predominantly thalamocortical fibres**, which go from the thalamus to all parts of the cerebral cortex (Figures 11.10 and 11.11).

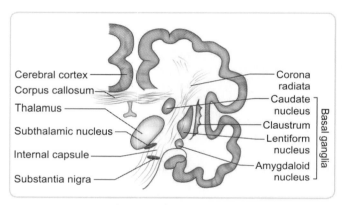

Figure 11.8: Coronal section through a cerebral hemisphere to show the location of internal capsule

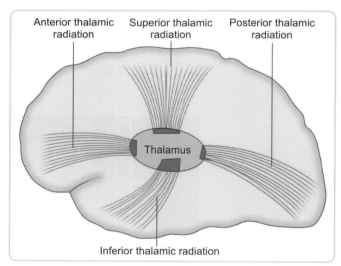

Figure 11.10: Ascending fibres passing through internal capsule—thalamic radiations

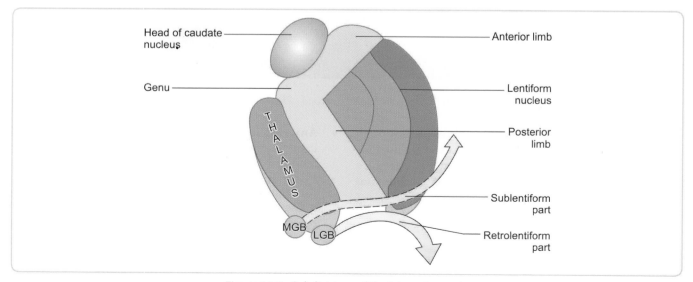

Figure 11.9: Subdivisions of the internal capsule

- **Anterior thalamic radiation**: Fibres to the frontal lobe constitute the anterior thalamic radiation. They pass through the anterior limb of the internal capsule. The fibres arise mainly from the medial and anterior nuclei of the thalamus. The anterior thalamic radiation also carries fibres from the hypothalamus and limbic structures to the frontal cortex.
- **Superior thalamic radiation**: Fibres travelling from the ventral group of nuclei (ventral anterior, ventral lateral, ventral posteromedial and ventral posterolateral) of the thalamus to the somatomotor and somatosensory areas constitute the superior thalamic radiation. These fibres occupy the genu and posterior limb of the capsule. It should be noted that these fibres are third-order sensory neurons responsible for conveying somaesthetic sensations to the cerebral cortex.
- **Posterior thalamic radiation**: Fibres from the thalamus to the occipital lobe constitute the posterior thalamic radiation. This includes the **optic radiation** from the lateral geniculate body to the visual cortex. These radiations lie in the retrolentiform part of the internal capsule. The retrolentiform part also contains some fibres passing from the thalamus to the posterior part of the parietal lobe.

- **Inferior thalamic radiation**: Fibres from the thalamus to the temporal lobe constitute the inferior thalamic radiation. It includes the **auditory radiation** from the medial geniculate body to the auditory area of the cerebral cortex. These fibres pass through the sublentiform part of the internal capsule.

DESCENDING FIBRES (CORTICOFUGAL FIBRES) (FIGURE 11.11)

- **Corticopontine fibres**: They originate from all four lobes of cerebral cortex and are named according to the lobe from which they arise:
  - **Frontopontine fibres** account for 55% of cortico-pontine fibres. Therefore, they pass through the anterior limb, genu and posterior limb of the internal capsule.
  - **Parietopontine fibres** pass mainly through the retrolentiform part. Some fibres pass through the sublentiform part.
  - **Temporopontine fibres** pass through the sublentiform part (Figure 11.12).
  - **Occipitopontine fibres** pass through the retrolentiform part.

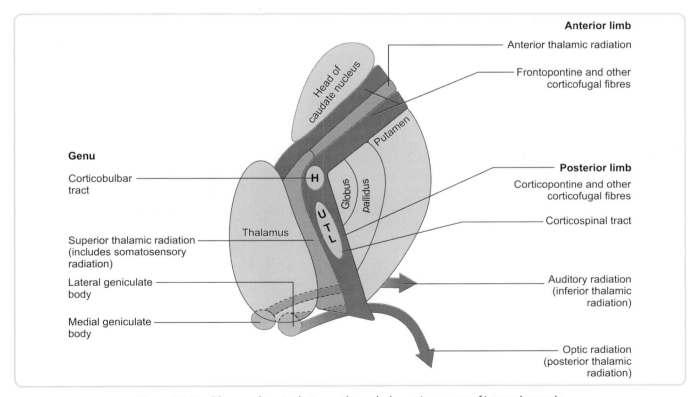

Figure 11.11: Fibres and tracts that pass through the various parts of internal capsule
(*Abbreviations*: H - Head and neck; U - Upper limb; T - Trunk; L - Lower limb)

- **Pyramidal fibres (corticospinal and corticonuclear fibres)**:
  - **Corticonuclear fibres** (for motor cranial nerve nuclei) pass through the genu of the internal capsule.
  - **Corticospinal fibres** form several discrete bundles in the posterior limb of the capsule. The fibres for the upper limb are most anterior followed (in that order) by fibres for the trunk and lower limb.
- **Corticothalamic fibres**: These pass from various parts of the cerebral cortex to the thalamus. They form part of the thalamic radiations described above.

- **Extrapyramidal fibres**:
  - **Corticostriate fibres** originating from all parts of cerebral cortex and terminating in caudate nucleus and putamen
  - **Corticorubral fibres** originating from the motor areas of the frontal lobe and terminating in the red nucleus
  - **Corticoreticular fibres** beginning from the motor cortex and the parietal lobe and terminating in reticular nuclei.

A summary of the various ascending and descending fibres passing through different parts of internal capsule are given in Table 11.1.

ARTERIAL SUPPLY OF INTERNAL CAPSULE

The main arteries supplying the internal capsule are the medial and lateral striate branches of the middle cerebral artery, the recurrent branch of the anterior cerebral artery and the anterior choroidal artery. The internal capsule may also receive direct branches from the internal carotid artery and branches from the posterior communicating artery (Figure 11.13).

- The **upper parts** of the anterior limb, the genu and the posterior limb are supplied by the medial and lateral striate branches of the middle cerebral artery. One of the lateral striate branches is larger and more frequently ruptured. It is often called

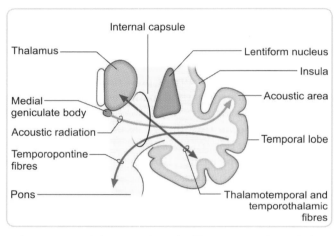

Figure 11.12: Scheme to show the fibres passing through the sublentiform part of the internal capsule

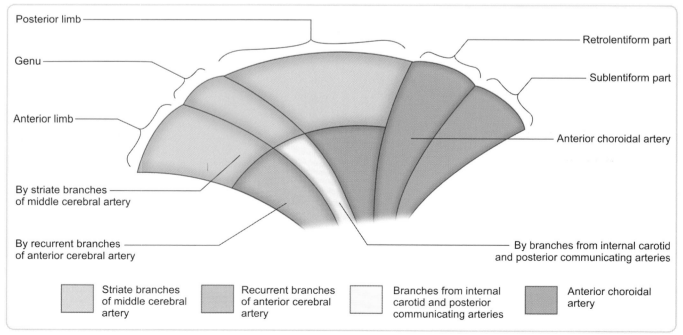

Figure 11.13: Arterial supply of the internal capsule

TABLE 11.1: Fibres in internal capsule

Part	Motor fibres (Descending fibres)	Sensory fibres (Ascending fibres)
Anterior limb	• Frontopontine fibres • Frontothalamic fibres	Anterior thalamic radiation
Genu	• Frontopontine fibres • Corticonuclear fibres • Corticoreticular fibres • Parietothalamic fibres	Superior thalamic radiation
Posterior limb	• Frontopontine fibres • Corticospinal fibres • Corticorubral fibres • Corticoreticular fibres • Parietothalamic fibres	Superior thalamic radiation
Retrolenti-form part	• Parietopontine fibres • Occipitopontine fibres • Corticotectal fibres • Occipitothalamic fibres	Posterior thalamic radiation including optic radiation
Sublentiform part	• Temporopontine fibres • Temporothalamic fibres	Inferior thalamic radiation including auditory radiation

Charcot's artery of cerebral haemorrhage. It enters through the anterior perforated substance and supplies the posterior limb of the internal capsule.
- The **lower parts** of these regions are supplied as follows:
  – The lower part of the anterior limb is supplied by the medial striate artery (also called **recurrent artery of Heubner**), branch of the anterior cerebral artery
  – The lower part of the genu is supplied by direct branches from the internal carotid and from the posterior communicating artery
  – The lower part of the posterior limb is supplied by the anterior choroidal artery and striate branch of posterior cerebral artery
- The retrolentiform part of the internal capsule is supplied by the anterior choroidal artery
- The sublentiform part is probably supplied by the anterior choroidal artery.

Clinical Anatomy

Cerebrovascular Accident or Stroke Syndrome
- When the blood vessel supplying the internal capsule is occluded by a thrombus or an embolus, the patient develops contralateral hemiplegia of sudden onset and aphasia, if dominant hemisphere is involved. There may be contralateral sensory loss and homonymous hemianopia, if retrolentiform part of internal capsule is involved.
- These signs and symptoms may also occur, if a blood vessel supplying the internal capsule ruptures suddenly and the blood vessel that often ruptures especially in a hypertensive patient is Charcot's artery of cerebral haemorrhage.
  As the tracts passing through the internal capsule are closely packed, even a small lesion can cause extensive paralysis.

Faciobrachial Monoplegia
Occlusion of anterior recurrent artery of Heubner affects the corticonuclear fibres for face and corticospinal fibres for the upper limb (as they are present in the genu and anterior part of posterior limb) and results in faciobrachial monoplegia.

MULTIPLE CHOICE QUESTIONS

Q1. The cortical areas of the same cerebral hemisphere are connected by:
A. Internal capsule
B. Association fibres
C. Corona radiata
D. Commissural fibres

Q2. Internal capsule is an example of which type of white fibres?
A. Long association
B. Projection
C. Commissural
D. Short association

Q3. The upper surface of the corpus callosum is related to:
A. Indusium griseum
B. Arcuate fasciculus
C. Fornix
D. Locus coeruleus

Q4. The fibres forming corona radiata intersect with the fibres of:
A. Anterior commissure
B. Cingulum
C. Inferior longitudinal fasciculus
D. Corpus callosum

Q5. **The structure related laterally to the internal capsule is:**
  A. Lentiform nucleus
  B. Thalamus
  C. Caudate nucleus
  D. Amygdaloid body

Q6. **The posterior limb of the internal capsule contains:**
  A. Corticospinal fibres
  B. Corticorubral fibres
  C. Superior thalamic radiation
  D. All of the above

Q7. **Which of the following parts of internal capsule lies between the head of the caudate nucleus and the lentiform nucleus?**
  A. Genu
  B. Anterior limb
  C. Posterior limb
  D. Sublentiform part

Q8. **Which part of the internal capsule is supplied by Charcot's artery of cerebral haemorrhage?**
  A. Anterior limb
  B. Genu
  C. Posterior limb
  D. Sublentiform part

Q9. **Anterior choroidal artery supplies which part of internal capsule?**
  A. Anterior limb
  B. Genu
  C. Upper part of posterior limb
  D. Retrolentiform part

ANSWERS

1. B	2. B	3. A	4. D	5. A	6. D	7. B	8. C	9. D

SHORT NOTES

1. Classify the white fibres of cerebrum and give two examples each
2. Define association fibres and name the association bundles
3. Define commissural fibres and name the commissures
4. Define projection fibres and name the projection fibre systems

LONG QUESTIONS

1. Describe the corpus callosum under the following headings: Parts, relations, fibre systems, functions and applied anatomy.
2. Describe the internal capsule under the following headings: Parts, relations, fibres and tracts present within each part, blood supply, applied anatomy.

Clinical Cases

11.1: A 60-year-old man, a known hypertensive, developed sudden inability to move his right upper and lower limbs. He was also not able to reply to the questions asked by the examining doctor. The angle of his mouth was deviated to the left side.
  A. What is this man suffering from?
  B. Which artery is likely to be affected?
  C. Explain the anatomical basis of his signs and symptoms.

11.2: A 15-year-old boy who was suffering from intractable epilepsy had undergone corpus callosotomy.
  A few months after this surgery, the boy was asked to throw a ball with his left hand and he was not able to do. He was asked to identify a Rs.10 coin kept in his left hand which he could not do.
  A. What are these conditions together termed as?
  B. Explain the anatomical pathways affected in each of them.

INTRODUCTION

The basal nuclei (or basal ganglia) are large masses of grey matter situated in the cerebral hemispheres.

Anatomically, the basal nuclei include large subcortical masses of grey matter located within each cerebral hemisphere developing from telencephalon. They include (Figure 12.1):
- **Caudate nucleus**
- **Lentiform nucleus**, which consists of two functionally distinct parts, the **putamen** and the **globus pallidus**
- **Amygdaloid nuclear complex**
- **Claustrum**

The caudate nucleus and the lentiform nucleus together constitute the **corpus striatum** (Figure 12.2). This consists of two functionally distinct parts. The caudate nucleus and the putamen form one unit called the **striatum** (also known as **neostriatum**), while the globus pallidus forms the other unit, the **pallidum** (also known as **paleostriatum**). Phylogenetically, **amygdaloid nuclear complex** and **claustrum** are considered as **archistriatum**.

Functionally, the basal nuclei comprise of structures, the lesion of which produces **dyskinesias** (abnormal involuntary purposeless movements). The structures included are:
- **Corpus striatum**
- The **subthalamic nucleus** (which is of diencephalic origin) is very closely linked to the basal nuclei and is regarded as belonging to this group.
- The **substantia nigra** (midbrain) is also closely linked, functionally, to the basal nuclei.
- Some masses of grey matter found just below the corpus striatum (near the anterior perforated substance) are described as the **ventral striatum**. The part of the globus pallidus, which lies below the level of

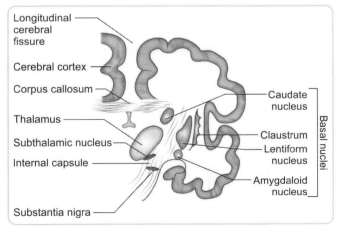

Figure 12.1: Coronal section of cerebrum showing basal nuclei

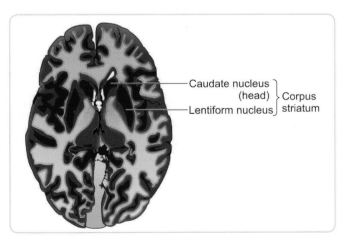

Figure 12.2: Plastinated horizontal section of the brain through interventricular foramen showing corpus striatum

the anterior commissure, is designated as the **ventral pallidum**.

CAUDATE NUCLEUS

The caudate nucleus is a C-shaped mass of grey matter (Figure 12.3). It consists of a large head, body and thin tail. The nucleus is intimately related to the lateral ventricle (Figures 12.4A and B). The head of the nucleus bulges into the anterior horn of the ventricle and forms the greater part of its floor. The body of the nucleus lies in the floor of the central part and the tail in the roof of the inferior horn of the ventricle. The anterior part of the head of the caudate nucleus is fused, inferiorly, with the lentiform nucleus. Fusion of these two results in strands of grey matter passing through the descending fibres of internal capsule giving a striated appearance and hence the name 'Corpus striatum' to denote caudate and lentiform nuclei. This region of fusion is referred to as the **fundus striati**. The fundus striati is continuous, inferiorly, with the anterior perforated substance. The anterior end of the tail of the caudate nucleus ends by becoming continuous with the amygdaloid nucleus.

The body of the caudate nucleus is related medially to the thalamus and laterally to the internal capsule, which separates it from the lentiform nucleus.

LENTIFORM NUCLEUS

The lentiform nucleus appears triangular (or wedge-shaped) in the coronal section.

Relations

The lentiform nucleus lies lateral to the internal capsule. Laterally, it is separated from the claustrum by fibres of the external capsule (Figure 12.5). (Note that these capsules are so called because they appear, to the naked eyes, to form a covering or capsule for the lentiform nucleus.) Superiorly, the lentiform nucleus is related to the corona

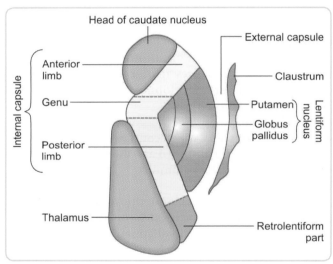

Figure 12.5: Horizontal section of the cerebral hemisphere showing corpus striatum, thalamus, claustrum and internal capsule

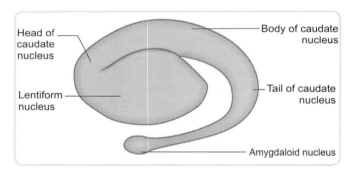

Figure 12.3: Corpus striatum viewed from the lateral aspect

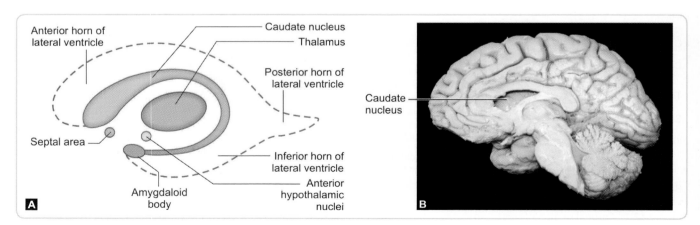

Figure 12.4A and B: Relations of caudate nucleus with the cavity of lateral ventricle and thalamus.
(A) Line diagram; and (B) specimen of brain

radiata and inferiorly, to the sublentiform part of the internal capsule.

Parts

It is divided by a thin lamina of white matter, known as external medullary lamina, into a lateral part, the **putamen** and a medial part, the **globus pallidus (Figure 12.6).** The globus pallidus is further subdivided into medial and lateral (or internal and external) segments, by the internal medullary lamina. Relation of corpus striatum to the internal capsule is shown in Figure 12.7.

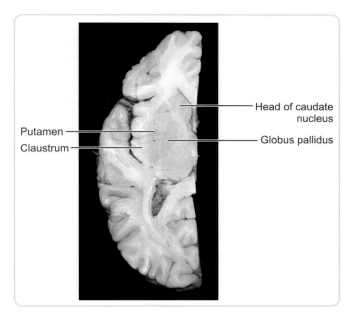

Figure 12.6: Horizontal section of cerebrum to show the basal nuclei

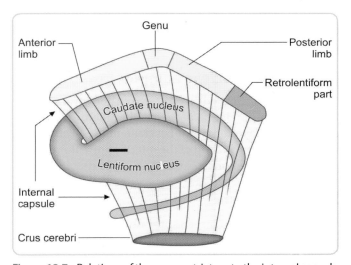

Figure 12.7: Relations of the corpus striatum to the internal capsule

CONNECTIONS OF CORPUS STRIATUM

Afferent Connections

The striatum (caudate and lentiform nuclei) receives afferents from the following (Figure 12.8):
- The entire cerebral cortex via **corticostriate** fibres. These fibres are glutamatergic.
- The intralaminar nuclei of the thalamus via **thalamostriate** fibres
- The pars compacta of the substantia nigra via **nigrostriate** fibres. These fibres are dopaminergic.
- Noradrenergic fibres are received from the locus coeruleus.
- Serotoninergic fibres are received from the raphe nuclei (in the reticular formation of the midbrain).

Efferent Connections

The main output of the striatum is concentrated upon the pallidum and on the substantia nigra (pars reticularis). The outflow from globus pallidus forms four separate bundles (Figure 12.9):
- **Fasciculus lenticularis** arises from the inner segment of the globus pallidus and enters the subthalamic region.
- **Ansa lenticularis** arises from both the inner and outer segments of the globus pallidus and enters the subthalamic region where it meets the

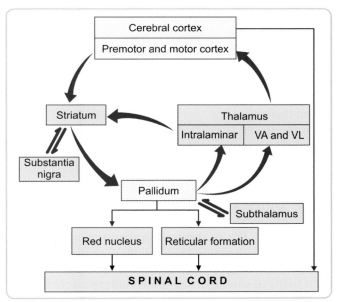

Figure 12.8: Major connections of basal nuclei. (*Abbreviations*: VA, ventral anterior; VL, ventral lateral)

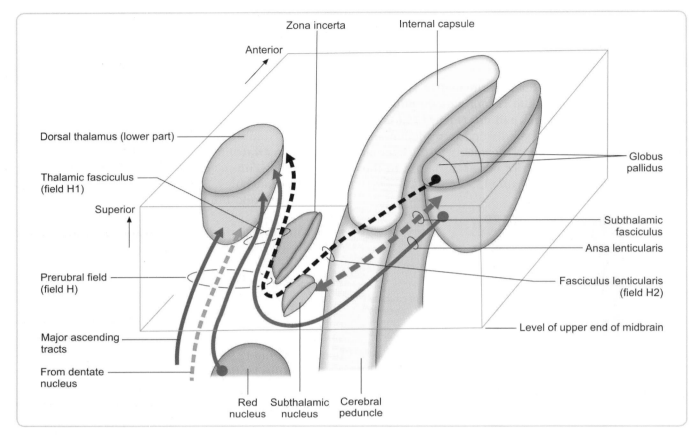

Figure 12.9: Efferent fibre systems from globus pallidus

dentatorubrothalamic fibres and the fasciculus lenticularis. The union of the three tracts is called the **thalamic fasciculus**, which terminates in the ventral anterior (VA), ventral lateral (VL) and centromedian nuclei of thalamus.

- **Subthalamic fasciculus** consists of reciprocal connections between the globus pallidus and nucleus subthalamicus.
- Some fibres from globus pallidus also pass to the substantia nigra (**pallidonigral fibres**).

Functions of Corpus Striatum

- The corpus striatum mediates enormous number of automatic activities involved in normal motor functions. For example, the maintenance of erect posture when sitting or standing, or swinging of arms during walking.
- It helps in smoothening the voluntary motor activity of the body.
- It helps in maintenance of muscle tone.
- It helps in prevention of involuntary movement.

Claustrum

This is a thin lamina of grey matter that lies lateral to the lentiform nucleus (Figure 12.1). It is separated from the latter by fibres of the external capsule (Figure 12.5). Laterally, it is separated by a thin layer of white matter from the cortex of the insula. It is functionally related probably to limbic system.

Amygdaloid Nuclear Complex

This complex (also called the amygdaloid body or amygdala) lies in the temporal lobe of the cerebral hemisphere and close to the temporal pole. It lies deep to the uncus and is related to the anterior end of the inferior horn of the lateral ventricle. It is functionally related to limbic system.

Substantia Nigra

Substantia nigra is a large motor nucleus present in the midbrain. The nucleus consists of two parts: (1) pars reticularis and (2) pars compacta. Pars reticularis is related functionally to the internal part of globus pallidus.

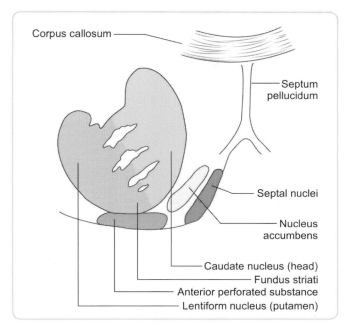

Figure 12.10: Coronal section passing through the anterior part of corpus striatum

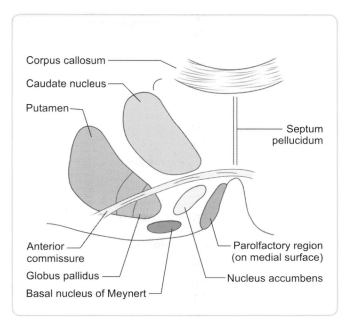

Figure 12.11: Composite diagram showing the region of the ventral striatum

Connections of Substantia Nigra

The **pars compacta** of the substantia nigra sends a dopaminergic projection to the striatum. The **pars reticularis** projects to the ventral anterior nucleus of the thalamus. These impulses are relayed to frontal lobe of the cerebral cortex. Other efferents of the pars reticularis reach the reticular formation of the medulla and to the spinal cord.

Clinical Anatomy

The main connections (both afferent and efferent) of substantia nigra are with the striatum (i.e. caudate nucleus and putamen). Dopamine produced by neurons in the substantia nigra (pars compacta) passes along their axons to the striatum (**mesostriatal dopamine system**). Dopamine is much reduced in patients with a disease called **Parkinsonism**, in which there is a degeneration of the striatum.

In summary:

- The cerebral cortex sends impulses to the corpus striatum, which forms a direct feedback loop.
- The substantia nigra, the subthalamic nucleus and the corpus striatum are integrated with the centromedian nucleus of thalamus.
- Descending fibres from the basal nuclei influence the red nucleus, the reticular formation of the medulla, and thus, the motor neurons of the spinal cord.

VENTRAL STRIATUM AND PALLIDUM

Inferiorly, the caudate nucleus and putamen fuse to form the **fundus striati** (Figure 12.10). Immediately below the fundus striati, there is the olfactory tubercle (in the anterior perforated substance). More medially, there is a mass of grey matter called the **nucleus accumbens**. The **ventral striatum** consists of the nucleus accumbens and the olfactory tubercle (Figure 12.11). The portion of globus pallidus below the anterior commissure is called **ventral pallidum**. The ventral striatum and pallidum connect to limbic lobe of cerebral cortex via anterior and medial nuclei of thalamus.

Thus,

- Dorsal striatum includes caudate nucleus and putamen.
- Ventral striatum includes nucleus accumbens and olfactory tubercle.
- Dorsal pallidum is formed by globus pallidus.
- Ventral pallidum is the part of globus pallidus below anterior commissure.

The reason for considering the nucleus accumbens and the olfactory tubercle as parts of the striatum is that their connections are very similar to those of the main part of the striatum (or dorsal striatum).

BLOOD SUPPLY OF BASAL NUCLEI

The basal nuclei are supplied by:
- Lenticulostriate branches of middle and anterior cerebral arteries
- Anterior choroidal branch of internal carotid artery

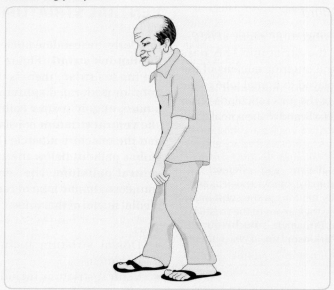

MULTIPLE CHOICE QUESTIONS

Q1. Which one of the following constitutes the basal nuclei of the cerebrum?
A. Habenular nucleus
B. Geniculate bodies
C. Claustrum
D. Subthalamus

Q2. The term "neostriatum" includes:
A. Caudate nucleus and putamen
B. Globus pallidus
C. Caudate nucleus and globus pallidus
D. Amygdaloid nucleus

Q3. The head of the caudate nucleus becomes continuous with the:
A. Lentiform nucleus
B. Amygdaloid body
C. Claustrum
D. Thalamus

Q4. The tail of the caudate nucleus ends in relation to:
A. Thalamus
B. Cerebral fornix
C. Amygdaloid body
D. Claustrum

Q5. The body of caudate nucleus is related to which part of the lateral ventricle?
A. Anterior horn
B. Posterior horn
C. Inferior horn
D. Central part

Q6. A lesion of the basal nuclei can produce:
A. Hypotonia
B. Intention tremor
C. Muscular atrophy
D. Aphasia

Q7. Parkinson's disease is due to a lesion of:
A. Amygdaloid body
B. Lentiform nucleus
C. Substantia nigra
D. Dorsal nucleus of thalamus

Q8. Which of the following neurotransmitters is deficient in Parkinson's disease?
A. GABA
B. Serotonin
C. Dopamine
D. Acetylcholine

ANSWERS

1. C   2. A   3. A   4. C   5. D   6. A   7. C   8. C

SHORT N

1. Enumerate the components of basal nuclei
2. Specify what constitute archistriatum, paleostriatum and neostriatum?
3. What is ventral striatum?
4. Define hemiballismus

LONG ANSWER QUESTIONS

1. Describe the corpus striatum under the following headings: Components, afferent connections, efferent connections, blood supply and applied anatomy
2. Classify abnormal movements that occur in lesions of basal nuclei and subthalamus and specify the differences between them.
3. Describe the features of paralysis agitans explaining the anatomicophysiological basis of the disease.

Clinical Cases

12.1: A middle-aged office goer found that his hands have started shaking uncontrollably over the past few days.
His relatives found him to be not expressive in his face of late, he also developed short-shuffling gait.
He was investigated and found to be developing Parkinsonism.
A. What other features characterize this disease?
B. How can one distinguish the tremors seen in this condition from those seen in cerebellar disease?

Chapter 13 | Limbic System and Reticular Formation

Specific Learning Objectives

At the end of learning, the student shall be able to:
➤ Enumerate the components of limbic system
➤ Describe the connections and functions of limbic system
➤ Describe the functions of reticular formation
➤ Correlate the relevant clinical anatomy

INTRODUCTION

The limbic system includes the limbic lobe and the structures connected to it. In 1878, Broca coined the term "limbic lobe" formed by structures present on the medial and inferior surface of the cerebral hemispheres which form a "border or ring" around the brainstem.

Limbic system consists of several cortical and subcortical structures, which form a ring-like structure around the upper end of brainstem.

The term **limbic system** has been applied in the past to certain regions of the brain that are believed to play an important role in the control of visceral activity. The olfactory system in man is not only concerned with smell but also activates other neural systems for emotional behaviour and hence included as a part of limbic system.

Functions of the Limbic System

Some of the functions attributed to limbic system are as follows:

- Integration of olfactory, visceral, and somatic impulses reaching the brain
- Control of activities necessary for survival of the animal, including procuring of food and eating behaviour
- Control of activities necessary for survival of the species, including sexual behaviour
- Emotional behaviour
- Retention of recent memory

Components of the Limbic System

The limbic system consists of **cortical** and **subcortical** structures. The cortical regions include limbic lobe, hippocampal formation, septal area and olfactory areas. The subcortical structures include amygdaloid nuclear complex, hypothalamus, anterior nucleus of thalamus, habenular nucleus and reticular formation (Flowchart 13.1).

Flowchart 13.1: Components of limbic system

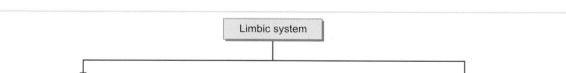

The limbic lobe consists of cingulate gyrus, isthmus, parahippocampal gyrus, and uncus (Figure 13.1).

Hippocampal formation includes hippocampus, dentate gyrus, gyrus fasciolaris, indusium griseum, and medial and lateral longitudinal striae (Figure 13.2).

AMYGDALOID NUCLEAR COMPLEX

This region is also called the amygdaloid body or amygdala. The complex lies in the temporal lobe of the cerebral hemisphere, close to the temporal pole.

It fuses with the anterior end of the tail of the caudate nucleus (Figure 13.3). Some relations of the amygdaloid complex are shown in Figure 13.4.

Connections

Afferent

The amygdaloid nuclear complex receives afferents mainly from primary olfactory cortex, hippocampus, hypothalamus, thalamus (medial dorsal nucleus), ventral striatum, ventral pallidum, cerebral cortex and brainstem reticular formation.

Efferent

Efferent fibres from amygdala pass through two major routes:
- Stria terminalis—to septal nuclei, olfactory areas
- Ventral amygdalofugal route

Connections with the Brainstem

- The amygdala receives fibres from and sends fibres to the reticular formation, particularly the parabrachial nucleus (Flowchart 13.2).
- Some fibres from the amygdala reach the nucleus of the solitary tract and the dorsal nucleus of the vagus.

Through these connections, the amygdala receives gustatory and visceral information and can influence cardiovascular and respiratory functions.

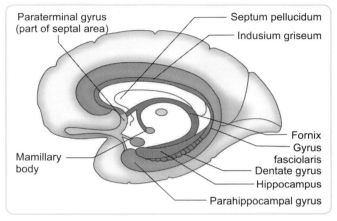

Figure 13.2: Sagittal section of the brain showing the structures forming hippocampal formation (viz. hippocampus, dentate gyrus, gyrus fasciolaris, and indusium griseum)

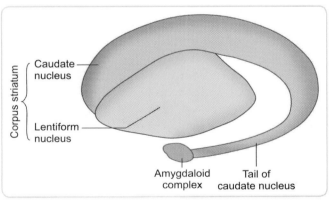

Figure 13.3: Structure and location of amygdaloid nuclear complex

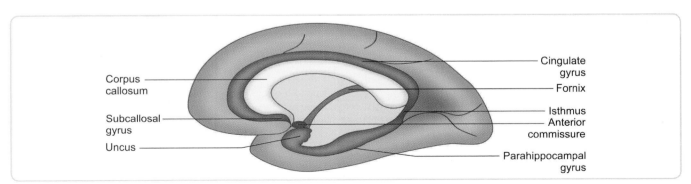

Figure 13.1: Sagittal section of the brain showing the location of the limbic lobe. The limbic lobe consists of cingulate gyrus, isthmus, parahippocampal gyrus, and uncus

Connections with the Diencephalon

- The amygdala sends a major projection to various nuclei in the hypothalamus. Some fibres are also received from the hypothalamus.

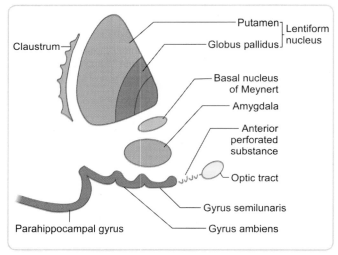

Figure 13.4: Relations of the amygdala as seen in a coronal section

- Fibres projecting to the thalamus end mainly in the medial dorsal nucleus. The impulses are relayed to the prefrontal cortex.

Connections with the Corpus Striatum

A prominent projection reaches the nucleus accumbens (which is a nucleus in the ventral striatum). Through the striatum, the amygdaloid complex indirectly influences the ventral pallidum, which in turn projects to the medial dorsal nucleus of the thalamus. The amygdaloid complex sends many fibres to the basal nucleus of Meynert (lying in the region ventral to the corpus striatum). This projection is cholinergic. The nucleus projects back to the amygdala.

Cortical Connections of Amygdala

It is now known that in addition to its connections to olfactory areas, entorhinal area, and hippocampus, the amygdaloid complex has numerous connections with widespread areas of neocortex. The areas include the cingulate gyrus and parts of the frontal, temporal, and occipital lobes, including the visual and auditory areas.

Flowchart 13.2: Main connections of the amygdala

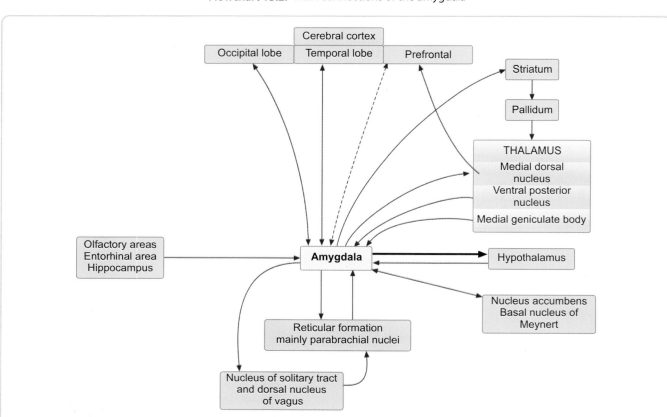

Functions

- On the basis of all the connections described above and experimental studies, amygdala plays an important role in the control of emotional behaviour.
- Since it receives olfactory inputs, it is believed that the amygdaloid body plays an important role in smell-mediated sexual behaviour.

Clinical Anatomy

Kluver-Bucy syndrome results due to bilateral temporal lobe lesion involving amygdala and adjacent structures. The amygdala is probably responsible for evaluating the significance of environmental events, for example, in recognizing what objects are edible, or in recognizing attributes of the opposite sex. This results in marked changes in ingestive behaviour, the animal ingests material (like fecal matter), not normally eaten. Abnormalities in sexual behaviour are also seen, probably because of the failure to distinguish between male and female animals.

SEPTAL REGION

These are certain masses of grey matter that lie immediately anterior to the lamina terminalis and the anterior commissure (Figure 13.5). They include the **paraterminal gyrus, prehippocampal rudiment** and **subcallosal area** (or **parolfactory gyrus).**

Phylogenetically, the septal region is divided into a **precommissural septum** and a **supracommissural septum.** The septal area is the precommissural septum. The supracommissural septum is represented by the septum pellucidum.

The septal area is continuous inferiorly with the medial olfactory stria. Superiorly, it is continuous with the indusium griseum (Figure 13.5).

Connections

Afferent

Septal area predominantly receives afferents from:
- Olfactory tract through medial olfactory stria
- Amygdala through stria terminalis
- Hippocampus through fornix

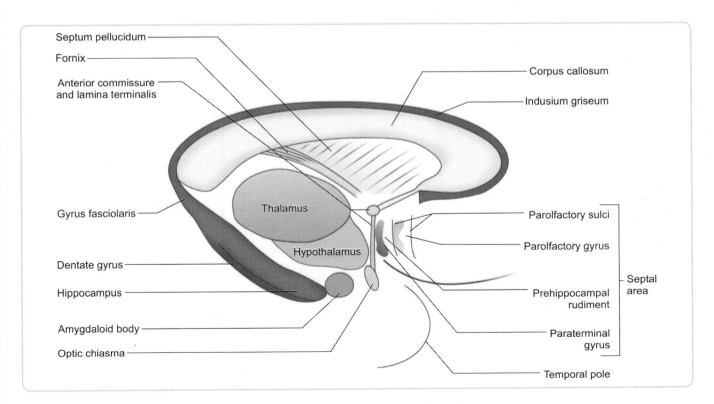

Figure 13.5: Hippocampal formation and septal areas

Efferent

Efferent corrections from septal nuclei are predominantly to habenular nuclei through stria medullaris thalami (stria habenularis).

HIPPOCAMPAL FORMATION

In the human embryo, the **hippocampal formation** is C-shaped. The upper part of the formation remains underdeveloped and lines the upper surface of the corpus callosum as **indusium griseum.**

Posteriorly, the indusium griseum is continuous with **splenial gyrus** or **gyrus fasciolaris.** The splenial gyrus runs forwards to become continuous with the **dentate gyrus.**

In the region of the inferior horn of the lateral ventricle, the **hippocampal formation** is best developed and forms the **hippocampus or cornu ammonis** and the **dentate gyrus.**

Subdivisions of the region are illustrated in Figure 13.6, which is a coronal section through the inferior horn of the lateral ventricle. The cerebral cortex that lies below the choroid fissure is S-shaped in cross-section.

The superior limb of the "S" forms the hippocampal formation (cornu ammonis and dentate gyrus). The middle limb of the "S" is called the **subiculum**. The lower lip of the "S" is parahippocampal gyrus.

The anterior end of hippocampus is expanded and notched and resembles a foot. It is, therefore, called the **pes hippocampi** (Figure 13.7).

The ventricular surface of the hippocampus is covered by a layer of nerve fibres that constitute the **alveus.** The fibres of the alveus pass medially and collect to form **fimbria** (Figures 13.6 and 13.8).

The fimbria runs backwards along the medial side of the hippocampus to become continuous with the fornix.

The medial margin of **dentate gyrus** is free and bears a series of notches that give it a teeth-like (dentate) appearance; hence, the name dentate gyrus (Figure 13.7).

The hippocampus is made up of three layers only (Figure 13.8). These are as follows:

- Superficial molecular layer
- Middle pyramidal cell layer
- Deep polymorphic cell layer

The subiculum is a transitional zone which has 4–5 layers.

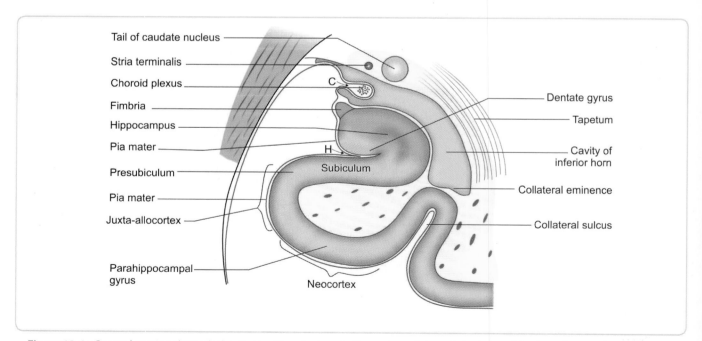

Figure 13.6: Coronal section through the cerebral hemisphere in the region of the inferior horn of the lateral ventricle to show the hippocampus and related structures (*Abbreviations*: C, choroid fissure; H, hippocampal fissure)

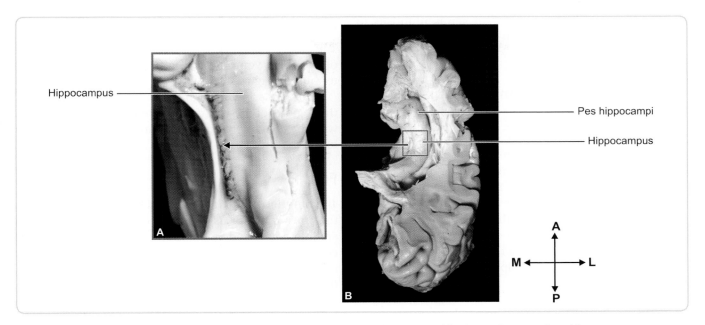

Figures 13.7A and B: (A) Enlarged view to show dentate gyrus; (B) Dissected brain specimen to show hippocampus

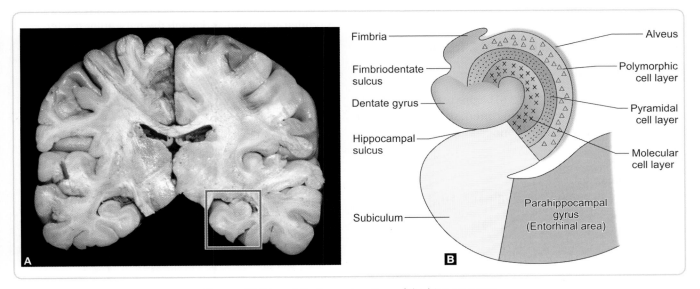

Figures 13.8A and B: Coronal section of the hippocampus

Connections of the Hippocampus

Afferent

Hippocampus receives fibres mainly from entorhinal area (area 28), olfactory cortex, amygdala, opposite hippocampus, parahippocampal gyrus.

Efferent

The fornix is the main efferent tract of the hippocampus. The fibres leaving the hippocampus pass:

- To the opposite hippocampus through the **commissure of fornix/hippocampal commissure**
- To the septal and anterior hypothalamic regions

- To the mamillary body, which sends impulses to cingulate gyrus through anterior nucleus of thalamus, through Papez circuit

Papez Circuit (Hippocampal Circuit)

It is a circular pathway that interconnects certain important structures in limbic system (Flowchart 13.3). It is concerned with short-term memory. Papez in 1937 described the circuit, beginning from the hippocampus projecting via the fornix to mamillary nucleus, the mamillary nucleus projecting via the mamillothalamic tract to the anterior nucleus of thalamus, anterior nucleus of thalamus projecting to the cingulate gyrus, and the cingulate gyrus projecting via the cingulum back to the parahippocampal gyrus and hippocampus.

Mamillothalamic Tract

Mamillothalamic tract (also called **bundle of Vicq d'Azyr**) is the bundle of fibres, which carries impulses from mamillary body to the anterior nucleus of thalamus.

FIBRE BUNDLES OF LIMBIC REGION

Stria Terminalis

This bundle of fibres (Figure 13.6) begins in the amygdaloid complex and runs backwards medial to the caudate nucleus. The stria terminalis connects amygdaloid nucleus to:

- Septal area
- Hypothalamus
- Habenular nuclei, through the stria medullaris thalami.

Flowchart 13.3: Scheme to show Papez circuit

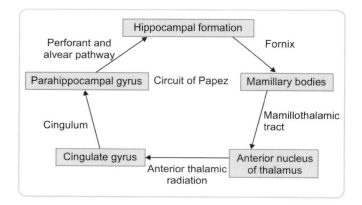

Anterior Commissure

The anterior commissure is situated in the anterior wall of the third ventricle at the upper end of the lamina terminalis (Figure 13.5).

Fibres passing through the commissure interconnect the regions of the two cerebral hemispheres concerned with the olfactory pathway and anterior part of temporal lobes.

Fornix

The fimbriae of the hippocampus run backwards. Then, they turn upwards as two crura of fornix. The two crura are interconnected by the **hippocampal commissure** or **commissure of the fornix** (Figure 13.9). Then the crura run forward as body of fornix which is suspended from the corpus callosum by the septum pellucidum. The body descends as columns of fornix to end in the mamillary bodies of hypothalamus.

Some fibres of the fornix that descend in front of the anterior commissure terminate in septal area.

Some of these fibres turn backwards to enter the stria medullaris thalami and reach the habenular nuclei.

Clinical Anatomy

Disorders of Memory and Behaviour

Some neurological disorders are associated with impairment of memory (amnesia-loss of memory). It is now known that discrete areas of the brain are involved in memory and different areas influence different modalities of memory. The best known "system" damage which leads to defects of memory, consists of the hippocampus (including the subiculum), the fimbria and fornix, the mamillary bodies, the mamillothalamic tract, the anterior nuclei of the thalamus, and the gyrus cinguli (and the fibres of the cingulum). It has been shown that damage anywhere along this pathway results in loss of memory of events, leaving general knowledge of the person intact. Bilateral transection of the fornix can lead to acute amnesic syndrome, in which an individual is unable to process his/her short-term memory into long-term memory.

Alzheimer's disease is a degenerative disorder of the brain affecting the limbic system. It is associated with loss of memory, initially short-term and later long-term memory. Cognitive deficit is due to reduced cholinergic inputs.

RETICULAR FORMATION OF THE BRAINSTEM

The reticular formation are areas of the central nervous system which are not occupied by well-defined nuclei or fibre bundles, but consist of a network of fibres within

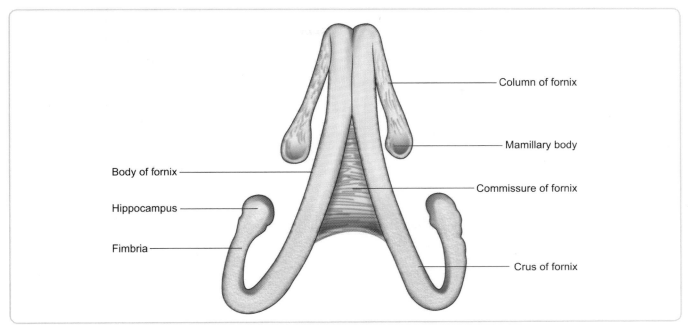

Figure 13.9: Dorsal view of hippocampus and fornix to show the commissure of fornix

which scattered neurons are situated. The reticular formation is best defined in the brainstem where it is now recognized as an area of considerable importance. Some centres in the cerebrum and cerebellum are regarded to be closely related, functionally, to this region.

The reticular formation extends throughout the length of the brainstem. In the medulla, it occupies the region dorsal to the inferior olivary nucleus. In the pons, it lies in the dorsal part, while in the midbrain it lies in the tegmentum.

The neurons seen in the reticular formation vary considerably in the size of their cell bodies, the length and ramifications of their axons, and the behaviour of their dendrites.

A number of reticular nuclei have been described:
- The **median column** lies next to the midline. The nuclei in it are called the **nuclei of the raphe,** or **paramedian nuclei.**
- The **medial column** (or **magnocellular** column) consists of nuclei having neurons of large or medium size.
- The nuclei of the **lateral column** are made up of small neurons. (Figure 13.10 and Table 13.1).

Connections of Reticular Formation

The reticular formation has numerous connections. Directly, or indirectly, it is connected to almost all parts of the nervous system. The better established afferents are shown in Flowchart 13.4 and the efferents in Flowchart 13.5.

The pathways involved are both ascending and descending, crossed and uncrossed, somatic and visceral. It has an important regulatory role, both facilitatory and inhibitory.

Corticoreticulospinal Pathways

The reticular formation receives impulses from the motor and other areas of the cerebral cortex and relays them to the spinal cord through the medial and lateral reticulospinal tracts. The corticoreticular fibres descend along with corticospinal fibres. The reticular formation also establishes connections with motor cranial nerve nuclei.

Cerebelloreticular Connections

The reticular formation has reciprocal connections with the cerebellum (Flowchart 13.6). Through these connections, the reticular formation connects the cerebral cortex, and the spinal cord, to the cerebellar cortex.

Ascending Reticular Activating System

The spinothalamic tracts, secondary trigeminal pathways and auditory pathways give collaterals to the reticular formation. Fibres arising here project to the intralaminar and reticular nuclei of the thalamus.

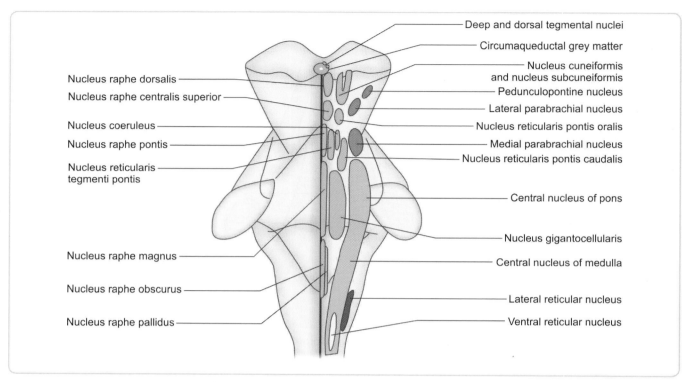

Figure 13.10: Nuclei of the reticular formation of the brainstem projected onto its posterior surface

TABLE 13.1: Nuclei of the reticular formation in the brainstem (Figure 13.10)		
	Median column (nuclei of raphe)	*Medial column (magnocellular)*	*Lateral column (parvocellular)*
Midbrain	Nucleus raphe dorsalis	Circumaqueductal grey matter Deep tegmental nucleus Dorsal tegmental nucleus Nucleus subcuneiformis Nucleus cuneiformis	Nucleus pedunculopontis Lateral parabrachial nucleus Medial parabrachial nucleus
Pons	Nucleus raphe centralis superior Nucleus raphe pontis Nucleus raphe magnus	Nucleus coeruleus Nucleus reticularis pontis oralis Nucleus reticularis tegmenti pontis Nucleus reticularis pontis caudalis Gigantocellular nucleus (pontine part)	Central nucleus of pons
Medulla	Nucleus raphe obscurus Nucleus raphe pallidus	Gigantocellular nucleus (medullary part)	Central nucleus of medulla Lateral reticular nucleus Ventral reticular nucleus

These nuclei, in turn, project to widespread areas of the cerebral cortex. These pathways form part of the ascending reticular activating system (ARAS) which is responsible for maintaining a state of alertness.

Serotoninergic Raphe System

They are also referred to as the paramedian reticular nuclei.

- Serotoninergic fibres descending from the raphe nuclei reach all levels of the spinal cord.
- Fibres descend to the locus coeruleus.

Locus Coeruleus and Noradrenergic System

The locus coeruleus is an area in the floor of the fourth ventricle, at the upper end of the sulcus limitans. The area has a bluish colour caused by the presence of pigment

Flowchart 13.4: Major afferents of the reticular formation

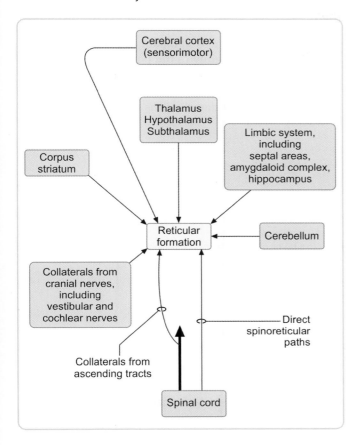

Flowchart 13.6: Cerebelloreticular connections

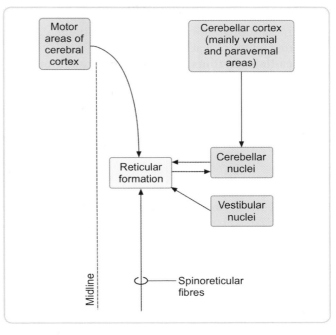

Flowchart 13.5 Major efferents of the reticular formation

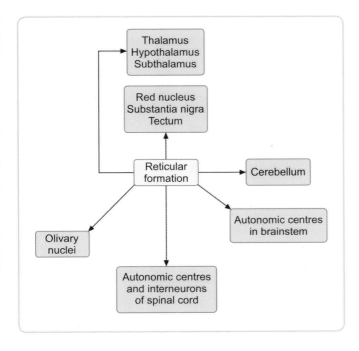

in the underlying neurons. These neurons constitute the nucleus coeruleus.

The locus coeruleus contains noradrenergic neurons.

Functions of the Reticular Formation

Because of its diverse connections, the reticular formation is believed to have a controlling or modifying influence on many functions. Some of them are given below:

- **Somatomotor control:** Through its direct connections with the spinal cord, and indirectly through the corpus striatum, the cerebral cortex and the cerebellum, the reticular formation has an influence on fine control of movements including those involved in postural adjustments, locomotion, skilled use of the hands, speech, etc. Ventrally descending fibres influence ventral horn cells to which they are facilitatory.

- **Somatosensory control:** The reticular formation influences conduction through somatosensory pathways. Similar effects may also be exerted on visual and auditory pathways.

- **Visceral control:** Stimulation of certain areas in the reticular formation of the medulla has great influence on respiratory and cardiovascular function. These effects are through connections between the reticular formation and autonomic centres in the brainstem and spinal cord. The "intermediate" fibres descending into the spinal cord influence sympathetic control of the cardiovascular system.

- **Neuroendocrine control:** Through its connections with the hypothalamus, the reticular formation influences the activity of the adenohypophysis and of the neurohypophysis. A similar influence is also exerted on the pineal body.
- **Circadian rhythms**: The reticular formation also influences other hypothalamic functions. These include a possible effect on circadian rhythms.
- **Arousal:** The reticular formation controls the arousal and the state of consciousness through the ARAS.

Ascending fibres also influence the activities of the limbic and related areas.
- **Pain control:** Fibres descending dorsally in the spinal cord forms part of a pain controlling pathway. They terminate mainly in the posterior grey column. The locus coeruleus plays a role in the control of cardiovascular, respiratory and gastrointestinal functions and in circadian rhythms (including the sleep-waking cycle).

MULTIPLE CHOICE QUESTIONS

Q1. The fibres of the column of the fornix end in
A. Mamillary body
B. Caudate nucleus
C. Hypothalamus
D. Collateral eminence

Q2. The following structures are included in the "Papez circuit" except
A. Fornix
B. Mamillary body
C. Medial nucleus of thalamus
D. Hippocampus

Q3. The hippocampal formation consists of
A. Dentate gyrus
B. Indusium griseum
C. Gyrus fasciolaris
D. All of the above

Q4. The fibres of the fornix arise from
A. Mamillary body
B. Hippocampus

C. Amygdaloid body
D. Collateral eminence

Q5. The layer of white fibres covering the ventricular surface of the hippocampus is known as
A. Pes hippocampi
B. Alveus
C. Fimbria
D. Stria terminalis

Q6. Cingulate gyrus is a part of
A. Hippocampal formation
B. Limbic lobe
C. Subcallosal area
D. Olfactory area

Q7. The functions of reticular formation are
A. Maintenance of alert state
B. Control of pain
C. Neuroendocrine control
D. All of the above

ANSWERS

1. A   2. C   3. D   4. B   5. B   6. B   7. D

SHORT NOTES

1. Specify the parts of limbic lobe
2. Specify the components of hippocampal formation
3. Papez circuit
4. Fornix
5. Connections of amygdala
6. Functions of limbic system
7. Functions of reticular formation

Clinical Cases

13.1: A 45-year-old male who used to be quite an outgoing and assertive person became calm and withdrawn and was not showing any emotions over the past few months. He also complained of headache and was investigated for the same.
Magnetic resonance imaging showed a tumour in the anterior part of temporal lobe.
A. Which structure is likely to be affected?
B. What is its role in causing a lack of emotion in this patient?

Chapter 14 — Autonomic Nervous System

Specific Learning Objectives

At the end of learning, the student shall be able to:

➤ Specify the location of the cell bodies and axonal course and termination of preganglionic sympathetic and parasympathetic neurons
➤ Specify the location of the cell bodies and axonal course and termination of postganglionic sympathetic and parasympathetic neurons
➤ Name the neurotransmitters that are released by preganglionic autonomic neurons, postganglionic sympathetic neurons, postganglionic parasympathetic neurons, and the chemicals released by adrenal medullary cells
➤ Specify the role of the autonomic nervous system at select organs and glands
➤ Describe the enteric nervous system

INTRODUCTION

The **autonomic nervous system (ANS)** is made up of nerves supplying the viscera (and blood vessels) along with the parts of the brain and spinal cord related to them. The ANS includes the following:

- **Areas for visceral function located in the cerebral hemispheres**: These are the structures in the limbic region of the brain. The hypothalamus, parts of the thalamus, and the prefrontal cortex are also involved in autonomic functions.
- **Autonomic centres in the brainstem**: These are located in the reticular formation and in the general visceral nuclei of cranial nerves.
- **Autonomic centres in the spinal cord**: These are located in the intermediolateral grey column.
- **Peripheral part of ANS**: This is made up of all autonomic nerves and ganglia throughout the body. Many of these are intimately related to cranial and spinal nerves.

Divisions of Autonomic Nervous System

The ANS is subdivided into three divisions:

- The sympathetic nervous system
- The parasympathetic nervous system
- The enteric nervous system

The ANS, like the somatic nervous system, contains efferent as well as afferent fibres. The efferent fibres supply smooth muscles throughout the body. The influence may be either to cause contraction or relaxation. In a given situation, the sympathetic and parasympathetic nerves generally produce opposite effects. For example, sympathetic stimulation causes dilatation of the pupil, whereas parasympathetic stimulation causes constriction. In hollow viscera like the stomach or urinary bladder, parasympathetic stimulation produces movement and inhibits the sphincters. An opposite sympathetic effect is usually described. In the case of blood vessels, the influence on smooth muscle may result in vasoconstriction or in vasodilatation.

In addition to supplying smooth muscle, autonomic nerves innervate glands. Such nerves are described as **secretomotor**. The secretomotor nerves to almost all glands are parasympathetic. One exception is the sweat gland, which has a sympathetic supply.

EFFERENT AUTONOMIC PATHWAY

The efferent autonomic pathway, for innervation of smooth muscle or gland, always consists of two neurons that synapse in a ganglion (Figure 14.1). The first neuron carries the nerve impulses from the central nervous system (CNS) to the ganglion and is called the **preganglionic neuron**. The second neuron carries impulses from the ganglion to smooth muscle or gland and is called the **postganglionic neuron**. The ANS, thus, has a general visceral efferent motor system, which controls and regulates smooth muscles and glands.

The location of cell bodies of ganglia in ANS is shown in Table 14.1.

The number of postganglionic sympathetic neurons (or fibres) is much greater than that of preganglionic neurons, each preganglionic fibre synapsing with many

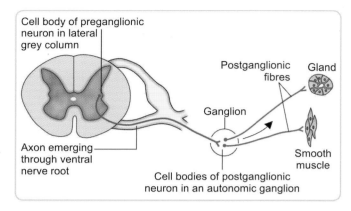

Figure 14.1: Typical arrangement of neurons in autonomic nervous system (general visceral efferent neurons)

TABLE 14.1: Location of cell bodies of ganglia in autonomic nervous system

Location	Sympathetic	Parasympathetic
Head	–	Ciliary, pterygopalatine, submandibular and otic
Neck	Superior, middle and inferior cervical	In the wall of the cervical viscera
Thorax	Paravertebral	Cardiac and pulmonary plexus
Abdomen	Paravertebral and prevertebral plexus along the abdominal aorta (e.g. coeliac plexuses)	In the wall of the viscera (myenteric and submucosal)
Pelvis	Paravertebral and plexus along the internal iliac artery (hypogastric plexuses)	In the wall of the viscera (myenteric, submucosal and vesical)

postganglionic neurons. This results in considerable dispersal of the nerve impulses. A similar, but much lesser, dispersal of impulses also takes place in the parasympathetic nervous system. This is to be correlated with the fact that sympathetic stimulation produces widespread effects, whereas the effects of parasympathetic stimulation are much more localized.

SYMPATHETIC NERVOUS SYSTEM

Sympathetic Preganglionic Neurons

The cell bodies of sympathetic preganglionic neurons are located in the intermediolateral grey column of the spinal cord in all the thoracic and upper two lumbar segments

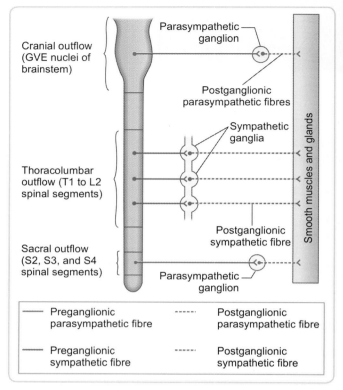

Figure 14.2: Craniosacral outflow (parasympathetic) and thoracolumbar outflow (sympathetic) (*Abbreviation:* GVE, general visceral efferent)

(Figure 14.2). Fibres arising from these neurons constitute the **thoracolumbar outflow**. Their axons leave the spinal cord through anterior nerve roots to reach the spinal nerves of the segments concerned. After a very short course in the ventral primary rami, these fibres enter the white rami communicantes to reach the sympathetic trunk (Figure 14.3).

On reaching the sympathetic trunk, these fibres behave in one of the following ways (Figures 14.3 and 14.4):
- They may terminate in relation to cells of the sympathetic ganglion at the level concerned.
- They may travel up or down the sympathetic trunk to terminate in ganglia at a higher or lower level.
- They may leave the sympathetic trunk through one of its branches to terminate in a peripherally situated ganglion in the peripheral autonomic plexus (Figure 14.3).

Sympathetic Postganglionic Neurons

The sympathetic trunks (right and left) with a number of enlargements placed along its length, called **sympathetic**

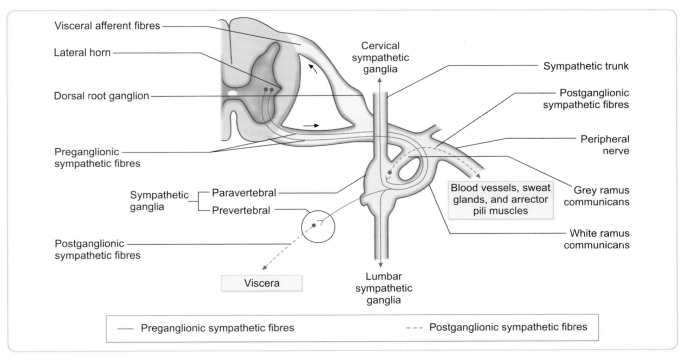

Figure 14.3: Grey and white rami connecting a spinal nerve to the sympathetic trunk and the fibres passing through them

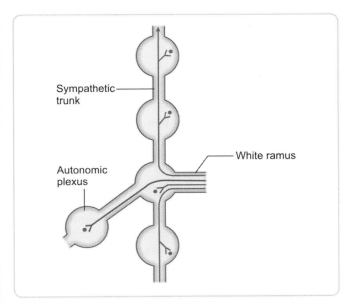

Figure 14.4: Mode of termination of sympathetic preganglionic neurons

ganglia, form the postganglionic neurons. They are placed on either side of the vertebral column. Above, they extend to the base of the skull and below, to the coccyx. The number of ganglia is variable. Generally, there are 3 (superior, middle, and inferior) in the cervical region; 11 in the thoracic region; 4 in the lumbar region; and 4 in the sacral region, so that in all there are 22 ganglia on each trunk (Figure 14.5). The inferior cervical ganglion and the first thoracic are often fused to form a large **stellate ganglion**.

The sympathetic trunks are connected to the spinal nerves by a series of communicating branches or **rami communicantes**. These are of two types: white and grey. The white rami consist of myelinated fibres, while the grey rami are made up of unmyelinated fibres. The white rami carry fibres (originating in the spinal cord) from the spinal nerve to the sympathetic trunks. They are present only in the thoracic and upper lumbar regions. The grey rami carry fibres from the sympathetic trunk to spinal nerves. All spinal nerves receive grey rami. The fibres of the grey rami are distributed to peripheral tissues through the spinal nerves. The sympathetic trunks also establish communications with several cranial nerves through branches arising from the superior cervical ganglion.

In addition to communicating branches, the sympathetic trunks give off branches for supply of blood vessels and viscera. The visceral branches are directed medially (Figure 14.3) and take part in forming a series of autonomic plexuses in the thorax, abdomen, and pelvis.

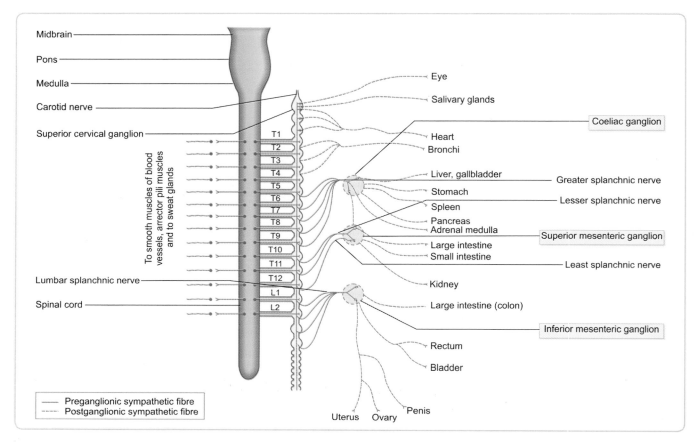

Figure 14.5: Sympathetic nervous system

Branches to peripheral parts of the body follow one of the two routes. Some branches from the sympathetic trunks reach blood vessels directly and form perivascular plexuses on them. One such branch arises from the cranial end of the superior cervical ganglion and forms a plexus around the internal carotid artery. Other sympathetic fibres reach blood vessels (especially in the limbs) after running for part of their course through spinal nerves and their branches (Figure 14.3).

Apart from supplying the blood vessels themselves, these sympathetic fibres innervate sweat glands and arrector pili muscles of the skin.

Axons arising from sympathetic postganglionic neurons behave in one of the following ways:

- The axons may pass through a grey ramus communicans to reach a spinal nerve. They then pass through the spinal nerve and its branches to innervate sweat glands and arrectores pilorum muscles of the skin in the region to which the spinal nerve is distributed.

- The axons may reach a cranial nerve through a communicating branch and may be distributed through it, as in the case of a spinal nerve.

- The axons may pass into a vascular branch and may be distributed to branches of the vessel. Some fibres from these plexuses may pass to other structures in the neighborhood of the vessel.

- Some axons, meant for innervation of blood vessels, travel for part of their course in spinal nerves or their branches and reach the vessels through vascular branches arising from these nerves. Many blood vessels in the peripheral parts of the limbs are innervated in this way.

- The axons of postganglionic neurons arising in sympathetic ganglia may travel through visceral branches and through autonomic plexuses to reach some viscera (for example, the heart).

- The axons of postganglionic neurons located in peripheral autonomic plexuses innervate neighboring

TABLE 14.2: Autonomic plexuses and their locations

Region	Autonomic plexuses
Thorax	Superficial and deep cardiac, pulmonary, and oesophageal
Abdomen	Coeliac, superior mesenteric, inferior mesenteric, and aortic
Pelvis	Superior and inferior hypogastric and pelvic

viscera. These fibres often travel to the viscera in plexuses along blood vessels. For example, fibres for the gut travel along plexuses surrounding the branches of the coeliac, superior mesenteric, and inferior mesenteric arteries.

AUTONOMIC PLEXUSES

The visceral branches of sympathetic trunks help form various plexuses in the thorax, abdomen, and pelvis. In addition to sympathetic fibres, these plexuses contain parasympathetic fibres derived either from the vagus nerve or from pelvic splanchnic nerves. They also contain collections of neurons, which are often referred to as ganglia. In the thorax, there are **superficial and deep cardiac plexuses** in relation to the heart and the **pulmonary plexus**es in relation to the lungs (Figure 14.6). In the abdomen, there is a prominent **coeliac ganglion** on either side of the aorta. The two ganglia are interconnected by numerous fibres that form the **coeliac plexus**. This plexus is closely related to the coeliac trunk and sends ramifications along its branches. Other plexuses (or ganglia) are related to the abdominal aorta, superior and inferior mesenteric arteries, and other branches arising from the aorta. The pelvis has a **superior hypogastric plexus** (often called the **presacral nerve**) situated near the bifurcation of the aorta. When traced downwards, it divides into two **inferior hypogastric plexuses** (or **hypogastric nerves**) related to each internal iliac artery (Table 14.2). Subsidiary plexuses run along branches of the internal iliac artery. Some plexuses are present in close relation to some viscera or even within their walls. The vesical plexus surrounds the urinary bladder. In the gut, there is a **myenteric plexus** (of Auerbach) between the muscle coats and a **submucosal plexus** (of Meissner).

PARASYMPATHETIC NERVOUS SYSTEM

Parasympathetic Preganglionic Neurons

The parasympathetic preganglionic neurons are located in two distinct situations:
1. The first group is located in the general visceral efferent nuclei of the brainstem. Axons arising in these nuclei constitute the **cranial parasympathetic outflow**

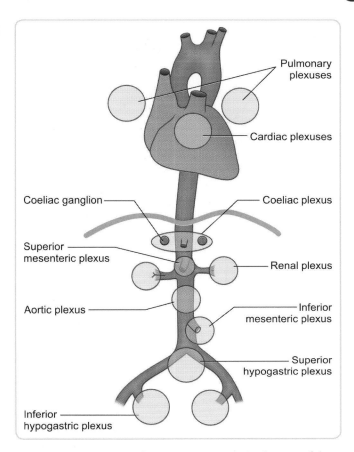

Figure 14.6: Location of important autonomic plexuses of the thorax and abdomen

(Figure 14.2). They pass through the third, seventh, ninth, and tenth cranial nerves to terminate in peripheral ganglia (Figure 14.7). The largest part of this outflow is constituted by the vagus nerve. Its fibres terminate in relation to postganglionic neurons located in cervical, thoracic and abdominal autonomic plexuses.
2. The second group of parasympathetic preganglionic neurons is located in the second, third, and fourth sacral segments of the spinal cord (Figure 14.2). Their axons constitute the **sacral parasympathetic outflow**. They emerge from the cord through the anterior nerve roots of the corresponding spinal nerves. The axons leave the spinal nerves to form the **pelvic splanchnic nerves,** which end in pelvic autonomic plexuses in the walls of the pelvic viscera (Figure 14.7).

Parasympathetic Postganglionic Neurons

- Postganglionic neurons related to the third, seventh, and ninth cranial nerves are located in the ciliary, submandibular, pterygopalatine, and otic ganglia.

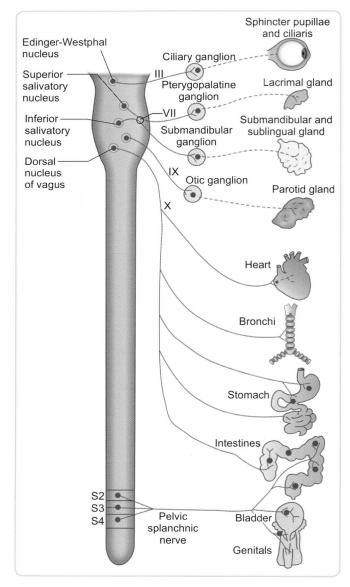

Figure 14.7: Craniosacral (parasympathetic) outflow

NEUROTRANSMITTERS OF AUTONOMIC NEURONS

- The neurotransmitter acetylcholine is liberated at the terminals of preganglionic neurons, both sympathetic and parasympathetic (Figure 14.8).
- Acetylcholine is also liberated at the terminals of parasympathetic postganglionic neurons.
- The neurotransmitter liberated at the terminals of sympathetic postganglionic neurons is noradrenalin. Cells of the adrenal medulla, which receive terminals of preganglionic sympathetic neurons and produce noradrenalin and adrenalin, may be regarded as **modified sympathetic postganglionic neurons**. It may be noted that cells of the sympathetic ganglia and of the adrenal medulla have a common embryological origin from the neural crest.
- Postganglionic sympathetic neurons innervating sweat glands and some blood vessels of skeletal muscles are exceptional in that their terminals liberate acetylcholine.

AFFERENTS ACCOMPANYING AUTONOMIC PATHWAYS

The sensory neurons related to the ANS are general visceral afferent neurons, and their arrangement is similar to that of afferent fibres in cerebrospinal nerves. The neurons concerned are located in spinal ganglia or in sensory ganglia of cranial nerves. They carry impulses arising in viscera and in blood vessels to the CNS. They may be associated with the parasympathetic as well as the sympathetic systems. Accordingly, the cell bodies of the neurons in question may be located in one of the following situations.

Afferents Related to the Cranial Part of Parasympathetic System

These are general visceral afferent fibres related to the glossopharyngeal and vagus nerves (Figure 14.9A). The cell bodies of the neurons concerned are located in sensory ganglia related to the cranial nerve in question. Their central processes terminate in the nucleus of the solitary tract.

Glossopharyngeal afferents carry sensations from the pharynx and posterior part of the tongue. They also innervate the carotid sinus and carotid body. Sensory fibres carried by the vagus innervate all organs to which its efferent fibres are distributed. The sensory fibres in the vagus are much more numerous than efferent fibres. Apart

- Postganglionic neurons related to the vagus are located in cervical, thoracic and abdominal autonomic plexuses, close to or within the viscera supplied (Figure 14.7). The axons arising from these postganglionic neurons innervate various thoracic and abdominal viscera, including the foregut and midgut.
- Postganglionic neurons related to the sacral parasympathetic outflow are located in pelvic autonomic plexuses. They innervate the pelvic viscera. They also supply the hindgut (rectum, the sigmoid colon, the descending colon and the left one-third of the transverse colon).

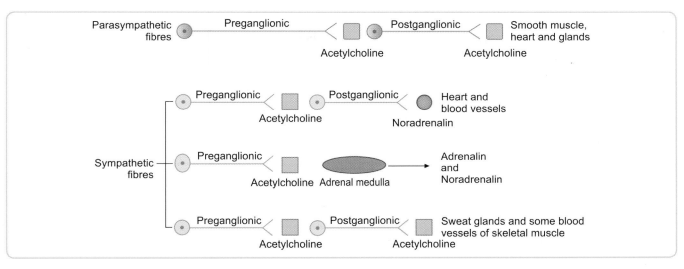

Figure 14.8: Neurotransmitters of autonomic neurons

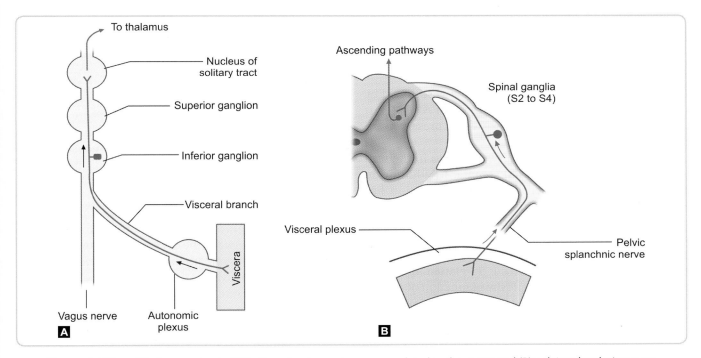

Figures 14.9A and B: Arrangement of (A) afferent autonomic neurons related to the vagus and (B) pelvic splanchnic nerves

from carrying sensations, afferent fibres are also involved in various reflexes related to the organs concerned.

Afferents Related to the Sacral Part of Parasympathetic System

These afferents are peripheral processes of unipolar neurons located in the dorsal nerve root ganglia of the second, third, and fourth sacral nerves (Figure 14.9B). These fibres run through the pelvic splanchnic nerves to innervate pelvic viscera. The central processes of these neurons enter the spinal cord.

Afferents Related to Sympathetic Nervous System

Afferent fibres accompany almost all efferent sympathetic fibres. These afferent fibres are peripheral processes of unipolar neurons located in the spinal ganglia of spinal nerves T1 to L2 (or L3) (Figure 14.10).

- Autonomic afferents are necessary for various visceral reflexes. Most of these impulses are not consciously perceived.
- Some normal visceral sensations that reach consciousness include those of hunger, nausea, distension of the urinary bladder or rectum, and sexual sensations. Sense of touch or pressure perceived by the tongue and pharynx and the sensation of taste are also visceral sensations.
- Under pathological conditions, visceral pain is perceived. This is produced by distension, by spasm of smooth muscle, or by ischaemia. The pain is projected (referred) to that part of the body wall that is innervated by the same spinal segment (dermatome) and is known as referred pain.
- Sensory impulses from the same organ may travel both along sympathetic and parasympathetic nerves. However, referred pain of cervical viscera is felt in the ear (glossopharyngeal and vagus); that of pelvic organs, including cervix, is referred to low back (S2, 3, 4). The thoracic and abdominal organs (including uterus) project their referred pain to the dermatome equivalent to their sympathetic innervation.

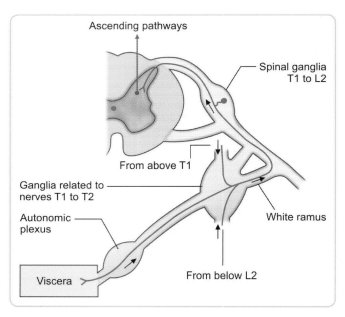

Figure 14.10: Afferent autonomic pathways involving sympathetic nerves

ENTERIC NERVOUS SYSTEM

The entire length of gastrointestinal tract is supplied by sympathetic and parasympathetic parts of ANS. Apart from these, two different nerve plexuses are present in the gut wall.

Although the presence of nerve plexuses in the wall of the gut containing neuronal somata, in addition to nerve fibres, has been well known, their function has been obscure. Recent researches using immunochemical methods have revealed the presence of a large number of neuroactive substances in these plexuses. It has even been claimed that almost every neuroactive substance to be found in the CNS is also present in relation to the gut, suggesting much greater complexity of function of enteric plexuses than hitherto believed. The nerve plexuses of the gut are, therefore, now regarded as third component of the ANS (the other two components being sympathetic and parasympathetic), which is referred to as the **enteric nervous system**.

The enteric nervous system is located within the wall of the digestive tract, from the oesophagus to the anus. It is comprised of two well-organized neural plexuses:

1. **Myenteric plexus (of Auerbach)** is located between longitudinal and circular layers of muscle. This is involved in control of gastrointestinal tract motility.
2. **Submucosal plexus (of Meissner)** is located between the circular muscle and the luminal mucosa. This innervates the muscularis mucosae and thus regulates blood flow to the mucosa, movement of mucosa,

absorption and secretive function of the lining epithelium.

The enteric nervous system contains sensory neurons, interneurons and motor neurons. It contains sensory neurons innervating receptors in the mucosa. Motor neurons control motility, secretion, and absorption. Interneurons integrate information from sensory neurons to the motor neurons.

Although the enteric nervous system can function autonomously, normal digestive function requires communication between the CNS and the enteric nervous system. It is the parasympathetic stimulation that increases overall degree of activity of the gastrointestinal tract. This also increases the rate of secretion of the gastrointestinal glands. Strong sympathetic stimulation inhibits peristalsis and increases the tone of the sphincters. This results in slowing of propulsion of food through the tract and decreased secretion as well.

AUTONOMIC NERVE SUPPLY OF SOME IMPORTANT ORGANS

The Eyeball

The **sphincter pupillae** is supplied by parasympathetic nerves. The preganglionic neurons concerned are located in the Edinger-Westphal nucleus. Their axons travel through the oculomotor nerve and terminate in the ciliary ganglion. Postganglionic neurons are located in this ganglion. Their axons supply the sphincter pupillae and the ciliaris muscle (Figure 14.11).

The **dilator pupillae** is supplied by sympathetic nerves. The preganglionic neurons concerned are located in the intermediolateral grey column of the first thoracic segment of the spinal cord. Their axons emerge through the anterior nerve root of the first thoracic nerve to reach the stellate ganglion. They, however, pass through this ganglion without relay and ascend in the sympathetic trunk to reach the superior cervical sympathetic ganglion. Postganglionic neurons are located in this ganglion. Their axons pass through the internal carotid nerve. In the cavernous sinus, they pass (through communicating twigs) to the ophthalmic division of the trigeminal nerve. They travel through the nasociliary nerve and its long ciliary branches to the dilator pupillae.

Some sympathetic fibres reach the eyeball after passing through the ciliary ganglion. These fibres do not relay in this ganglion but merely pass through it. They supply the blood vessels of the eyeball. Apart from the dilator pupillae and blood vessels, sympathetic fibres also supply the orbitalis muscle, (Müller's muscle III),

and superior and inferior tarsal muscles of the eyelid (Müller's muscles I and II, respectively).

> **Clinical Anatomy**
>
> **Horner's Syndrome**
> Interruption of sympathetic supply to the head and neck results in Horner's syndrome. This consists of the following:
> - Constriction of the pupil (**miosis**)
> - Drooping of the upper eyelids (**ptosis**)
> - Reduced prominence of the eyeball (**enophthalmos**)
> - Absence of sweating on the face and neck (**anhidrosis**)
> - Loss of ciliospinal reflex (pinching of nape of neck **does not** cause dilatation of pupils)

Salivary Glands

Submandibular and Sublingual Glands

The secretomotor supply to the salivary glands is parasympathetic. Preganglionic neurons for the submandibular and the sublingual glands are located in the superior salivatory nucleus (Figure 14.12). Their axons pass through the facial nerve, its chorda tympani

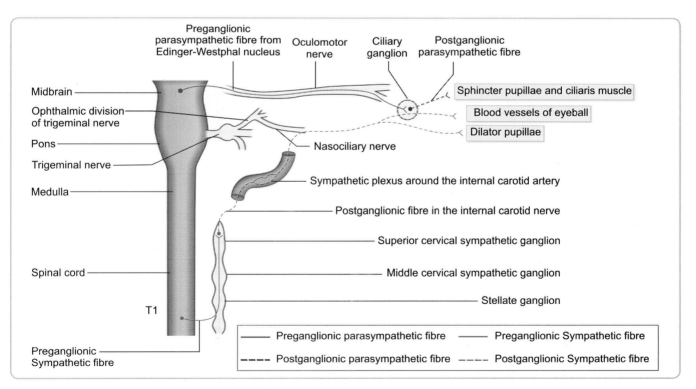

Figure 14.11: Innervation of the pupil

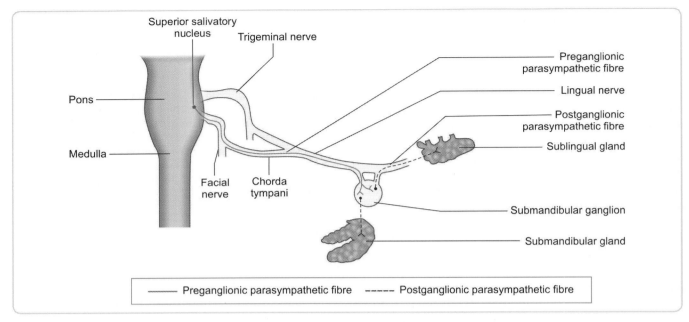

Figure 14.12: Secretomotor pathway to submandibular and sublingual salivary glands

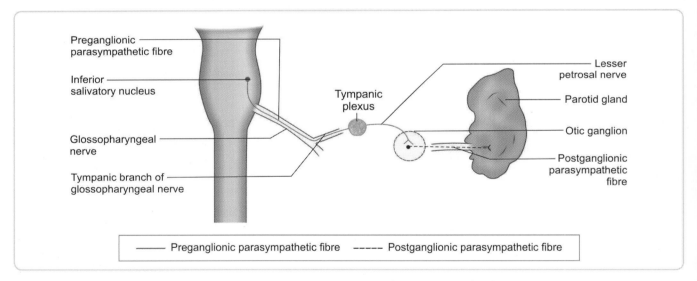

Figure 14.13: Secretomotor pathway for the parotid gland

branch, and then through the lingual nerve, to reach the submandibular ganglion. The postganglionic neurons are located in this ganglion. Their axons reach the submandibular gland through branches from the ganglion to the gland. Some postganglionic neurons may be located in the hilum of the submandibular gland.

Fibres meant for the sublingual gland re-enter the lingual nerve and pass through its distal part to reach the gland.

Parotid Gland

The preganglionic neurons for the parotid gland are located in the inferior salivatory nucleus. Their axons pass through the glossopharyngeal nerve and its tympanic branch, the tympanic plexus, and the lesser petrosal nerve to terminate in the otic ganglion (Figure 14.13). Postganglionic fibres arising in this ganglion reach the gland through the auriculotemporal nerve.

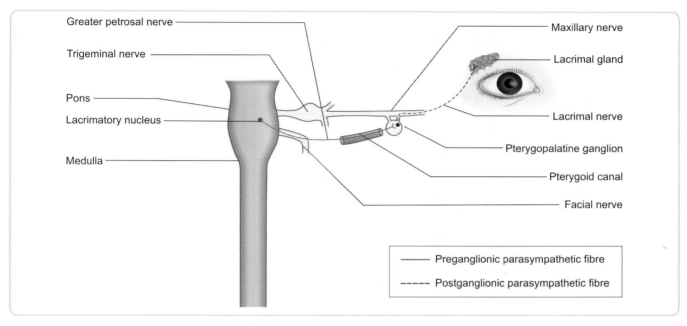

Figure 14.14: Innervation of the lacrimal gland

Sympathetic fibres travel to salivary glands along the blood vessels which cause vasoconstriction and therefore produce a thick, viscous saliva.

Lacrimal Gland

Preganglionic neurons for the lacrimal gland are located in the lacrimatory nucleus near the superior salivatory nucleus. Their axons pass through the facial nerve, its greater petrosal branch, and through the nerve of the pterygoid canal to reach the pterygopalatine ganglion (Figure 14.14). Postganglionic fibres arising in this ganglion pass successively through the maxillary nerve, its zygomatic branch, the zygomaticotemporal nerve, a communicating branch from the zygomaticotemporal nerve to the lacrimal branch of the ophthalmic nerve, and finally, through the lacrimal branch itself to reach the gland.

Heart

Parasympathetic preganglionic neurons for the heart are located in the dorsal nucleus of the vagus. They reach the heart through cervical cardiac branches of the vagus. The postganglionic neurons are located within the superficial and deep cardiac plexuses. Their axons are distributed to the sinoatrial (SA) node, the atria, the atrioventricular (AV) node, and the AV bundle.

Preganglionic sympathetic neurons are located in segments T1–T5 of the spinal cord (Figure 14.15). On reaching the sympathetic trunks, their axons synapse with postganglionic neurons in the upper thoracic ganglia. Some fibres run upwards in the sympathetic trunk to end in cervical sympathetic ganglia. Postganglionic fibres leave these ganglia through their cardiac branches, and join the vagal fibres in forming the cardiac plexuses.

Contraction of cardiac muscle is not dependent on nerve supply. It can occur spontaneously. The nerves supplying the heart, however, influence heart rate. Sympathetic stimulation increases heart rate and parasympathetic stimulation reduces it. Sympathetic nerves supplying the coronary arteries cause vasodilatation increasing blood flow through them.

Afferent fibres from the heart travel through both sympathetic and parasympathetic pathways. Afferent fibres running along the vagus are concerned with reflexes controlling the activity of the heart.

Clinical Anatomy

Impulses of pain arising in the heart, due to ischaemia, are carried mainly by the sympathetic cardiac branches and enter the spinal cord through spinal nerves T1–T5. These pathways are important as they convey impulses of pain produced as a result of anoxia of heart muscle (angina). The pain is predominantly retrosternal (T2–T5), but it may be referred to the inner side of the left arm (T1).

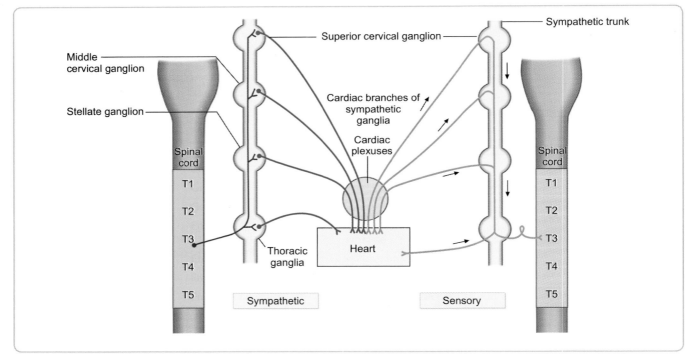

Figure 14.15: Sympathetic innervation of the heart—afferent fibres traveling along the sympathetic nerves

Bronchi

Parasympathetic preganglionic neurons, that supply the bronchi, are located in the dorsal vagal nucleus. The fibres travel through the vagus and its branches, to reach the anterior and posterior pulmonary plexuses. Postganglionic neurons are located near the roots of the lungs. Their axons run along the bronchi and supply them.

Preganglionic sympathetic neurons are located in the second to fifth thoracic segments of the spinal cord. Their axons terminate in the corresponding sympathetic ganglion. Postganglionic fibres arising in these ganglia reach the bronchi through branches from the sympathetic trunks to the pulmonary plexuses.

Parasympathetic stimulation causes broncho-constriction, while sympathetic stimulation causes bronchodilatation. Parasympathetic stimulation also has a secretomotor effect on glands in the bronchi. Sympathetic stimulation causes vasoconstriction.

Gastrointestinal Tract

- The parasympathetic nerve supply of the greater part of the gastrointestinal tract (from the pharynx to the junction of the right two-thirds of the transverse colon with the left one-third) is through the vagus.

The preganglionic neurons are situated in the dorsal nucleus of the vagus.

- The hindgut is supplied by the sacral part of the parasympathetic system. The preganglionic neurons concerned are located in the second, third and fourth sacral segments of the spinal cord. They emerge through the ventral nerve roots of the corresponding nerves, and pass into their pelvic splanchnic branches. The fibres to the rectum and the upper part of the anal canal pass through the inferior hypogastric plexus. The remaining fibres pass through the superior hypogastric plexus and are distributed along the inferior mesenteric artery.

- The postganglionic parasympathetic neurons are located in the myenteric and submucosal plexuses in the region to be supplied.

- Preganglionic sympathetic neurons for the gut are located in the thoracolumbar region of the spinal cord (Figure 14.16). Their axons pass through the sympathetic trunks without relay. They travel through the splanchnic nerves to terminate in plexuses (and ganglia) related to the coeliac artery, the superior mesenteric artery and the inferior mesenteric artery. Postganglionic neurons are located in these plexuses. They travel along these blood vessels to reach the gut.

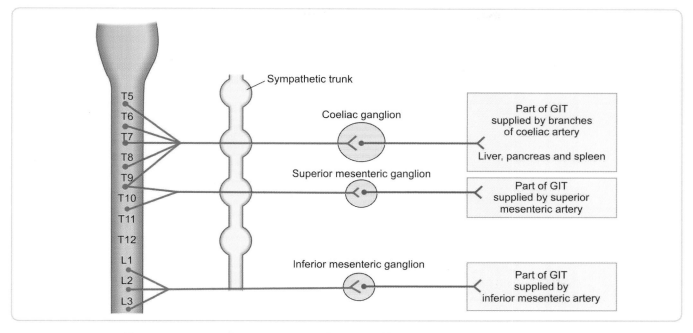

Figure 14.16: Sympathetic innervation of the gut (*Abbreviation:* GIT, gastrointestinal tract)

Parasympathetic nerves stimulate intestinal movement and inhibit the sphincters. They are secretomotor to the mucosal glands. Sympathetic fibres are distributed chiefly to blood vessels.

Afferent fibres travel both along sympathetic and parasympathetic pathways. Pain from most of the gastrointestinal tract travels along sympathetic nerves. However, pain from the pharynx and oesophagus is carried by the vagus and that from the rectum and lower part of the pelvic colon by pelvic splanchnic nerves.

Urinary Bladder

The parasympathetic nerves to the urinary bladder are derived from the sacral outflow. The preganglionic fibres pass through the pelvic splanchnic nerves and the inferior hypogastric plexuses to reach the vesical plexus. Parasympathetic postganglionic neurons are located in the vesical plexus. Parasympathetic stimulation is motor to the detrusor muscle and inhibitory to the sphincter (Figure 14.17).

Sympathetic preganglionic neurons are located in spinal segments L1, L2. Their axons terminate in the inferior mesenteric, superior hypogastric and inferior hypogastric plexuses. Postganglionic neurons are located in these plexuses. Sympathetic stimulation has an effect opposite to that of the parasympathetic.

> ### Clinical Anatomy
>
> Sensory fibres carry impulses of distension and of pain from the urinary bladder. They run through both sympathetic and parasympathetic pathways. In the spinal cord, fibres carrying the two types of sensation follow different routes. Fibres carrying pain are located in the anterior and lateral white columns while fibres carrying the sensation of bladder filling travel through the posterior column. As a result, intractable bladder pain (such as that may occur because of carcinoma) can be relieved by cutting the anterior and lateral white columns of both sides (bilateral anterolateral cordotomy) without abolishing the sensation of bladder filling.
>
> The medial frontal cortex of both sides controls the bladder centre in pons (pontine paramedian reticular formation). Lesions involving both medial frontal cortices (superior sagittal sinus thrombosis/meningioma of falx cerebri/occlusion of unpaired anterior cerebral artery) interrupt normal initiation of micturition (hesitancy), and stoppage of micturition when circumstances are unfavourable (urgency and precipitancy). This triad is called as **uninhibited bladder**.
>
> Severe lesions of the spinal cord above the sacral segments, involving the pontine reticulospinal tract, interfere with both afferent and efferent pathways. Normal micturition becomes impossible. However, the bladder empties reflexly when it is full (**automatic bladder**).
>
> Lesion of sacral segments of spinal cord or the corresponding spinal nerves (conus-cauda syndrome) results in loss of spinal reflex for bladder emptying. Urinary bladder when it is filled beyond its capacity causes dribbling of urine called as overflow incontinence (**autonomous bladder**).

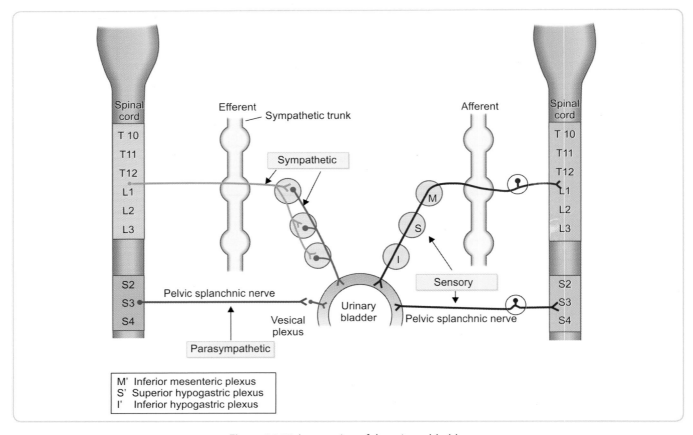

M' Inferior mesenteric plexus
S' Superior hypogastric plexus
I' Inferior hypogastric plexus

Figure 14.17: Innervation of the urinary bladder

Ureter

Autonomic nerves to the ureter are predominantly sensory in function. They are derived mainly from segments T12, L1 of the cord and also from segments S2–S4. Distension by a stone causes severe pain (incorrectly called, renal colic). This is referred to a severe, radiating pain from loin (T12) to groin (L1).

Upper Limb

The arteries of the upper limb are innervated by sympathetic nerves. The preganglionic fibres arise from T2 and T8 (vasomotor fibres mostly from T2 and T3) segments of the spinal cord. The postganglionic fibres join brachial plexus and are distributed to the arteries. The sympathetic nerves are responsible for vasoconstriction of cutaneous arteries and vasodilatation of arteries that supply skeletal muscle (Figure 14.18).

Lower Limb

The arteries of the lower limb are innervated by sympathetic nerves. The preganglionic fibres arise from

T10 to L2 segments of the spinal cord. The postganglionic fibres reach the arteries through branches of lumbar and sacral plexuses (Figure 14.19).

Clinical Anatomy

Raynaud's Disease (or Phenomenon)
In all persons, exposure to cold can cause vasoconstriction. In some persons, this response is abnormally high and vasoconstriction of arterioles in the distal part of the limb may seriously impair blood supply to the hands. In such cases, a series of events may be observed. When the hand is cooled first, there is a loss of colour (blanching) and the hand becomes pale. After an interval, the arterioles dilate and blood starts flowing into the hand, but this blood is deoxygenated (because of stagnation in arteries). The hand becomes swollen and dark. As more blood flows into the hand, the deoxygenated blood is washed off (with oxygenated blood) and the hand becomes red in colour.

Basically, the condition is caused by abnormally active sympathetic nerves. It can be controlled with drugs. In more severe cases, sympathetic denervation of blood vessels of the limb is necessary. This can be achieved by surgical removal of the upper thoracic sympathetic ganglia (**preganglionic cervicodorsal sympathectomy**). Care has to be taken not to damage the stellate ganglion or the fibres entering or leaving it; else it would result in Horner's syndrome.

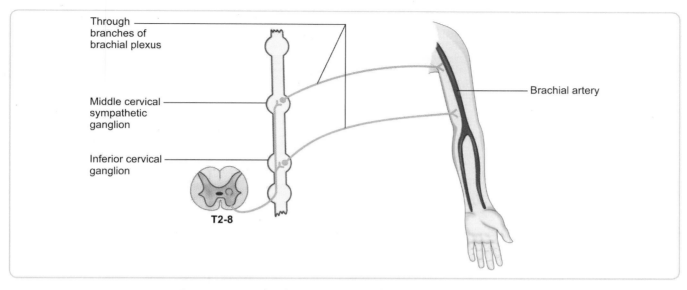

Figure 14.18: Sympathetic innervation of the arteries of upper limb

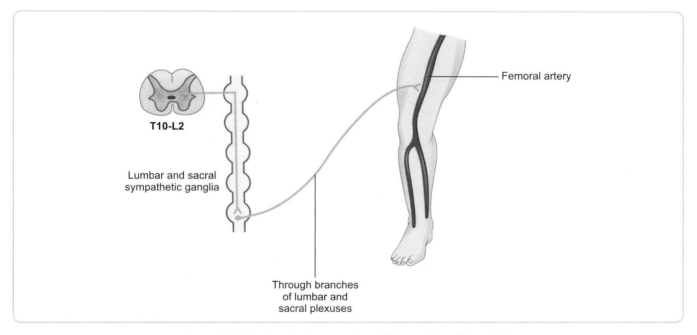

Figure 14.19: Sympathetic innervation of the arteries of lower limb

Thromboangiitis Obliterans (Buerger's Disease)
In this condition, arteries of the leg and foot are narrowed, and there is thrombophlebitis of veins. The condition is seen only in male smokers. Localized inflammatory changes are present in the walls of arteries and veins. Symptoms of arterial insufficiency are present. Gangrene of toes can occur. The condition can sometimes be controlled by complete abstinence from smoking and may benefit from lumbar sympathectomy which will result in vasodilation. Care has to be taken not to damage the first lumbar ganglion; else it would result in absence of ejaculation.

A comparison between sympathetic and parasympathetic nervous systems, and their effects on organs, have been summarized in Tables 14.3 and 14.4, respectively.

TABLE 14.3: Comparison between the sympathetic and parasympathetic nervous system

Components	Sympathetic system	Parasympathetic system
Highest modulators	Limbic region	Limbic region
Hypothalamus	Caudal	Rostral
Brain stem control	Reticular formation	Reticular formation
Supraspinal fibres	Hypothalamospinal fibres	Dorsal longitudinal fasciculus and hypothalamospinal fibres
Preganglionic neurons (connector neurons)	Intermediolateral grey column of T1 to L2	General visceral efferent nuclei of cranial nerves III, VII, IX and X and intermediolateral grey column of spinal segments S2 to S4
Preganglionic fibres	Along with ventral nerve roots of thoracolumbar nerves	Along with cranial nerves III, VII, IX, X and ventral nerve roots of sacral nerves
Myelination of preganglionic fibres	Myelinated (white ramus communicans)	Myelinated
Length of preganglionic fibres	Relatively short	Relatively long
Preganglionic neuron terminal (and receptor)/neurotransmitter	Acetylcholine (nicotinic receptor)	Acetylcholine (nicotinic receptor)
Ganglia of relay (Effector neuron)	Paravertebral and plexus along the abdominal aorta and internal iliac artery	Ciliary, pterygopalatine, submandibular, otic, cardiopulmonary plexus and in the wall of the viscera
Ratio of preganglionic fibres to neurons of ganglia	One is to many (therefore mass discharge)	One is to a few (therefore localized effect)
Postganglionic fibres	Along spinal nerves, blood vessels and visceral branches of paravertebral chain	Through branches of trigeminal in head region; and direct ganglionated branches
Myelination of postganglionic fibres	Unmyelinated	Unmyelinated
Length of postganglionic fibres	Relatively long	Relatively short
Postganglionic neuron terminal (and receptor)/neurotransmitter	Noradrenaline (α and β adrenergic receptor) and acetylcholine (muscarinic receptor to sweat gland and some blood vessels of skeletal muscle)	Acetylcholine (muscarinic receptor)
Effect	Response as in "fright-flight-fight" response	Responsible for homeostasis
Metabolism	Catabolic	Anabolic

TABLE 14.4: Response of organs to sympathetic and parasympathetic nervous system

Organs	Sympathetic system	Parasympathetic system
Eye	Dilatation of pupils and contraction of orbitalis and smooth muscles of tarsals	Constriction of pupils and ciliaris muscle for accommodation
Lacrimal gland	–	Secretion
Salivary glands	Thick, viscous secretion	Profuse, watery secretion
Heart	Increases heart rate, increases contractility	Decreases heart rate, decreases contractility
Lung	Bronchial smooth muscle relaxation	Bronchial smooth muscle contraction
Gastrointestinal tract	Decreases motility, contraction of sphincters and inhibition of secretion	Increases motility, relaxation of sphincters and stimulation of secretion
Urinary bladder	Relaxation of detrusor and contraction of involuntary sphincter vesicae	Contraction of detrusor and relaxation of involuntary sphincter vesicae
Male sex organs	Ejaculation	Erection
Skin	Contraction of arrector pili and secretion of sweat glands	–
Blood vessels	Vasoconstriction, dilation in some vessels	–

MULTIPLE CHOICE QUESTIONS

Q1. Which of the following exocrine glands gets secretomotor innervation from the sympathetic part of the autonomic nervous system?
A. Bronchial
B. Anal
C. Sweat
D. Bartholin's gland

Q2. The "stellate ganglion" is formed by the fusion of which of the following ganglia?
A. Middle and inferior cervical
B. Inferior cervical and first thoracic
C. First and second thoracic
D. Second and third thoracic

Q3. The usual number of pairs of thoracic ganglia is:
A. 8
B. 9
C. 10
D. 11

Q4. The white rami communicantes contain fibres from:
A. Paravertebral sympathetic ganglia to spinal nerves
B. Paravertebral sympathetic ganglia to viscera
C. Spinal cord to paravertebral sympathetic ganglia
D. Viscera to paravertebral sympathetic ganglia

Q5. The grey rami communicates entering the spinal nerves function as:
A. Vasomotor
B. Pilomotor
C. Sudomotor
D. All of the above

Q6. The internal carotid nerve is a branch of:
A. Vagus
B. Glossopharyngeal
C. Superior cervical ganglion
D. Stellate ganglion

Q7. Which of the following autonomic nerve plexuses is situated near the bifurcation of the abdominal aorta?
A. Superior hypogastric
B. Inferior hypogastric
C. Superior mesenteric
D. Inferior mesenteric

Q8. The control of the parasympathetic part of the autonomic nervous system is which part of hypothalamus?
A. Caudal
B. Lateral
C. Medial
D. Rostral

Q9. Where are the cell bodies that convey painful impulses from the heart located?
A. Ganglia located in cardiac plexus
B. Upper thoracic dorsal root ganglia
C. Substantia gelatinosa of thoracic spinal cord
D. Upper thoracic sympathetic ganglia

Q10. The receptors of postganglionic autonomic nerve endings at sudoriferous glands are:
A. Muscarinic
B. Nicotinic
C. α adrenergic
D. β adrenergic

ANSWERS

1. C	2. B	3. D	4. C	5. D	6. C	7. A	8. D	9. B	10. A

SHORT NOTES

1. Autonomic ganglia
2. Sacral outflow of parasympathetic system
3. Horner's syndrome
4. Automatic bladder
5. Autonomous bladder
6. Autonomic innervation of salivary glands

LONG QUESTIONS

1. Describe the enteric nervous system.
2. Parasympathetic nervous system.
3. Sympathetic nervous system.
4. Differentiate between sympathetic and parasympathetic systems.

Clinical Cases

14.1: A patient presents with history of sudden exposure to cold resulting in cold fingers, pain, numbness and change in colour of skin, suggesting extreme vasospasm of the upper limb. A diagnosis of Raynaud's disease is made and surgery is planned.
   A. Surgical sympathectomy should be done at which level? Why?
   B. In vasospasm of lower limb, if surgery is planned, surgical removal of sympathetic trunk should include which ganglia?

14.2: The peristaltic movement of the gut is retained even after autonomic denervation. Explain.

14.3: A patient suffering from syphilis on examination is found to have a fixed constricted pupil not reacting to light but contracting with accommodation.
   A. What is this condition known as?
   B. Which are the fibres affected in this patient?

Chapter 15 | Ventricles of the Brain and CSF Circulation

Specific Learning Objectives

At the end of learning, the student shall be able to:
➢ Describe the features of lateral, third and fourth ventricles
➢ Describe the circulation of cerebrospinal fluid (CSF) and the blood-CSF barrier
➢ Describe the relevant clinical anatomy

INTRODUCTION

The interior of the brain contains a series of cavities (Figure 15.1). The cerebrum contains a median cavity, the **third ventricle,** and two **lateral ventricles**, one in each hemisphere. Each lateral ventricle opens into the third ventricle through an **interventricular foramen**.

The third ventricle is continuous caudally with the **cerebral aqueduct,** which traverses the midbrain and opens into the fourth ventricle.

The **fourth ventricle** is situated dorsal to the pons and medulla and ventral to the cerebellum. It communicates inferiorly, with the **central canal,** which traverses the lower part of the medulla and the spinal cord. The entire ventricular system is lined by an epithelial layer called the **ependyma.**

LATERAL VENTRICLES

The lateral ventricles are two cavities, one situated within the telencephalic part of each cerebral hemisphere. Each ventricle is a C-shaped cavity, consisting of **four parts**, i.e. a **central part (body)**, in the parietal lobe, from which three extensions are given off-one each in the frontal, occipital and temporal lobes, called the **anterior, posterior** and **inferior horns** (Figure 15.2). The **atrium (trigone)** of the lateral ventricle is the site of confluence of the body, posterior and inferior horns. It is the most dilated part of the lateral ventricle.

Central Part

The central part of the lateral ventricle is elongated anteroposteriorly. Anteriorly, it becomes continuous

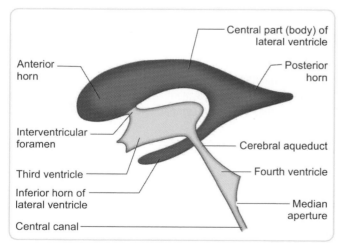

Figure 15.1: Ventricular system of the brain seen from the lateral side

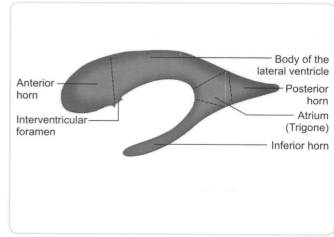

Figure 15.2: Parts of the lateral ventricle

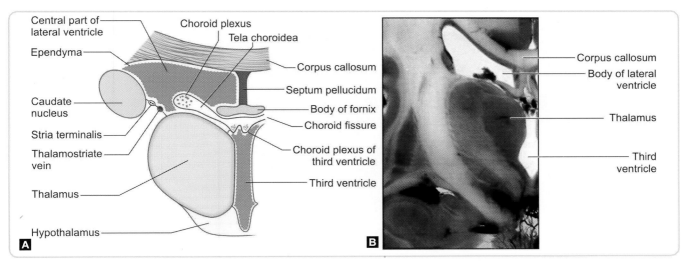

Figures 15.3A and B: (A) Boundaries of the central part of the lateral ventricle and of the third ventricle (Note the relationship of the tela choroidea and the choroid plexuses to these ventricles); (B) Plastinated coronal section specimen of the brain

with the anterior horn at the level of the interventricular foramen. Posteriorly, the central part reaches the splenium of the corpus callosum.

The central part is triangular in cross section (Figures 15.3A and B). It has a roof, a floor, and a medial wall. The roof and floor meet on the lateral side. The **roof** is formed by the trunk of the corpus callosum. The **medial wall** is formed by the septum pellucidum and by the body of the fornix. It is common to the two lateral ventricles. The **floor** is formed mainly by the superior surface of the thalamus, medially and by the caudate nucleus, laterally. Between these two structures, there are the stria terminalis, laterally and the thalamostriate vein, medially. There is a space between the fornix and the upper surface of the thalamus (Figure 15.4). This is the **choroid fissure** which is "C" shaped. The inferior part of choroid fissure is bounded by tail of caudate nucleus above and by fimbria and hippocampal gyrus below.

Anterior Horn

The anterior horn of the lateral ventricle lies anterior to its central part; the two being separated by an imaginary vertical line drawn at the level of the interventricular foramen (Figure 15.1). This horn is triangular in section. It has a roof, a floor, and a medial wall (Figures 15.5 and 15.6). It is closed anteriorly by the genu and rostrum of the corpus callosum.

The **roof** is formed by the most anterior part of the trunk of the corpus callosum. The floor is formed mainly by the head of the caudate nucleus. A small part of the

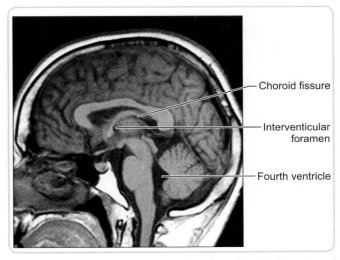

Figure 15.4: Magnetic resonance imaging of sagittal section of brain showing interventricular foramen (*Courtesy:* Dr HD Deshmukh, Professor and Head, Department of Radiology, Seth GS Medical College and KEM Hospital, Mumbai)

floor, near the middle line, is formed by the upper surface of the rostrum of the corpus callosum. The **medial wall** (common to the two sides) is formed by the septum pellucidum. It may be noted that the tela choroidea and the choroid plexus **do not** extend into the anterior horn.

Posterior Horn

The posterior horn of the lateral ventricle extends backwards into the occipital lobe. It has a roof, a lateral wall, and a medial wall (Figures 15.7A and B).

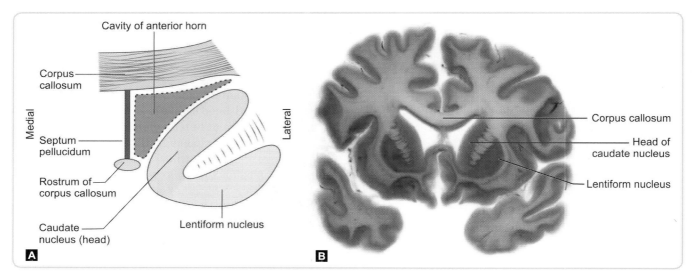

Figures 15.5A and B: (A) Boundaries of the anterior horn of the lateral ventricle; (B) Plastinated specimen of the brain showing anterior horns of lateral ventricles in a coronal section

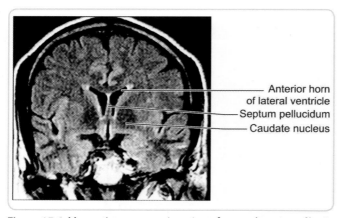

Figure 15.6: Magnetic resonance imaging of coronal section of brain showing anterior horn of lateral ventricle (*Courtesy:* Dr HD Deshmukh, Professor and Head, Department of Radiology, Seth GS Medical College and KEM Hospital, Mumbai)

The **roof** and **lateral wall** are formed by the tapetum (a sheet of fibres from the splenium of the corpus callosum). The **medial wall** shows two elevations. The uppermost of these is the **bulb of the posterior horn**, which is produced by fibres of the forceps major, as they run backwards from the splenium of the corpus callosum. The lower elevation is called the **calcar avis**. It represents white matter "**pushed in**" by formation of the calcarine sulcus.

Inferior Horn

The inferior horn of the lateral ventricle begins at the posterior end of the central part. It runs downwards and forwards into the temporal lobe, its anterior end reaching close to the uncus.

In considering the structures to be seen in the walls of the inferior horn, it is useful to note that the anterior horn, the central part, and the inferior horn form one continuous C-shaped cavity. From Figure 15.1, it will be obvious that the floor of the central part of the ventricle is continuous with the roof of the inferior horn. It is also useful to recall that the body of the fornix divides posteriorly into two crura, which become continuous with the fimbriae and hippocampi.

In the central part of the ventricle, the choroid fissure lies below the fornix. When traced into the inferior horn, the fissure lies **above** the fimbria and hippocampus. The choroid plexus extends into the inferior horn through the choroid fissure.

In cross section, the inferior horn is seen to be a narrow cavity (Figures 15.8A and B). The cavity is bounded above and laterally by the **roof** and below and medially by the **floor.** Because of this orientation, the lateral part of the roof is sometimes called the **lateral wall** and the medial part of the floor, the **medial wall.**

The lateral part of the roof is formed by fibres of the tapetum. The medial part of the roof is formed by the tail of the caudate nucleus, laterally and the stria terminalis, medially. These structures are continued into the roof of the inferior horn from the floor of the central part. Anteriorly, the tail of the caudate nucleus and the stria terminalis end in relation to the amygdaloid complex, which lies in the most anterior part of the roof.

The floor of the inferior horn is formed mainly by the hippocampus (Figures 15.8 and 15.9). The fibres of hippocampus form a thin sheet of white matter called **alveus** that covers its ventricular surface. The fibres of

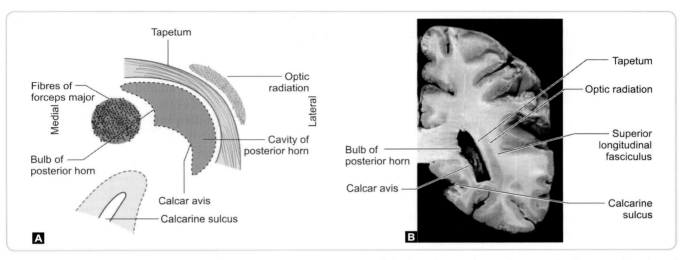

Figures 15.7A and B: (A) Coronal section passing through posterior horn of the lateral ventricle; (B) Photograph of a coronal section of the brain through left posterior horn, viewed from the anterior aspect

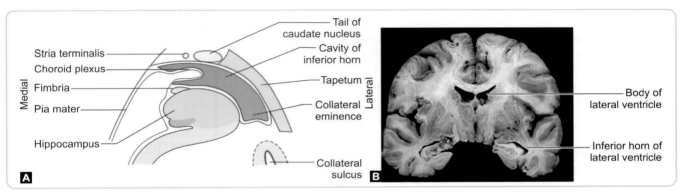

Figures 15.8A and B: (A) Boundaries of the inferior horn of the lateral ventricle (coronal section); (B) Photograph of the coronal section of brain showing the body and inferior horn of lateral ventricle

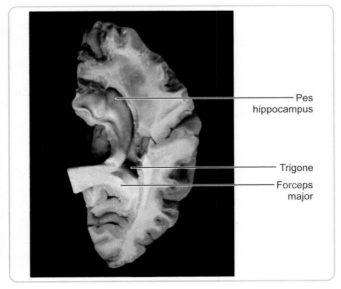

Figure 15.9: Photograph of the right inferior horn of the lateral ventricle viewed from above in a dissected brain

alveus converge medially to form a ridge called **fimbria.** In the lateral part of the floor, there is an elevation, the **collateral eminence**, produced by inward bulging of the white matter by the collateral sulcus.

Communications

Each lateral ventricle communicates with the third ventricle through the interventricular foramen (of Monro). Interventricular foramen is bounded by the column of fornix anteriorly and by the anterior end of thalamus posteriorly (Figures 15.4 and 15.10).

Choroid Plexus

The choroid plexus of third ventricle formed by medial and lateral posterior choroidal arteries extends into the central part of each lateral ventricle through the upper part of choroid fissure. The choroid plexus of inferior horn of lateral ventricle is formed by the branches of anterior choroidal artery which enters through the inferior part of choroid fissure. In the trigone, the choroid plexus is formed by the anastomoses of anterior and posterior choroidal arteries.

THIRD VENTRICLE

The third ventricle is the cavity of the diencephalon. It is a median cavity situated between the right and left thalami.

Boundaries

The third ventricle has an anterior wall, a posterior wall, two lateral walls, floor, and roof.

Each **lateral wall** is marked by the **hypothalamic sulcus** (Figure 15.10), which follows a curved course from the interventricular foramen to the aqueduct. Above the sulcus, the wall is formed by the medial surface of the thalamus. The two thalami are usually connected by a band of grey matter called the **interthalamic adhesion,** which passes through the ventricle. The lateral wall, below the hypothalamic sulcus, is formed by the medial surface of the hypothalamus. A small part of the lateral wall, above and behind the thalamus, is formed by the epithalamus.

The interventricular foramen is seen on the lateral wall, just behind the column of the fornix.

The **anterior wall** of the third ventricle is formed mainly by the lamina terminalis. Its upper part is formed by the anterior commissure and columns of the fornix, as they diverge from each other.

The **posterior wall** is formed by the epithalamus consisting of the pineal body, posterior commissure and the habenular commissure.

The **floor** is formed by the optic chiasma, tuber cinereum, infundibulum, mamillary bodies, posterior perforated substance, and the tegmentum of the midbrain.

The **roof** of the ventricle is formed by the ependyma that stretches across the two thalami (Figure 15.3). Above the ependyma, there is the tela choroidea. Within the tela choroidea, there are two plexuses of blood vessels (one on either side of the middle line), which bulge downwards into the cavity of the third ventricle. These are the choroid plexuses of the third ventricle (Figure 15.11).

Communications

The cavity of third ventricle communicates on either side with the lateral ventricle through the interventricular foramen (Figures 15.1 and 15.4). Posteriorly, it continues

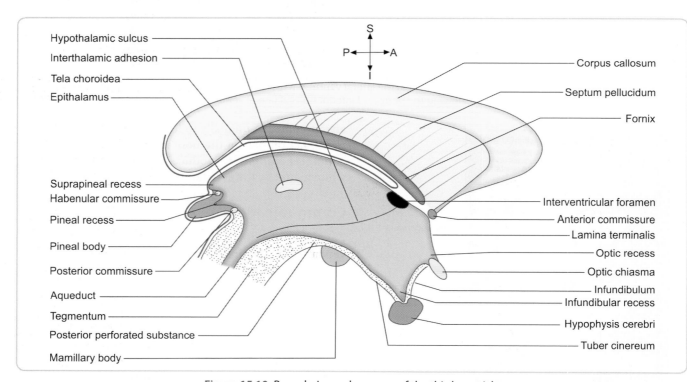

Figure 15.10: Boundaries and recesses of the third ventricle

into the cerebral aqueduct, which connects it to the fourth ventricle.

Extensions

The cavity of the third ventricle shows a number of prolongations or recesses (Figure 15.10). The **infundibular recess** extends into the infundibulum. The **optic recess** lies just above the optic chiasma. The **pineal recess** lies between the superior and inferior laminae of the stalk of the pineal body. The **suprapineal recess** lies above the pineal body in relation to the epithalamus.

Choroid Plexus

The choroid plexus of the third ventricle is formed by the medial and lateral posterior choroidal branches of posterior cerebral artery.

FOURTH VENTRICLE

Fourth ventricle is the cavity of rhombencephalon. Ventrally, it is related to the pons and the medulla and dorsally, it is related to the cerebellum.

The upper part of the ventricle is related to the **superior (or anterior) medullary velum** (Figure 15.12). When traced inferiorly (and posteriorly), the velum merges into the white matter of the cerebellum. The lower part of the ventricle is related to the nodule (Figure 15.12). It will be recalled that the nodule forms the anterior-most part of the inferior vermis. Immediately lateral to the nodule, there is the tonsil of the cerebellum. If the tonsil is lifted away, the nodule is seen to be continuous laterally with a membrane called the **inferior (or posterior) medullary velum** (Figure 15.13). Posteriorly, the inferior velum merges into the white matter of the cerebellum. The inferior medullary velum has a thickened free edge, which connects the nodule to the flocculus. This edge is the peduncle of the flocculus. In the intact brain, this peduncle is very near the

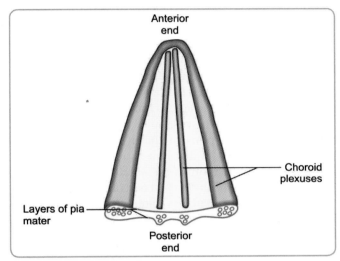

Figure 15.11: Schematic diagram of the tela choroidea removed and viewed from above

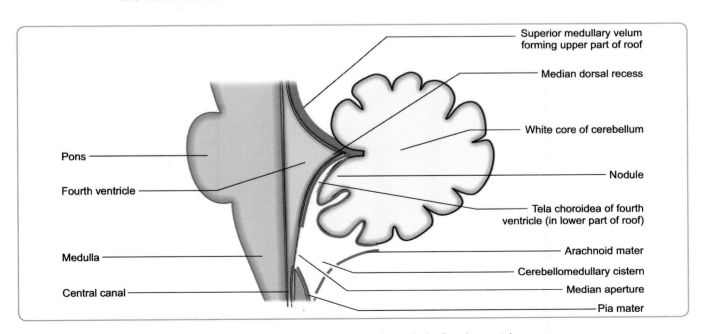

Figure 15.12: Sagittal section passing through the fourth ventricle

posterior surface of the medulla and is separated from the inferior cerebellar peduncle only by a narrow interval.

Boundaries

The cavity of fourth ventricle is bounded by a floor, a roof, and lateral walls.

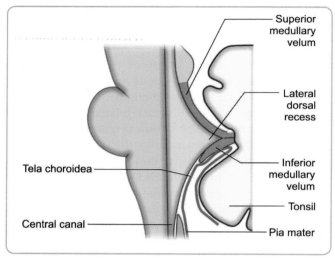

Figure 15.13: Parasagittal section passing through the fourth ventricle lateral to the nodule

Floor

Because of its shape, the floor of the fourth ventricle is often called the **rhomboid fossa** (Figure 15.14). It is divisible into an upper triangular part formed by the posterior surface of the pons, a lower triangular part formed by the upper part of the posterior surface of the medulla, and an intermediate part at the junction of the medulla and pons. The intermediate part is prolonged laterally over the inferior cerebellar peduncle as the floor of the lateral recess. Its surface is marked by the presence of delicate bundles of transversely running fibres. These bundles are the **striae medullares.**

The entire floor is divided into right and left halves by a **median sulcus.** On either side of the median sulcus, there is a longitudinal elevation called the **medial eminence.** The eminence is bounded laterally by the **sulcus limitans.** The region lateral to the sulcus limitans is the **vestibular area,** which overlies the vestibular nuclei. The vestibular area lies partly in the pons and partly in the medulla.

The pontine part of the floor shows some features of interest in close relation to the sulcus limitans and the medial eminence. The uppermost part of the sulcus limitans overlies an area that is bluish in colour and is called the **locus coeruleus.** Deep to the locus coeruleus, there is the nucleus

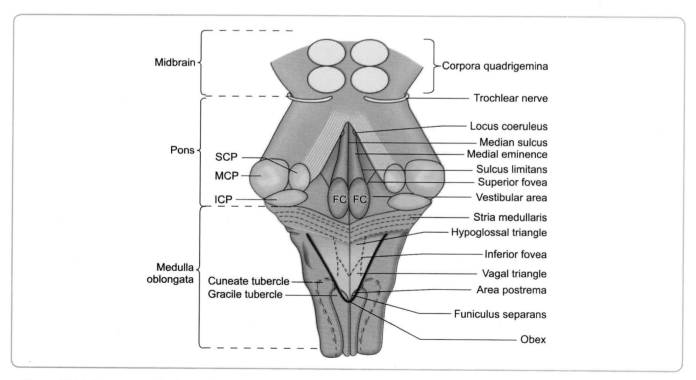

Figure 15.14: Structures in the floor of the fourth ventricle (*Abbreviations:* SCP, superior cerebellar peduncle; MCP, middle cerebellar peduncle; ICP, inferior cerebellar peduncle; FC, facial colliculus)

coeruleus, which extends upwards into the tegmentum of the midbrain. It is regarded as part of the reticular formation.

Somewhat lower down, the sulcus limitans is marked by a depression, the **superior fovea.** At this level, the medial eminence shows a swelling, the **facial colliculus,** deep to which are the abducent nucleus and the internal genu of the facial nerve.

The medullary part of the floor also shows some features of interest in relation to the medial eminence and the sulcus limitans. The sulcus limitans is marked by a depression, the **inferior fovea.** Descending from the fovea, there is a sulcus that runs obliquely towards the middle line. This sulcus divides the medial eminence into two triangles. These are the **hypoglossal triangle**, medially and the **vagal triangle,** laterally. The hypoglossal nucleus lies deep to the hypoglossal triangle and the dorsal vagal nucleus lies deep to the vagal triangle. Between the vagal triangle (above) and the gracile tubercle (below), there is a small area called the **area postrema.** The lower part of the floor of the fourth ventricle is called the **calamus scriptorius,** because of its resemblance to a nib of a pen. Each inferolateral margin of the ventricle is marked by a narrow white ridge or **taenia.** The right and left taeniae meet at the inferior angle of the floor to form a small fold called the **obex.** The term obex is often used to denote the inferior angle itself.

Roof

The roof of the fourth ventricle is tent-shaped and can be divided into upper and lower parts, which meet at an apex (Figure 15.15). The apex extends into the white core of the cerebellum. The upper part of the roof is formed by the superior cerebellar peduncles and the superior medullary velum (Figure 15.12). The inferior part of the roof is devoid of nervous tissue in most of its extent. It is formed by a membrane consisting of ependyma and a double fold of pia mater, which constitutes the **tela choroidea of the fourth ventricle** (Figure 15.15). Laterally, on each side, this membrane reaches and fuses with the inferior cerebellar peduncles. The lower part of the membrane has a large aperture in it. This is the **median aperture** of the fourth ventricle through which the ventricle communicates with the subarachnoid space in the region of the cerebellomedullary cistern. In the region of the lateral recess, the membrane is prolonged laterally and helps form the wall of the recess. The inferior medullary velum forms a small part of the roof in the region of the lateral dorsal recess (Figure 15.16). It may be noted that some authors describe the entire membranous structure, forming the lower part of the roof of the fourth ventricle,

as the inferior medullary velum. The nodule is intimately related to the roof of the ventricle in the region of the median dorsal recess.

Lateral Walls

The upper part of each lateral wall is formed by the superior cerebellar peduncle (Figure 15.15B). The lower part is formed by the inferior cerebellar peduncle and by the gracile and cuneate tubercles (Figures 15.15C and D).

Communications

The cavity of the ventricle is continuous inferiorly with the central canal and superiorly with the cerebral aqueduct. It communicates with the subarachnoid space through three apertures, one median (foramen of Magendie) and two lateral (Figure 15.15). The median opening is a large opening in the lower part of the roof. Through this midline opening, it communicates with the cerebellomedullary cistern. Two lateral openings (foramina of Luschka), one on each side, lie in the lateral angle of the ventricle between the inferior cerebellar peduncle and flocculus. Through this opening, the cerebrospinal fluid (CSF) escapes into the subarachnoid space. The choroid plexus of the fourth ventricle also protrudes through this opening.

Extensions

A number of extensions from the main cavity are described in Figure 15.16. The largest of these are two **lateral recesses,** one on either side. Each lateral recess passes laterally in the interval between the inferior cerebellar peduncle, ventrally and the peduncle of the flocculus, dorsally (Figure 15.15). The lateral extremity of the recess reaches the flocculus. At this extremity, the recess opens into the subarachnoid space as the **lateral aperture.** Another recess present in the midline is called the **median dorsal recess.** It extends into the white core of the cerebellum and lies just cranial to the nodule (Figures 15.12 and 15.13). Immediately lateral to the nodule, another recess projects dorsally, on either side, above the inferior medullary velum. These are the **lateral dorsal recesses** (Figures 15.13 and 15.16).

Choroid Plexuses of the Fourth Ventricle

The **choroid plexuses of the fourth ventricle** are similar in structure to those of the lateral and third ventricles. Each plexus (right or left) consists of a vertical limb lying next to the midline and a horizontal limb extending into

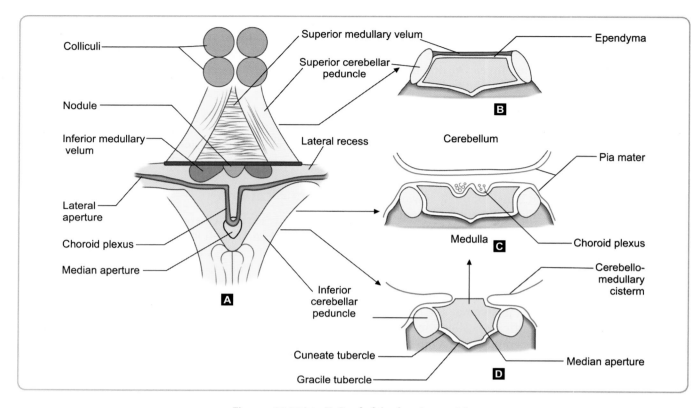

Figures 15.15A to D: Roof of the fourth ventricle

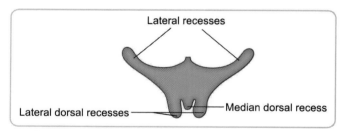

Figure 15.16: Various recesses of the cavity of the fourth ventricle

- The **area postrema** in the floor of fourth ventricle is the site of the vomiting centre.
- **Tumours** (medulloblastomas) are common near the roof of the fourth ventricle which may block the median aperture and lateral apertures and may result in hydrocephalus.
- In **Arnold-Chiari malformation**, the medulla and the tonsils of the cerebellum herniate through the foramen magnum and come to lie in the vertebral canal. Apertures in the roof of the fourth ventricle are blocked, leading to obstruction to flow of CSF and internal hydrocephalus. Cranial nerves arising from the medulla are stretched. This is a congenital anomaly. It is often associated with syringomyelia.

the lateral recess. The vertical limbs of the two plexuses lie side by side, so that the whole structure is T-shaped (Figure 15.15). The lower ends of the vertical limbs reach the median aperture and project into the subarachnoid space through it. The lateral ends of the horizontal limbs reach the lateral apertures and can be seen on the surface of the brain, near the flocculus. This choroid plexus is formed by posterior inferior cerebellar artery.

CEREBROSPINAL FLUID

The CSF fills the ventricles of the brain and the central canal of the spinal cord and extends into the subarachnoid space.

Site of Production

The choroid plexuses are highly vascular structures that are responsible for the formation of CSF. The surface of each plexus is lined by a membrane formed by fusion of the ventricular ependyma with the pia mater of the tela choroidea. Deep to this membrane, there is a plexus of blood vessels.

Circulation of Cerebrospinal Fluid

The CSF formed in each lateral ventricle flows into the third ventricle through the interventricular foramen (Figure 15.17). From the third ventricle, it passes through the aqueduct into the fourth ventricle. From the fourth ventricle, the CSF flows through the central canal of the medulla and the central canal of the spinal cord and reaches the terminal ventricle. From the terminal ventricle, it ascends up to reach the fourth ventricle again. Here, it passes through the median and lateral apertures in the roof of this ventricle to enter the part of the subarachnoid space, which forms the cerebellomedullary cistern. From here, the fluid enters other parts of the subarachnoid space, including the spinal subarachnoid space. In passing from the posterior cranial fossa into the upper (supratentorial) part of the cranial cavity, the CSF traverses the narrow interval between the free margin of the tentorium cerebelli and the brainstem. It leaves the subarachnoid space by entering the venous sinuses through arachnoid villi (Figure 15.17). The route of CSF circulation is given in the form of a flow chart in Flowchart 15.1.

Characteristic Features of Cerebrospinal Fluid

- The total volume of CSF is about 140 ml of which about 25 ml is in the ventricles. Daily production of CSF is around 500 ml; this indicates that the CSF is constantly replaced.
- The normal pressure in supine position in lumbar subarachnoid space is 50–200 mm of water and in sitting position 200–250 mm of water.
- Its specific gravity ranges from 1.003 to 1.008.
- Glucose level is half of that of blood (40–60 mg%).
- Protein content is very low compared to plasma proteins (20–40 mg%) (Table 15.1).

TABLE 15.1: Comparison of the composition of CSF and blood plasma

Substance	CSF	Plasma
Protein	20–40 mg%	600 mg%
Glucose	40–60 mg%	100 mg%
Chloride	120 mEq/l	100 mEq/l
Calcium	2.5 mEq/l	4.5 mEq/l

Abbreviation: CSF, cerebrospinal fluid

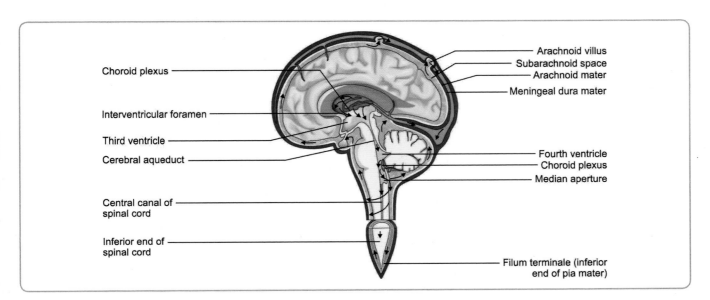

Figure 15.17: Circulation of cerebrospinal fluid

Flowchart 15.1: Route of cerebrospinal fluid (CSF) circulation

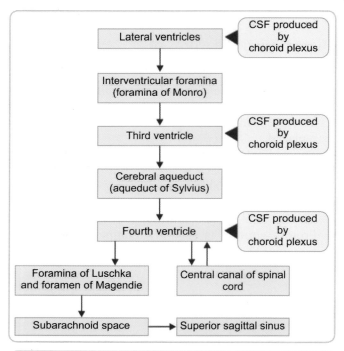

BLOOD-CEREBROSPINAL FLUID BARRIER

The tight junctions of the ependyma and other tissues of the choroid plexuses form an effective barrier between the blood and the CSF.

Blood-CSF barrier (Figure 15.18) is formed by:

- Capillary endothelium
- Basement membrane of capillary endothelium
- Basement membrane of ependymal cells
- Ependyma

This blood-CSF barrier allows selective passage of substances from blood to CSF, but not in the reverse direction. The arachnoid villi provide a valvular mechanism for flow of CSF into blood, without permitting back-flow of blood into the CSF.

Tanycytes and Specialized Areas of Ependyma

At some isolated sites in the walls of the third and fourth ventricles, there are patches of ependyma where the ependymal cells are tall, columnar, and ciliated and possess special histochemical properties. These cells are called **tanycytes.** Some areas where these patches are found (in the human brain) are as follows:

- The **subcommissural organ,** located over the dorsal wall of the aqueduct, just behind the posterior commissure
- The **subfornical organ,** present in relation to the roof of the third ventricle, just below the body of the fornix
- The **intercolumnar tubercle** or the **organum vasculosum,** present in relation to the anterior wall of the third ventricle (in the region where the columns of the fornix diverge)
- In the floor of the fourth ventricle, the hypoglossal triangle is separated from the **area postrema** by a narrow ridge called the **funiculus separans.** This ridge and the area postrema are lined by tanycytes.

Similar areas have been identified at various other sites in other species.

The functions attributed to tanycytes are:

- Secretion of neurochemical substances into CSF
- Secretion of CSF itself
- Transport of substances from CSF to underlying neurons or blood vessels
- They may also act as chemoreceptors.

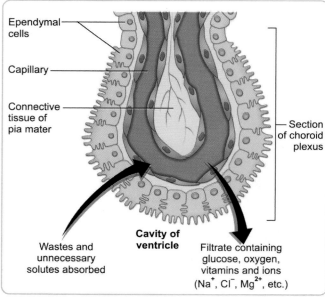

Figure 15.18: Blood-cerebrospinal fluid barrier

Functions of Cerebrospinal Fluid

The CSF provides a fluid cushion, which protects the brain from injury. It also probably helps to carry nutrition to the brain and remove waste products.

Clinical Anatomy

Lumbar Puncture
Samples of CSF are often required to assist in clinical diagnosis. They are obtained most easily by **lumbar puncture**. This procedure is explained in Chapter 2.
Cerebrospinal fluid may also be obtained by **cisternal puncture,** in which a needle is passed into the cerebellomedullary cistern. This procedure is explained in Chapter 4.

Papilloedema
The subarachnoid space extends up to the back of retina. An increased CSF pressure will result in backpressure on the retinal vessels, resulting in congestion and causing bulging of the optic disc, i.e. papilloedema.

Queckenstedt's Sign
It is positive when there is a block in the subarachnoid space. When the internal jugular vein in the neck is compressed, the cerebral venous pressure in increased and absorption of CSF is inhibited. When there is a CSF block, there is no rise in manometer reading and Queckenstedt's is said to be positive.

Hydrocephalus (Figure 15.19)
An abnormal increase in the quantity of CSF can lead to enlargement of the head in children. This condition is called **hydrocephalus.** Abnormal pressure of CSF leads to degeneration of brain tissue. Hydrocephalus may be caused by excessive production of CSF, by obstruction to its flow, or by impaired absorption through the arachnoid villi. It is classified as **obstructive or noncommunicating hydrocephalus,** when there is obstruction to flow of CSF from the ventricular system to the subarachnoid space or as **communicating hydrocephalus,** when such obstruction is not present. Obstruction is most likely to occur where CSF has to pass through narrow passages, for example, the interventricular foramina, the aqueduct, and the apertures of the fourth ventricle. In each of the above instances, dilatation is confined to cavities proximal to the obstruction. Occasionally, meningitis may lead to obstruction of the narrow interval between the tentorium cerebelli and the brainstem. Meningitis may also lead to hydrocephalus by affecting the arachnoid villi, thus, hampering the reabsorption of CSF.

Cerebrospinal Fluid and Injuries to the Skull
The skull is frequently injured by blows with a heavy object and frequently in automobile accidents. Injury can be avoided by wearing a protective helmet.
- Direct injury leading to fractures of the skull can damage any area of the brain. CSF can flow out and parts of brain can herniate out of the skull.
- Even in the absence of a fracture, direct injury can throw the brain against the opposite wall of the skull injuring it. This is contrecoup injury.
- In fractures of the base of the skull, CSF may flow into the nose. Haemorrhage may take place into brain tissue or into extradural space raising intracranial tension.

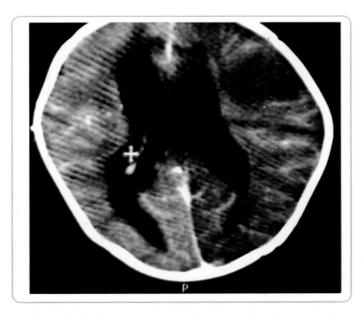

Figure 15.19: Noncommunicating hydrocephalus. The quadarrow indicates the choroid plexus. (*Courtesy:* Dr HD Deshmukh, Professor & Head, Department of Radiology, Seth GS Medical College & KEM Hospital, Mumbai.)

MULTIPLE CHOICE QUESTIONS

Q1. The lateral ventricle communicates with the third ventricle through:
A. Foramen of Magendie
B. Foramen of Luschka
C. Foramen of Monro
D. Aqueduct of Sylvius

Q2. Which of the following lobes of the cerebrum is related to the inferior horn of the lateral ventricle?
A. Frontal
B. Parietal
C. Temporal
D. Occipital

Q3. The choroid plexus of which part of lateral ventricle is formed by posterior choroidal artery?
A. Anterior horn
B. Posterior horn
C. Inferior horn
D. Central part (body)

Q4. The bulb of the posterior horn is produced by:
A. Forceps minor
B. Tapetum
C. Forceps major
D. Optic radiation

Q5. The roof of the inferior horn is formed by:
A. Optic radiation
B. Stria terminalis
C. Inferior longitudinal fasciculus
D. Body of the fornix

Q6. The anterior wall of the third ventricle is formed by:
A. Optic chiasma
B. Tuber cinereum
C. Lamina terminalis
D. Habenular commissure

Q7. The invagination of the pia mater forming the tela choroidea of the third ventricle occurs through the:
A. Median longitudinal fissure
B. Transverse fissure
C. Callosal sulcus
D. Stem of lateral sulcus

Q8. Which of the following structures forms a part of the roof of the fourth ventricle?
A. Stria medullaris
B. Facial colliculi
C. Vestibular area
D. Inferior medullary velum

Q9. Which of the following forms a part of the floor of the fourth ventricle?
A. Stria terminalis
B. Facial colliculus
C. Frenulum veli
D. Foramen of Magendie

Q10. The facial colliculus is formed by:
A. Facial nucleus with its fibres
B. Abducent nucleus with its fibres
C. Facial nucleus with fibres of abducent nerve
D. Abducent nucleus with fibres of the facial nerve

ANSWERS

| 1. C | 2. C | 3. D | 4. C | 5. B | 6. C | 7. B | 8. D | 9. B | 10. D |

SHORT NOTES

1. Specify the parts of lateral ventricle and boundaries of each part
2. Specify the boundaries of third ventricle
3. Draw and label the floor of fourth ventricle
4. Specify the arteries forming the choroid plexus of each ventricle
5. Specify the route of CSF circulation
6. Blood-CSF barrier

LONG QUESTIONS

1. Describe the lateral ventricle under the following headings: parts, boundaries of each part, communications, choroid plexus, and applied anatomy.
2. Describe the third ventricle under the following headings: boundaries, communications, choroid plexus, and applied anatomy.
3. Describe the fourth ventricle under the following headings: boundaries, communications, choroid plexus, and applied anatomy.

CLINICAL CASE

15.1: A six-month-old female child presented with herniation of cerebellum and medulla oblongata through the foramen magnum. A CT scan revealed that the lateral ventricles, third ventricle and fourth ventricle were dilated.
A. Specify the malformation that the child is suffering from.
B. Explain the anatomical basis of the enlarged ventricles.

Chapter 16 — Meninges and Blood Supply of Brain

Specific Learning Objectives

At the end of learning, the student shall be able to:
➢ Describe the meningeal coverings of brain
➢ Describe the dural venous sinuses
➢ Describe the arterial supply of brain
➢ Describe the anatomical basis of clinical syndromes due to lack of blood supply
➢ Describe the venous drainage of brain
➢ Describe the blood-brain barrier

INTRODUCTION

The brain and the spinal cord are covered by three layers of meninges; the outermost toughest layer is known as **dura mater**, the next layer is known as **arachnoid mater** and the innermost thin layer is known as **pia mater**. The dura mater, derived from mesoderm, is made up of dense fibrous tissue and hence it is also known as pachymeninx. It lines the bony cage in which the brain and the spinal cord are lodged. The arachnoid mater and the pia mater are derived from neural crest cells and are quite thin. Hence, these two inner layers are known as leptomeninges.

The space outside the dura mater in the cranial cavity is called **extradural space**. The space outside the spinal dura is called as **epidural space**. The space between the dura mater and the arachnoid mater is known as the **subdural space**. The space between the arachnoid mater and the pia mater is known as the **subarachnoid space** and the space between the pia mater and the brain is known as the **subpial space**.

MENINGES

Dura Mater

In the cranial cavity, the dura mater covering the brain almost fuses with the periosteum of the bones covering the brain so much so that it is described that the cranial dura mater has two layers, an **outer endosteal dura** and an **inner meningeal dura**. At certain places, the endosteal and the meningeal layers separate enclosing an endothelium-lined space filled with venous blood, the **dural venous sinus**. Since, the cranial dura mater fuses with the endosteal layer, there is normally **no extradural space** in the cranial cavity. Only when there is a rupture of the meningeal artery, there is collection of blood between the endosteal dura and the bone causing an **extradural haematoma.**

Specializations of Dura Mater

The cranial dura mater forms specific dural folds (Figure 16.1), which occupy major fissures on the surface of the brain. These are:
- **Falx cerebri** in the median longitudinal fissure of the cerebrum
- **Tentorium cerebelli** in the transverse fissure
- **Falx cerebelli** in the posterior cerebellar notch
- **Diaphragma sellae** bridging the interpeduncular fossa

Falx cerebri: It is a sickle-shaped dural fold present in the median longitudinal fissure of the cerebrum. It has an apex, a base, an upper convex border and a lower concave border. The apex is attached to the crista galli of the anterior cranial fossa and the base is attached to the superior surface of the tentorium cerebelli in the midline. The upper convex border is attached in front to the frontal crest, in the middle to the lips of superior sagittal sulcus and at the posterior end to the internal occipital protuberance. The lower concave border is free and lies in the floor of the median longitudinal fissure between the two cerebral hemispheres.

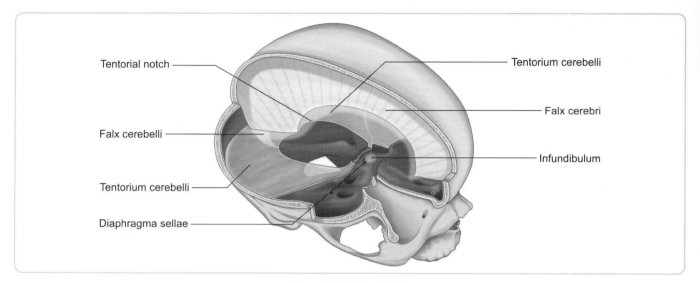

Figure 16.1: Dural folds

Venous sinuses in relation to falx cerebri:
- Superior sagittal sinus at the upper border
- Inferior sagittal sinus at the lower border
- Straight sinus at the base
- Confluence of venous sinuses (torcular herophili) at the posterior end of the base

Tentorium cerebelli: It is a semilunar-shaped fold of dura mater forming a roof over the cerebellum in the posterior cranial fossa and separates the cerebellum from the inferior surface of the occipital lobes of the cerebrum. It has a posterior attached border and an anterior free border. The posterior border is attached to the internal occipital protuberance, margins of transverse sulci, superior border of the petrous temporal bone and the posterior clinoid processes. The anterior free border forms a "U-shaped" gap called as tentorial notch through which the midbrain connects forebrain to the hindbrain. The free border crosses the anterior end of the attached border and anchors to the anterior clinoid processes.

Venous sinuses in relation to tentorium cerebelli:
- Right and left transverse sinuses at the posterior border
- Superior petrosal sinuses at the anterolateral part of attached border
- Straight sinus at the superior surface
- Confluence of venous sinuses at the posterior midline

Clinical Anatomy

Herniation of brain: A **mass effect** such as brain tumour, extradural or subdural haematoma, or abscesses in the supratentorial space can push the cerebrum beneath the falx cerebri (**subfalcine herniation**) to the opposite side.

If the pressure remains unabated or when there is a sudden drop in the pressure in subtentorial space, the uncus in the temporal lobe can be pushed beneath the tentorial notch (**uncal herniation**). This will also irritate and compress the oculomotor nerve, hence pupillary changes will be observed. A sudden uncal herniation can compress the brainstem vital centres and may result in death.

Further pressure can cause the tonsils of the cerebellum to herniate through foramen magnum (**tonsillar herniation**). This may obstruct the flow of ventricular fluid to the subarachnoid space and also compress the vertebral and/or the spinal arteries.

Falx cerebelli: It is a small sickle-shaped dural fold presents in the posterior cerebellar notch between the two cerebellar hemispheres. The apex is attached to the vermian fossa at the foramen magnum. The base is attached to the inferior surface of the tentorium cerebelli in the midline. The anterior border is concave and free. The posterior convex border is attached to the internal occipital crest.

Venous sinuses in relation to falx cerebelli:
- Occipital sinus between the two layers
- Confluence of sinuses at the base

Diaphragma sellae: It is a quadrangular sheet of dura mater, which stretches across the sella turcica. Its anterior ends are attached to the anterior clinoid processes and its posterior ends are attached to the posterior clinoid processes. It is pierced by the infundibular stalk of the pituitary gland.

Venous sinuses in relation to diaphragma sellae:
- Anterior intercavernous sinus at its anterior border
- Posterior intercavernous sinus at its posterior border

Nerve Supply of Dura Mater

The dura mater of anterior cranial fossa is supplied by branches of ophthalmic division of trigeminal nerve. The dura of middle cranial fossa is supplied by branches of maxillary and mandibular divisions of trigeminal nerve. The dura of posterior cranial fossa is supplied by upper three cervical nerves in the infratentorial part.

Clinical Anatomy

Headache as referred pain: Any inflammation/infection in the dura supplied by ophthalmic division of trigeminal nerve can manifest as a referred pain in the forehead.
Similarly, since the dura of the posterior cranial fossa is supplied by cervical nerves, any inflammation can manifest as occipital headache.

Blood Supply of Dura Mater

The dura mater of the anterior cranial fossa is supplied by meningeal branches of ophthalmic artery. The dura of the middle cranial fossa is supplied by the middle meningeal artery. The dura of the posterior cranial fossa is supplied by a branch of the occipital artery and the meningeal branch of ascending pharyngeal artery.

Clinical Anatomy

Extradural haematoma: In a case of head injury, if there is a tear of the middle meningeal artery, it results in bleeding in the space between the endosteal dura and the skull bone resulting in an extradural haematoma. The bleeding site is usually at pterion (a site where frontal, parietal, temporal and sphenoid bones meet). An initial spell of unconsciousness (due to cerebral concussion) may be interrupted by a lucid interval before the terminal unconsciousness (due to cerebral compression). A burr hole at the pterion to ligate the middle meningeal artery will arrest the bleed.

Dural Venous Sinuses

Dural venous sinuses are specialized veins that drain blood from the brain and cranium. They lie between the endosteal dura and meningeal dura, (some are between two layers of meningeal dura), e.g. inferior sagittal sinus. Like any veins, they are lined by endothelium but have no valves, and their walls are devoid of muscular tissue (no tunica media). They communicate with extracranial veins through numerous emissary veins.

Clinical Anatomy

Venous sinus thrombosis: Superior sagittal sinus communicates with veins in the loose areolar tissue of the scalp through parietal emissary foramina. So, infection from scalp in the loose areolar tissue (**dangerous area of scalp**) can result in superior sagittal sinus thrombosis.
Infections from the **dangerous area of face** (lower nose and upper lip) spread through ophthalmic veins and pterygoid venous plexus (via deep facial vein). Ophthalmic veins drain into cavernous sinus and pterygoid venous plexus communicates with cavernous sinus via emissary veins through foramen ovale. Both can cause **cavernous sinus thrombosis.**

The dural venous sinuses may be classified into a **posterosuperior** group and an **anteroinferior** group. The **posterosuperior group** includes (Figure 16.2):
- Superior sagittal
- Inferior sagittal
- Straight
- Transverse
- Occipital sinuses
- Confluence of sinuses (torcular herophili)

The **anteroinferior group** includes (Figure 16.3):
- Sigmoid
- Cavernous
- Sphenoparietal
- Superior petrosal
- Inferior petrosal
- Anterior and posterior intercavernous

Although, the sinuses are valveless and allow bidirectional flow of blood, if the need arises, blood

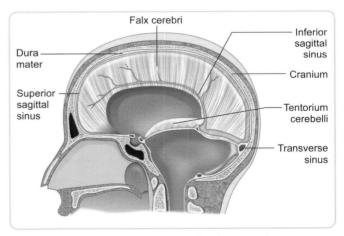

Figure 16.2: Posterosuperior dural venous sinuses

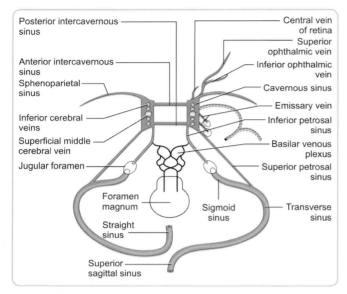

Figure 16.3: Anteroinferior dural venous sinuses

flows predominantly through them only in one direction. Flowchart 16.1 shows the direction of flow of blood in them. Confluence of sinuses (torcular herophili) and intercavernous sinuses allow blood flow through them only to equalize the pressure on both right and left sides.

Extradural Space

This is the space between the dura mater and the surrounding bone. In the cranial cavity, since the meningeal dura fuses with the endosteal dura and endosteal dura to the bone, this space is nonexistent, physiologically.

Subdural Space

This is a capillary space between the dura mater and the arachnoid mater.

> **Clinical Anatomy**
>
> **Subdural haematoma**: In a case of head injury, if there is tear of the cerebral veins or the dural venous sinuses, it results in bleeding deep to the dura mater and causes subdural haematoma. Subdural haematoma compresses upon the brain rapidly, hence there is no lucid interval (unlike extradural haematoma).

Arachnoid Mater

It is a thin membrane present deep to the dura mater covering the entire surface of the brain. Between this and the underlying pia mater there are delicate processes, which connect the two layers. The adhesions look like cobweb and hence the name for this membrane is arachnoid (arachnoid means "spider") membrane.

Flowchart 16.1: Direction of flow of blood

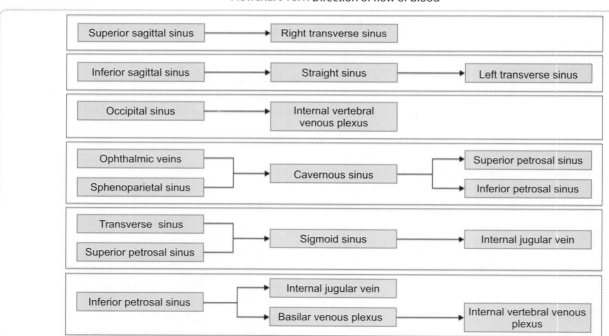

Specializations of Arachnoid Mater

Arachnoid membrane in the region of dural venous sinuses modifies into small finger-like projections called as **arachnoid villi**, which protrude into the sinus. Many such villi are grouped together and are known as **arachnoidal granulations.** Cerebrospinal fluid (CSF) produced in the ventricles circulates and reaches the subarachnoid space through the foramina in the roof of fourth ventricle. 75% of the CSF then ascends up and drains through the arachnoid villi into the superior sagittal sinus.

Clinical Anatomy

Monro-Kellie doctrine: The Monro-Kellie doctrine states that the cranial compartment is incompressible. The volume inside the cranium is fixed. The constituents of the compartment (i.e. blood, CSF and brain) are such that **any increase in volume of one will be compensated by a decrease in volume of another.**

Any generalized oedema of the brain either due to **increase in CSF production or decreased drainage** (due to superior sagittal sinus thrombosis) causes signs and symptoms of raised intracranial **pressure** (headache, vomiting and papilloedema).

Subarachnoid Space

This is a very well-developed important space between the arachnoid mater and the pia mater containing CSF. Since, the pia mater is intimately applied to the brain and the arachnoid stretches over it, there are areas where the pia and the arachnoid are widely separated and in these areas pools of CSF accumulate. These are called as subarachnoid cisterns (Figure 16.4). There are some important blood vessels present in these cisterns (Table 16.1).

Major blood vessels pass through the subarachnoid space and then give branches to the brain.

Clinical Anatomy

Cisternal puncture: Since, the spinal cord extends up to L3 vertebra in a newborn, collection of CSF for diagnostic procedure through lumbar puncture is too risky. A cisternal puncture through the suboccipital region may be chosen.

The needle is placed in the midline, and made to pass just under the occipital bone, into the cisterna magna. However, if the needle is pushed too far, it can enter the medulla oblongata. This may cause sudden respiratory arrest and death. Hence, a needle with a guard is used and the guard restricts the entry of the needle. Alternatively, the procedure must be done under fluoroscopic guidance.

TABLE 16.1: Subarachnoid cisterns

Subarachnoid cistern	Location	Blood vessel present
Interpeduncular	Base of brain—interpeduncular fossa	Circle of Willis
Cerebello-medullary (cisterna magna)	Angle between the cerebellum and medulla	Posterior inferior cerebellar artery (site for cisternal puncture)
Cisterna ambiens	Dorsal aspect of midbrain	Great cerebral vein of Galen
Basilar (pontine)	Ventral surface of pons	Basilar artery
Supracallosal	Superior surface of corpus callosum	Pericallosal branch of anterior cerebral artery
Sylvian	Over lateral sulcus	Middle cerebral artery
Lumbar	Below conus medullaris of spinal cord	No artery (site for lumbar puncture)

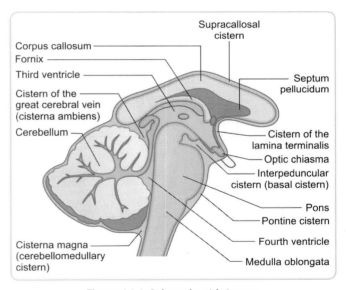

Figure 16.4: Subarachnoid cisterns

Pia Mater

Pia mater is the innermost delicate membrane, which fits each and every crevice on the surface of the brain and is closely applied to it. Arteries entering from the subarachnoid space into the brain take a sheath of pia mater with them. Along with that a sleeve of subpial space also is present around these vessels.

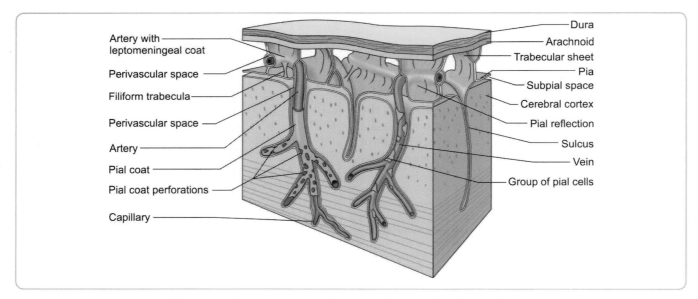

Figure 16.5: Perivascular space (Virchow-Robin space) and subpial space

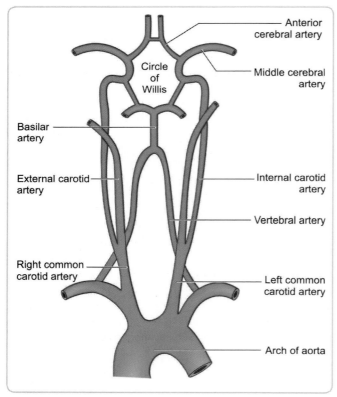

Figure 16.6: Major arteries supplying the brain

Subpial Space

This is a capillary space between the pia mater and the brain. When branches of blood vessels enter the substance of brain, they carry a sleeve of pia with them and this sleeve is closed at the proximal end by a septum effectively cutting off this perivascular space of Virchow-Robin from the subarachnoid space. As the vessels pierce the pia mater and enter the brain substance, a tube of subpial space is taken along (Figure 16.5).

ARTERIES SUPPLYING BRAIN

The brain is supplied by two sets of arteries: (1) **internal carotid** and (2) **vertebrobasilar arteries** (Figure 16.6).

Internal Carotid Arteries

Each internal carotid artery arises as one of the two terminal branches at the bifurcation of the common carotid artery in the neck at the level of C4 vertebra. The artery then ascends up in the carotid sheath and enters the cranial cavity through the carotid canal and upper part of foramen lacerum.

The course of the internal carotid artery is divisible into four parts: (1) cervical, (2) petrous, (3) cavernous and (4) cerebral.

1. **Cervical part**: This part of the artery is from its origin till it enters the carotid canal. This part lies entirely within the carotid sheath along with the internal jugular vein and the vagus nerve.

2. **Petrous part**: This part of the artery traverses the carotid canal in the petrous temporal bone.

3. **Cavernous part**: From the carotid canal, the artery enters the cavernous sinus through the upper part of the foramen lacerum. Here, the artery has a sinuous

course and is separated from the blood in the cavernous sinus by the endothelium. This part of the artery is also called as the "carotid siphon". The abducent nerve is related to the internal carotid artery closely in this course.

4. **Cerebral part**: At the anterior end of the cavernous sinus, the artery pierces the dura mater of the roof of the cavernous sinus and enters the subarachnoid space.

> **Clinical Anatomy**
>
> Trauma to the **internal carotid artery** in cavernous sinus leads to the formation of arteriovenous fistula causing pulsating exophthalmos.
> The internal carotid artery shows multiple bends, which produce S-shaped shadow called the **carotid siphon** on an angiogram. The carotid siphon helps in damping down its pulsations in the cranial cavity.

Branches of the Cerebral Part

- **Ophthalmic artery**: It supplies the orbit and its contents.
- **Anterior choroidal artery**: It runs backwards close to the optic tract and supplies the visual pathway, internal capsule and midbrain and forms the choroid plexus of the inferior horn of lateral ventricle.
- **Posterior communicating artery**: This also runs backwards and anastomoses with the posterior cerebral artery, a branch of the basilar artery.
- **Anterior cerebral artery**: This supplies the medial surface of cerebrum and upper strip of the superolateral surface except occipital lobe.
- **Middle cerebral artery**: This supplies the superolateral surface of cerebrum except occipital lobe and upper and lower strips each of the superolateral surface**.**

Vertebrobasilar Arteries

Each vertebral artery is a branch of the first part of the subclavian artery in the neck. The course of the vertebral artery is divisible into four parts: (1) cervical, (2) vertebral, (3) suboccipital, and (4) cerebral.

1. **Cervical part**: This is the part of the artery from its origin till it enters the foramen transversarium of C6 vertebra. Here, the artery lies in the scalenovertebral triangle.
2. **Vertebral part**: This is the part of the artery traversing the foramina transversaria of upper six cervical vertebrae.
3. **Suboccipital part**: This is the horizontal part of the artery lying in the suboccipital triangle.

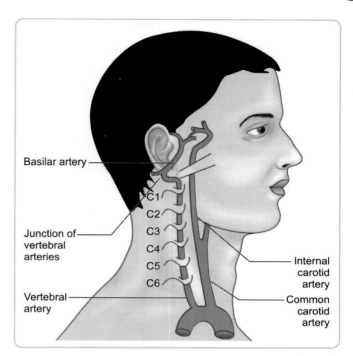

Figure 16.7: Origin and course of internal carotid and vertebral arteries

4. **Cerebral part:** The artery enters the cranial cavity by passing through the foramen magnum. It then pierces the dura mater to enter the subarachnoid space (Figure 16.7). This is the intracranial part of the artery lying in the subarachnoid space lateral to the medulla oblongata.

Branches of the Cerebral Part

- **Anterior spinal artery**: It supplies the medial part of the medulla oblongata and then fuses with the opposite anterior spinal artery and descends to supply the spinal cord.
- **Posterior spinal artery**: It descends to supply the spinal cord.
- **Posterior inferior cerebellar artery**: It supplies the dorsolateral part of the medulla oblongata, postero-inferior part of the cerebellum and the choroid plexus of the fourth ventricle.
- **Medullary branches**: These branches supply directly anterolateral part of the medulla oblongata.
- **Meningeal branches**: They supply the meninges of the posterior cranial fossa.

The two vertebral arteries ascend up and unite at the pontomedullary junction to form the basilar artery. The basilar artery runs in the basilar sulcus of the pons and at the pontomesencephalic junction divides into two posterior cerebral arteries.

Branches of Basilar Artery (Figure 16.8)

- **Anterior inferior cerebellar artery**: It supplies the anteroinferior part of the cerebellum.
- **Labyrinthine artery**: It supplies the inner ear.

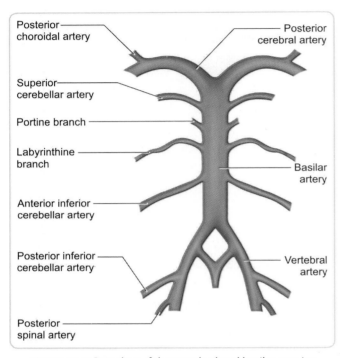

Figure 16.8: Branches of the vertebral and basilar arteries

- **Pontine branches**: These paramedian branches dip into the pons and supply the basilar part of the pons.
- **Superior cerebellar artery**: It supplies the superior surface of the cerebellum and midbrain.
- **Posterior cerebral arteries**: They supply the occipital lobes of the cerebrum, inferior surface of tentorial part of cerebrum and a lower strip of superolateral surface of cerebrum. Its posterior choroidal branches form the choroid plexus of the third ventricle and the central part of the lateral ventricle.

Circle of Willis (Circulus Arteriosus)

The circle of Willis is an arterial anastomotic circle present in the interpeduncular cistern. It is polygonal in shape and extends between the superior border of pons and median longitudinal fissure. It is closely related to the optic chiasma, tuber cinereum, mamillary bodies and posterior perforated substance. The arterial circle is an anastomosis between the internal carotid and the vertebrobasilar system of arteries (Figure 16.9).

Formation

- The **anterior communicating artery**, which connects the right and left anterior cerebral arteries and forms anterior part of the circle of Willis.
- The **anterior cerebral artery** forms the anterolateral part on each side.

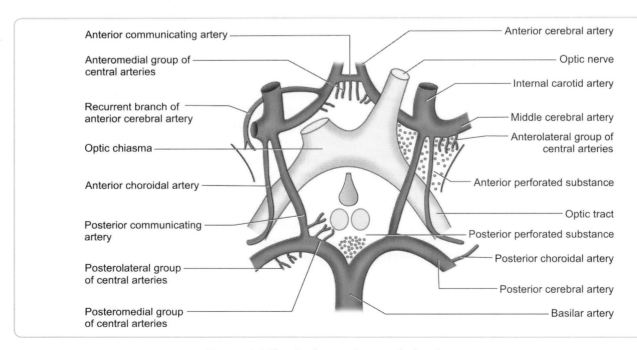

Figure 16.9: The circulus arteriosus and related structures

- The lateral part is formed by the termination of **internal carotid artery** on each side.
- Posterolaterally, the **posterior communicating artery** is the connecting link between the internal carotid and posterior cerebral arteries.

The circle is completed posteriorly by the bifurcation of basilar artery into the right and left **posterior cerebral arteries.**

> **Clinical Anatomy**
>
> **Berry aneurysm:** Berry aneurysm is a localized dilatation on one of the arteries of the circle of Willis due to congenital muscular weakness. The most common sites of berry aneurysm are the junction of anterior cerebral and anterior communicating arteries and at the bifurcation of internal carotid arteries. Rupture of berry aneurysm may cause life-threatening **subarachnoid haemorrhage.**

Functional Importance

- This arterial circle equalizes the pressure of the blood flow to the two sides of the brain, as it is the main collateral channel.
- The arterial anastomosis provides an alternative route through which blood entering the internal carotid artery or the basilar artery may be distributed to any part of the cerebral hemisphere.

Branching Pattern of the Circle of Willis

Anterior, middle and posterior cerebral arteries give origin to two types of branches:
1. Central
2. Cortical

Central branches: The central arteries arise in the region of arterial circle of Willis and are end arteries.

They pass deep into the substance of the cerebral hemisphere to supply structures within it and consist of six main groups:
1. Anteromedial
2. Posteromedial
3. Right and left anterolateral
4. Right and left posterolateral

The anteromedial group arises from the anterior cerebral and anterior communicating arteries and passes through the medial part of the anterior perforated substance.

> **Clinical Anatomy**
>
> **Recurrent artery of Heubner:** Recurrent branch of the anterior cerebral artery (also called the **artery of Heubner**) is one of the anteromedial group of arteries. It supplies the caudate nucleus, anterior limb and genu of the internal capsule. Thrombosis in the artery of Heubner results in contralateral paralysis of the face and upper extremity (**faciobrachial monoplegia**).

The arteries of the **anterolateral group** are the so-called **striate arteries** or **lenticulostriate arteries**. They arise mainly from the middle cerebral artery. Some of them arise from the anterior cerebral artery. The anterolateral group of perforating arteries enters the anterior perforated substance through its lateral part.

The anteromedial and anterolateral groups supply caudate nucleus, internal capsule and lentiform nucleus.

> **Clinical Anatomy**
>
> **Charcot's artery of cerebral haemorrhage:** One of the lateral striate arteries is usually larger than the others. It is called **Charcot's artery of cerebral haemorrhage**. Rupture of this artery, in elderly hypertensive individuals, results in loss of blood supply to internal capsule leading to contralateral spastic hemiplegia, paralysis of lower half of face and altered sensorium (due to involvement of genu and posterior limb of internal capsule).

The **posteromedial group** of central arteries arises from the posterior communicating artery and the proximal part of the posterior cerebral artery. They enter the posterior perforated substance in the interpeduncular region. They are also called as **thalamoperforators.** They supply the hypophysis, hypothalamus, anterior and medial groups of thalamic nuclei, subthalamic region and tegmentum of midbrain.

The central branches of the **posterolateral group** arise from the lateral part of the posterior cerebral artery, as it winds around the cerebral peduncle. They are also called as **thalamogeniculate arteries.** They supply the caudal half of thalamus, pulvinar, medial and lateral geniculate bodies, the lateral and the large ventral groups of thalamic nuclei.

Cortical branches: The **cortical branches** ramify on the surface of the cerebral hemispheres and supply the cortex. They give off branches that run perpendicularly into the substance of the cerebral hemisphere. Some of these are short and end within the grey matter of the cortex. Others are longer and penetrate into the subjacent white matter.

While cortical branches may anastomose with each other on the surface of the brain, the perpendicular branches (both long and short) behave as terminal or end arteries. Each branch supplies a limited area of brain tissue and does not anastomose with neighboring arteries. As a result, blockage of such a branch leads to death (necrosis) of brain tissue in the region of supply.

Anterior Cerebral Artery

This artery arises from the internal carotid artery below the anterior perforated substance and lateral to the optic chiasma. It crosses the optic chiasma to reach the median longitudinal fissure. At the anterior end of the longitudinal fissure, the anterior communicating artery connects the right and left anterior cerebral arteries. Inside the longitudinal fissure, the anterior cerebral artery winds around the genu of the corpus callosum and then runs posteriorly on the superior aspect of the body of corpus callosum.

Cortical branches (Figure 16.10):
- **Orbital branches**: Supply olfactory system and medial half of orbital surface of frontal lobe
- **Frontopolar branch**: Supplies frontal pole
- **Callosomarginal branch**: Supplies medial frontal gyrus, paracentral lobule and precuneus

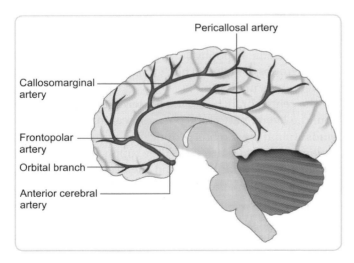

Figure 16.10: Branches of anterior cerebral artery

- **Pericallosal branch**: Supplies corpus callosum and cingulate gyrus

> **Clinical Anatomy**
>
> **Effects of occlusion of anterior cerebral artery:**
> - Paralysis (or weakness) of muscles of the leg and foot of the opposite side (by involvement of the upper part of the motor area).
> - Loss or diminution of sensations from the leg and foot of the opposite side (by involvement of the upper part of the sensory area).
> - Sense of stereognosis is impaired (by involvement of parietal lobe).
>
> Personality changes by involvement of frontal lobe usually do not occur unless there is involvement of both prefrontal cortices (one old standing lesion and one new lesion).

Middle Cerebral Artery

It is one of the terminal branches of the internal carotid artery. It turns laterally on the anterior perforated substance to enter the stem of the lateral sulcus, where it divides into four to five cortical branches.

Cortical branches (Figure 16.11):
Branches to frontal lobe:
- **Orbitofrontal branch**: Supplies lateral half of orbital surface of frontal lobe
- **Pre-Rolandic or precentral branch**: Supplies premotor area and Broca's area (in left cerebral cortex)
- **Rolandic or central branch**: Supplies primary motor cortex and primary sensory cortex

Branches to parietal lobe:
- **Anterior parietal branch**: Supplies anterior part of parietal lobe
- **Posterior parietal branch**: Supplies posterior part of parietal lobe and anastomoses with posterior cerebral artery to supply macular region of visual field of occipital lobe

Branches to temporal lobe:
- **Anterior temporal branch**: Supplies temporal pole and anterior part of temporal lobe
- **Posterior temporal branch**: Supplies posterior part of temporal lobe and Wernicke's area (in left cerebral cortex)

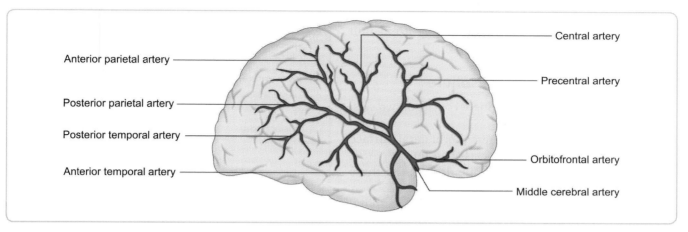

Figure 16.11: Branches of middle cerebral artery

Clinical Anatomy

Effects of occlusion of middle cerebral artery:
- Hemiplegia and loss of sensations on the opposite half of the body. The face and arms are most affected. Foot and leg may show mild weakness.
- Aphasia (by involvement of Broca's and Wernicke's areas), especially if the thrombosis is in the left hemisphere in a right-handed person.
- Homonymous quadrantanopia on the opposite side (by involvement of Meyer's loop passing superficially in the temporal lobe).

Hearing is never totally affected due to compensation by the opposite hemisphere.

Posterior Cerebral Artery

The right and left posterior cerebral arteries are the terminal branches of basilar artery. Each passes laterally around the crus cerebri of the midbrain, where it receives the posterior communicating artery. It continues along the lateral aspect of the midbrain and enters the supratentorial compartment through the tentorial notch. Then, it courses on the tentorial surface of the brain giving out its branches.

Cortical branches (Figure 16.12):
- **Temporo-occipital branch**: Supplies inferior surface of temporal lobe and lateral surface of the occipital lobe
- **Internal occipital branch:** Divides into parieto-occipital branch and calcarine branch and supplies cuneus and the rest of medial surface of the occipital lobe

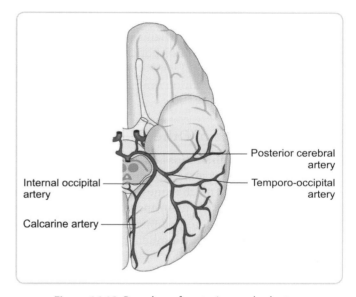

Figure 16.12: Branches of posterior cerebral artery

Clinical Anatomy

Effects of occlusion of posterior cerebral artery:
- The loss of cortical supply results in contralateral homonymous hemianopia with macular sparing.
- Damage to association cortex of visual area causes visual hallucinations (distortion of colour vision).

VENOUS DRAINAGE OF BRAIN

The veins draining the brain are valveless and thin walled because their walls are devoid of muscles. The veins draining the brain open into the nearby dural venous sinuses. Most of these sinuses ultimately drain into internal jugular vein.

Veins of the Cerebral Hemisphere

The veins of the cerebral hemisphere consist of two sets: (1) superficial and (2) deep.

The superficial veins on the superolateral surface of the cerebral hemisphere are classified into superior, superficial middle and inferior. The drainage of these veins is seen in Figure 16.13 and Table 16.2.

The superficial veins on the base of the cerebral hemisphere are the basal veins. Basal veins are formed by the union of deep middle cerebral vein and anterior cerebral vein. Basal veins drain into great cerebral vein (Figure 16.14).

The deep veins comprise of the septal veins, the choroidal vein and thalamostriate vein on each side. All these veins drain into the corresponding internal cerebral vein. Two internal cerebral veins join to form the great cerebral vein of Galen, which drains into straight sinus (Figure 16.14).

Venous Drainage of Other Parts of the Brain

The upper part of the **thalamus** is drained by the tributaries of the internal cerebral vein (including the thalamostriate vein). The lower part of the thalamus and the hypothalamus are drained by veins that run downwards to end in a plexus of veins present in the interpeduncular fossa. This plexus drains into the cavernous and sphenoparietal sinuses and into the basal veins.

TABLE 16.2: Superficial veins of the cerebrum on the superolateral surface	
Superficial cerebral veins	Drains into
Superior cerebral veins	Superior sagittal sinus
Superficial middle cerebral vein	Anteriorly, cavernous sinus
	Posteriorly, superior anastomotic vein to superior sagittal sinus
	Posteriorly, inferior anastomotic vein to transverse sinus
Inferior cerebral veins	Transverse sinus, straight sinus, superior petrosal sinus, cavernous sinus

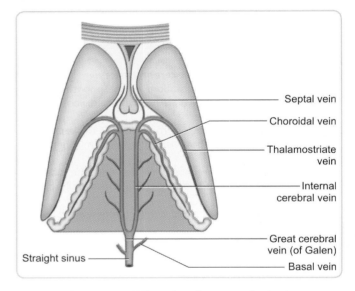

Figure 16.14: Tributaries of great cerebral vein

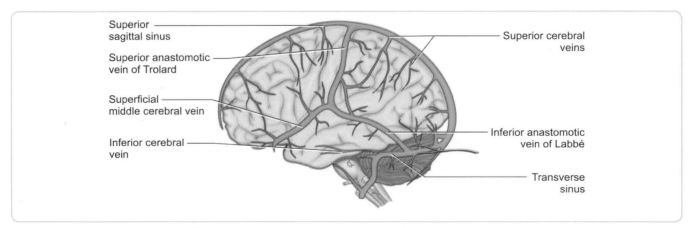

Figure 16.13: Superficial cerebral veins on the superolateral surface of the cerebrum

The **corpus striatum** and **internal capsule** are drained by two sets of striate veins. The **superior striate veins** run dorsally and drain into tributaries of the internal cerebral vein. The **inferior striate veins** run vertically downwards and emerge on the base of the brain through the anterior perforated substance. Here, they end in the basal vein.

Veins of the Cerebellum and Brainstem

The veins from the upper surface of the **cerebellum** drain into the straight, transverse and superior petrosal sinuses. Veins from the inferior surface drain into the right and left sigmoid sinuses, inferior petrosal sinuses, occipital sinus and straight sinus.

The veins of the **midbrain** drain into the great cerebral vein or into the basal vein. The **pons** and **medulla** drain into the superior and inferior petrosal sinuses, transverse sinus and occipital sinus. Inferiorly, the veins of the medulla are continuous with the veins of the spinal cord.

BLOOD-BRAIN BARRIER

It has been observed that while some substances can pass from the blood into the brain with ease, others are prevented from doing so. This has given rise to the concept of a selective barrier between blood and the brain.

Structure of Blood-brain Barrier

Anatomically, the structures that constitute the barrier are as follows (Figure 16.15).
- Capillary endothelium
- Basement membrane of the endothelium

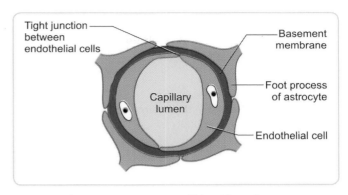

Figure 16.15: Structure of blood-brain barrier

- Closely applied to the vessels, there are numerous foot processes of astrocytes. It has been estimated that these processes cover about 85% of the capillary surface.

Areas of the Brain Devoid of Blood-brain Barrier

Some areas of the brain appear to be devoid of a blood-brain barrier. These include:
- Pineal body
- Neurohypophysis
- Organum vasculosum of lamina terminalis (OVLT)
- Median eminence (hypothalamus)
- Subcommissural organ
- Subfornical organ
- Area postrema

These are also called as circumventricular organs (CVOs), as these are specialized areas in the walls of third and fourth ventricles.

Clinical Anatomy

The **blood-brain barrier** can breakdown following ischaemia or infection of the brain. The barrier can also breakdown in trauma and through the action of toxins. Some drugs, including some antibiotics, can pass through the barrier while others cannot. In infants, bilirubin can pass through the barrier. There is a danger of encephalitis, if bilirubin levels are high (seen as jaundice in the newborn or **kernicterus**).

MULTIPLE CHOICE QUESTIONS

Q1. The venous sinus that is present at the base of falx cerebri is:
A. Occipital
B. Straight
C. Inferior sagittal
D. Cavernous

Q2. The branch of internal carotid artery that supplies the optic tract is:
A. Anterior choroidal
B. Middle cerebral
C. Posterior cerebral
D. Posterior communicating

Q3. **Which artery lies in the pontine cistern?**
 A. Superior cerebellar
 B. Basilar
 C. Posterior cerebral
 D. Anteroinferior cerebellar

Q4. **The vessel that lies in the cisterna ambiens is:**
 A. Superior cerebellar artery
 B. Basal vein
 C. Anterior choroidal artery
 D. Great cerebral vein

Q5. **The medial surface of the cerebral hemisphere up to parieto-occipital sulcus is supplied by which artery?**
 A. Anterior cerebral
 B. Middle cerebral
 C. Medial striate
 D. Posterior cerebral

Q6. **Which of the following areas of the brain show blood-brain barrier?**
 A. Median eminence of hypothalamus
 B. Hypophysis cerebri
 C. Choroid plexus of ventricles
 D. Tectum of midbrain

Q7. **Which of the following veins is related to the transverse fissure of the brain?**
 A. Basal
 B. Superficial middle cerebral
 C. Great cerebral
 D. Deep middle cerebral

Q8. **Which of the following cerebral veins unite to form the great cerebral vein?**
 A. Superficial middle
 B. Deep middle
 C. Internal
 D. Inferior

Q9. **The superficial middle cerebral vein ends in which of the following dural venous sinuses?**
 A. Superior sagittal
 B. Inferior sagittal
 C. Transverse
 D. Cavernous

ANSWERS

1. B   2. A   3. B   4. D   5. A   6. D   7. C   8. C   9. D

SHORT NOTES

1. Circle of Willis
2. Cisternal puncture
3. Anterior cerebral artery
4. Middle cerebral artery
5. Posterior cerebral artery
6. Blood-brain barrier

Clinical Cases

16.1: Following a head injury, a neurologist was explaining to his students how to differentiate a subdural haematoma from an extradural haematoma based on their shape on a computed tomography (CT) scan. What would be the shape of the haematoma, if it is:
 A. Subdural
 B. Extradural

16.2: Extracranial infections can spread to dural venous sinuses through vessels that are valveless. Trace the pathway of infection to the cavernous sinus from:
 A. Root of nose
 B. Upper lip

16.3: Angiograms are done to detect the site of block in the blood vessels. The vessels are identified by their area of distribution. How will a vertebral angiogram differ from an internal carotid angiogram in:
 A. Frontal view
 B. Lateral view

Answers to Clinical Cases

Chapter 1

1.1   A   Neurotmesis
      B   Neurapraxia or Axonotmesis

Chapter 2

2.1   A   Tenth thoracic spinal segment
      B   From umbilicus downward
2.2   A   Biceps jerk will be normal; knee jerk will be exaggerated
      B   Plantar reflex will show Babinski sign positive; cremasteric reflex will be lost
2.3   A   Skin, superficial fascia, supraspinous ligament, interspinous ligament, ligamentum flavum, areolar tissue
      B   The space between adjoining laminae in the lumbar region is increased to a maximum

Chapter 3

3.1   A   Pain sensations travel up ipsilaterally for 2 to 3 segments in the dorsolateral tract of Lissauer
      B   Left sided (ipsilateral) intrinsic muscles of hand
3.2   A   Lower motor neuron
      B   L3, L4
3.3   A   T1
      B   Cervical fibres are most medial, followed by thoracic, lumbar and sacral
3.4   A   Fasciculus gracilis, fasciculus cuneatus and corticospinal tracts
      B   Upper motor neuron

Chapter 4

4.1   A   Locked-in syndrome
      B   Short circumferential branches of basilar artery
4.2   A   Crossed diplegia
      B   Anterolateral part of lower medulla on the left side (beyond crossing of upper limb fibers, but before crossing of lower limb fibers)

Chapter 5

5.1   A   Involvement of corticospinal tract on the right side (before crossing); involvement of hypoglossal nerve fibres on the right side causing intact left genioglossus pulling the tongue to the right
      B   Medial part of medulla oblongata on the right side
5.2   A   Involvement of corticospinal tract on the left side (before crossing); involvement of facial nerve fibres on the left side causing left sided facial paralysis. Unopposed pull of normal muscles of the face pulled the angle of the mouth to the right
      B   Left lower pons; Millard-Gubler syndrome
5.3   A   Involvement of left spinal lemniscus (carrying pain sensation from contralateral half of the body); involvement of the left spinal nucleus of trigeminal nerve (carrying pain sensation from ipsilateral half of the face); involvement of vestibular nucleus
      B   Lateral part of medulla oblongata on the left side
5.4   A   Right corticospinal tract and right oculomotor nerve fibres
      B   Right half of midbrain at the level of superior colliculi; Weber syndrome

Chapter 6

6.1   A   Lower motor neuron type in both
      B   Right stylomastoid foramen in the first person; right cerebellopontine angle in the second
6.2   A   Right LMN lesion of hypoglossal nerve; left LMN lesion of mandibular nerve
      B   Left genioglossus; right lateral pterygoid
6.3   A   Right cerebellopontine angle
      B   Greater petrosal branch of facial nerve; relays in pterygopalatine ganglion
6.4   A   Skin over the angle of mandible is supplied by great auricular nerve, and not by trigeminal
      B   Pain
6.5   A   Right oculomotor nerve
      B   Optic nerve
6.6   A   At the lingula of mandible, before it enters the mandibular foramen
      B   Chorda tympani fibres carrying taste sensations joins the lingual nerve below base of the skull

Chapter 7

7.1 A Middle cerebral artery
    B Meyer's loop
7.2 A Bitemporal hemianopia
    B Pituitary tumour

Chapter 8

8.1 A Left side
    B Involvement of left vestibulocochlear nerve results in tinnitus and vertigo; involvement of left facial nerve results in decreased lacrimation in the left eye and deviation of angle of the mouth to the right side due to unopposed pull of right sided facial muscles
8.2 A Cerebrocerebellum
    B Vestibulocerebellum

Chapter 9

9.1 Pineal shifts to the contralateral side in a supratentorial space-occupying-lesion (SOL)
9.2 Olfactory sensation. Olfactory nerve is a direct extension of telencephalon (cerebrum)
9.3 Thalamogeniculate branch of posterior cerebral artery

Chapter 10

10.1 A Paracentral lobule of both sides
    B Anterior cerebral artery
10.2 A Astereognosis
    B Superior parietal lobule (Areas 5 and 7 of Brodmann)

Chapter 11

11.1 A Right sided hemiplegia with aphasia and right sided upper motor neuron type of facial paralysis
    B Striate branches of left middle cerebral
    C Involvement of uncrossed corticospinal tracts in the internal capsule of the left side; aphasia due to involvement of dominant hemisphere; involvement of left corticonuclear fibres to lower face results in deviation of angle of the mouth to the left side due to pull of left sided facial muscles
11.2 A Callosal syndrome

    B Inability of the senses perceived by the right hemisphere to go to left hemisphere through corpus callosum

Chapter 12

12.1 A Cog-wheel rigidity, stooping posture, difficulty in speech
    B Tremors are seen at rest in Parkinsonism; cerebellar tremors are seen during action

Chapter 13

13.1 A Amygdaloid nucleus
    B Amygdaloid nucleus with its limbic cortical connection is responsible for aggression

Chapter 14

14.1 A Surgical sympathectomy should be below the stellate ganglion or it would result in Horner's syndrome
    B Surgical sympathectomy should be below the first lumbar ganglion or it would result in absence of ejaculation
14.2 The enteric nervous system contains sensory neurons, interneurons and motor neurons. The motor neurons control motility, secretion, and absorption.
14.3 A Argyll-Robertson pupil
    B Fibres of optic tract joining pretectal nucleus

Chapter 15

15.1 A Arnold-Chiari malformation
    B Apertures in the roof of the fourth ventricles (foramina of Magendie and Luschka) are blocked causing accumulation of CSF in the ventricles

Chapter 16

16.1 A Crescentic
    B Biconvex
16.2 A Angular vein → Ophthalmic vein → Cavernous sinus
    B Deep facial vein → Pterygoid venous plexus → Emissary vein → Cavernous sinus
16.3 A Vertebral angiogram will show bilateral distribution
    B Vertebral angiogram shows distribution of blood to posterior fossa contents

Glossary

Greek / Latin term	English meaning
Abducens	Lead away
Abulia	Without willpower
Accumbens	Reclining
Acetylcholine	Vinegar bile
Acoustic	To hear
Adenohypophysis	Gland hypophysis (q.v.)
Adrenalin	Near the kidney
Afferent	To carry towards
Aganglionic	Without ganglion
Ageusia	Without taste
Agnosia	Without knowledge
Agraphia	Without ability to write
Akinesia	Without movement
Ala	Wing
Alexia	Inability to read
Allocortex	Other cortex (q.v.)
Allodynia	Other pain
Alveus	Canal, trough
Amacrine	Without long fibre
Ambiens	Both
Ambiguus	Doubtful
Ammonis	Egyptian deity with ram's head
Amnesia	Without remembrance
Ampulla	Small bottle
Amygdala	Almond
Amygdaloid	Almond-like
Anaesthesia	Without sensation
Analgesia	Without pain
Anastomotic	Communication between
Anencephaly	Without encephalon (q.v.)

Greek / Latin term	English meaning
Aneurysm	Widening
Angiogram	Vessel writing
Angular	Bend
Ansa	Looped handle
Antidromic	Against race course
Aphasia	Without speech
Apraxia	Without able to do
Aprosodia	Without song sung to rhythm
Aqueduct	Water canal
Arachnoid	Spider web-like
Arbor	Tree
Archicerebellum	Ancient cerebellum (q.v.)
Arcuate	Bow shaped
Astigmatism	Without point
Astrocyte	Star-like cell
Asynergia	Without coordination
Ataxia	Without orderliness
Athetosis	Without fixed position
Atrium	Main room
Atrophy	Without nourishment
Auditory	To hear
Autonomic	Self governed
Axolemma	Plasma membrane of axon (q.v.)
Axon	Axis
Axoplasm	Cytoplasm of axon (q.v.)
Basilar	Base
Bifida	Split
Bipolar	Two poles
Brachium	Arm
Bradykinesia	Slow movement

Greek / Latin term	English meaning
Bulb	Oval shaped
Calamus	Reed/stalk
Calcar	Spur
Calcarine	Spur-shaped
Callosum	Hard/tough
Capsule	Small box
Carotid	To put to sleep
Cauda	Tail
Caudate	Tail
Cavernous	Being in a large hollow space
Cephalic	Head
Cerebellum	Small brain
Cerebrum	Brain
Cervical	Neck
Chemoreceptor	Receive chemical
Chiasma	Cross
Chorea	Dance
Choroid	Like a membrane
Chromatolysis	Breakdown of colour
Ciliary	Eyelash
Cinereum	Ash grey
Cingulate	Belt
Cingulum	Belt
Circulus	Circle
Cistern	Reservoir or container
Clasp-knife	Foldable pocket knife
Claustrum	Barrier
Cleft	Space made by split
Cochlea	Snail shell
Coeliac	Belly
Coeruleus	Blue
Cogwheel	Toothed wheel
Collateral	Together by the side
Colliculus	Small hill
Coma	Deep sleep
Commissure	Joining together
Conjugate	Together yoke (neck)
Conjunctivum	Join

Greek / Latin term	English meaning
Connexus	Connection
Contra-coup	Opposite blow
Contralateral	Opposite side
Conus	Cone
Corneal	Horny tissue
Cornu	Horn
Corona	Crown
Corpus	Body
Corpuscle	Small corpus (q.v.)
Cortex	Outer layer (bark)
Cranial	Head
Crus	Leg
Culmen	Summit
Cuneus	Wedge
Cutaneous	Skin
Decussation	Crossing
Declive	Sloping downward
Dendrites	Tree
Dentate	Having teeth
Denticulate	Having small teeth
Diabetes	To pass through
Diencephalon	In between (dia) encephalon (q.v.)
Diplopia	Double vision
Dura	Hard
Dysarthria	Difficulty in articulation (speech)
Dysdiadochokinesisa	Difficulty in succeeding movement
Dyskinesia	Difficulty in movement
Dysmetria	Difficulty in measurement
Efferent	Carry away
Emboliform	Plug-like
Encephalogram	Encephalon (q.v.) writing
Encephalon	Organ inside the head (brain)
Enophthalmos	Inside eyeball
Enteric	Intestine

Greek / Latin term	English meaning
Entorhinal	Inside nose
Ependyma	Upper garment
Epithalamus	Above thalamus
Equina	Horse
Exteroceptor	External receiver
Extrafusal	Outside spindle
Facial	Face
Falx	Sickle
Fasciculus	Small bundle
Fasciolaris	Flat worm
Fastigial	Top of a gabled roof
Filum	Thread
Fimbria	Fringe
Fissure	Cleft or slit
Flaccid	Lacking firmness
Folium	Leaf
Forceps	Tongs/pincers
Fornix	Arch
Fossa	Trench/channel
Fovea	Pit/depression
Fundus	Bottom
Funiculus	Little cord
Fusiform	Spindle-shaped
Ganglion	Knot/swelling
Gelatinosa	Jelly
Gemmule	Small bud
Geniculate	Bent like a knee
Genu	Knee
Gliosis	Glue
Globose	Ball
Globus	Ball
Glomeruli	Small ball of thread
Glossopharyngeal	Tongue and throat
Gracile	Slender
Granule	Small grain

Greek / Latin term	English meaning
Gravis	Severe
Griseum	Grey
Gustatory	Taste
Gyrus	Ring, circle
Habenula	Rein
Haematoma	Swelling of blood
Haemorrhage	To burst forth with blood
Hemianopia	Half loss of vision
Hemiballisms	Half jumping
Hemiplegia	Half strike/blow
Hemisphere	Half sphere
Herpes	To creep
Hippocampus	Sea horse
Hydrocephalus	Water in the head
Hyperacusis	Loud hearing
Hypertrophy	Excess nourishment
Hypoglossal	Under the tongue
Hypophysis	Down growth
Hypothalamus	Under thalamus (q.v.)
Hypotonia	Decreased hold/grasp
Indusium	To put on/adorn
Infundibulum	Funnel
Insipidus	Tasteless
Insula	Island
Interoceptor	Between receiver
Interpeduncular	In between peduncle (q.v.)
Intersegmental	In between segments
Interstitial	In between placed
Interthalamic	In between thalamus (q.v.)
Intracerebellar	Inside cerebellum (q.v.)
Intrafusal	Within spindle
Intrinsic	Interior
Ipsilateral	Same side
Ischaemic	Stop blood
Isocortex	Equal cortex (q.v.)
Juxta-restiform	Next to restiform (q.v.)
Kernicterus	Yellowish-green nut
Laminae	Layer/thin plate

Greek / Latin term	English meaning
Leptomeninges	Slender meninges (q.v.)
Lemniscus	Woolen band or filet (ribbon)
Lenticularis	Shaped like a lens
Lentiform	Like a lens
Ligamentum	To bind
Limbic	Border/hem/fringe
Limen	Threshold
Limitans	To limit
Lingula	Little tongue
Locus	Location
Lumbar	Loin
Lunate	Moon
Lutea	Yellow
Macula	Spot, stain
Magna	Large
Mamilla	Small breast
Mater	Mother
Medulla	Innermost, marrow
Megacolon	Enlarged large intestine
Melatonin	Black serotonin (q.v.)
Meninges	Membranes
Meningocoele	Hernia of meninges (q.v.)
Meningo-encephalocoele	Hernia of meninges (q.v.) and encephalon (q.v.)
Meniscus	Crescent, moon
Mesencephalon	Middle encephalon (q.v.)
Metathalamus	After thalamus (q.v.)
Metencephalon	After encephalon (q.v.)
Microglia	Small glue
Mitral	Bishop's turban
Monoplegia	One strike/blow
Multipolar	Many poles
Myasthenia	Muscle lack of strength
Myelencephalon	Marrow encephalon (q.v.)
Myelin	Marrow
Myelon	Organ within (the vertebrae) – spinal cord
Myopia	To shut eye
Neocerebellum	New cerebellum (q.v.)

Greek / Latin term	English meaning
Neocortex	New cortex (q.v.)
Neostriatum	New striatum (q.v.)
Neuralgia	Neuron (q.v.) pain
Neurites	Branch of neuron (q.v.)
Neurobiotaxis	Neuron (q.v.) life law
Neuroglia	Nerve glue
Neurohypophysis	Neuron (q.v.) hypophysis (q.v.)
Neurolemma	Neuron (q.v.) husk
Neuron	Nerve
Neuropil	Neuron (q.v.) felt
Neurotransmitter	Neuron (q.v.) send accross
Nigra	Black
Node	Knot
Nodule	Small node (q.v.)
Nucleus	Small nut
Nystagmus	Nodding, drowsiness
Obex	Barrier
Oblongata	Rather long
Oculomotor	Eye movement
Olfactory	To smell
Oligodendrocytes	Few tree cell
Operculum	Cover, lid
Ophthalmic	Eyeball
Optic	For sight
Otic	Ear
Oxytocin	Sharp birth
Pachymeninx	Thick membrane
Paleocerebellum	Old cerebellum (q.v.)
Paleocortex	Old cortex (q.v.)
Paleostriatum	Old striatum (q.v.)
Pallidus	Pale
Pallium	Cloak
Parahippocampal	Beside, beyond hippocampus (q.v.)
Paralysis	To loosen
Paraplegia	Beside, beyond blow or stroke
Parastriate	Beside, beyond striate (q.v.)
Parasympathetic	Beside, beyond consoling, comforting

Greek / Latin term	English meaning
Paraterminal	Beside, beyond end
Parolfactory	Beside, beyond olfactory (q.v.)
Peduncle	Stem-like
Pellucidum	Translucent
Peristriate	Around striate (q.v.)
Pes	Foot
Petrosal	Stony hard
Pia	Soft
Pineal	Pine cone
Piriform	Pear-shaped
Pituitary	Slime, mucous
Plexus	A braid
Poliomyelitis	Inflammation of Grey matter of spinal cord
Pons	Bridge
Positron	Positive electron.
Pretectal	Before tectum (q.v.)
Proprius	One's own
Proprioceptor	Receiver
Prosencephalon	Before encephalon (q.v.)
Prosopagnosia	Inability to recognize faces
Ptosis	Fall
Pulvinar	Cushion, pillow, couch
Pupil	Doll, little girl
Putamen	Shell
Pyramis	Pyramid
Quadrigemina	Four twins
Quadriplegia	Four blow or stroke
Rachischisis	Main axis split
Radicularis	Small root
Ramus	Branch
Raphe	Seam
Receptor	Receiver
Reciprocal	Done in return
Rectus	Straight
Restiform	Rope-like
Reticular	Net-like
Retina	Net

Greek / Latin term	English meaning
Rhinal	Nose
Rhinencephalon	Nose encephalon (q.v.)
Rhombencephalon	Rhonbus encephalon (q.v.)
Rhomboid	Rhombus-like
Rigidity	Being stiff
Rostrum	Beak
Rubro	Red
Satellite	Attendant
Sclerosis	Hard
Scriptorius	Writing
Separans	Separating
Septal	Partition
Serotonin	Tonic inside serum
Siphon	Pipe, tube for drawing off fluid
Solitary	Alone
Somatotopic	Body place
Spastic	Drawing, pulling, stretching
Splenium	Bandage
Squint	Eyes askew
Stellate	Star
Strabismus	Eyes askew
Stria	Striped
Striate	Striped
Striatum	Striped
Subiculum	Small layer
Substantia	Substance
Subthalamus	Below thalamus (q.v.)
Sympathetic	Consoling, comforting
Synapse	Junction
Syndrome	The act of running together
Syringomyelia	Pipe / tube marrow (spinal cord)
Tabes	Emaciation
Tactile	Touch
Tanycyte	Stretched cell
Tapetum	Carpet
Tectum	Roof
Tegmental	Covering
Telencephalon	End encephalon (q.v.)

Greek / Latin term	English meaning
Tetanus	Muscle spasm
Thalamus	Inner chamber
Trabecula	Trabecula
Trapezoid	Trapezium-like
Tremor	Shake
Trigeminal	Triplet
Trigone	Three angles
Trochlear	Pulley
Tuber	Swelling
Tubercle	Small swelling
Uncus	Hook
Unipolar	One pole
Uvula	Little grape

Greek / Latin term	English meaning
Vagus	Wandering
Vallecula	Small valley
Vasocorona	Crowning vessel
Vasopressin	Vessel pressure
Velum	Covering
Ventricle	Small belly
Vermis	Worm
Vesicles	Blister, bladder
Vestibular	Entrance court
Vitae	Of life
Zona incerta	Belt uncertain
Zoster	Belt or girdle

Eponyms

Name of the scientist / discoverer	Nationality	Anatomical structure named after
Adamkiewicz, Albert	Polish Pathologist	Artery supplying lumbar segments of spinal cord
Alzheimer, Alois	German Neuropsychiatrist	Presenile and senile dementia
Argyll Robertson	Scottish Ophthalmologist	Pupillary constriction in accommodation, but not in response to light
Arnold, Julius	German Pathologist	Arnold-Chiari malformation
Auerbach, Leopold	German Anatomist	Myenteric plexus in the gastrointestinal tract
Babinski, Joseph François Félix	French Clinical Neurologist	Up-turning of the great toe and spreading of the toes on stroking the sole
Baillarger, Jules Gabriel François	French Psychiatrist	Bands of Baillarger in the cerebral cortex
Bell, Sir Charles	Scottish Anatomist, Clinical Neurologist, and Surgeon	Bell's palsy (facial paralysis) and Bell-Magendie law (dorsal roots are sensory, ventral roots are motor)
Benedikt, Moritz	Viennese Neurologist	Oculomotor nerve palsy and ataxia including tremors
Betz, Vladimir A	Russian Anatomist	Giant pyramidal cells in the motor cortex
Broca, Pierre Paul	French Pathologist and Anthropologist	Motor speech area; and diagonal band of Broca in the anterior perforated substance
Brodmann, Korbinian	German Neuropsychiatrist	Brodmann's area of the cerebral cortex
Brown-Séquard, Charles Edouard	Physiologist and Clinical Neurologist	Sensory and motor abnormalities in hemisection of the spinal cord
Bucy, Paul Clancy	American Neurosurgeon	Klüver-Bucy syndrome is caused by extensive bilateral lesions of the temporal lobes
Buerger, Leo	American Physician and Urologist	Chronic inflammatory disease of the peripheral vessels
Burdach, Karl Friedrich	German Physiologist	Fasciculus cuneatus (tract of Burdach)
Cajal, Santiago Felipe Ramón y	Spanish Histologist	Interstitial nucleus of midbrain; Neuron Doctrine on the basis of his observations with silver staining methods
Charcot, Jean-Martin	French Neurologist	Lenticulostriate branch of the middle cerebral artery
Chiari, Hans	Czech Physician	Arnold-Chiari malformation
Clarke, Jacob Augustus Lockhard	English Anatomist and Clinical Neurologist	Nucleus dorsalis (thoracicus) of the spinal cord
Corti, Marchese Alfonso	Italian Histologist	Sensory epithelium of the cochlea (organ of Corti)
Darkschewitsch, Liverij Osipovich	Russian Clinical Neurologist	One of the accessory oculomotor nuclei in the midbrain
Deiters, Otto Friedrich Karl	German Anatomist	Lateral vestibular nucleus,

Name of the scientist / discoverer	Nationality	Anatomical structure named after
Dejerine, Joseph Jules	French Neurologist	Hypoglossal alternating hemiplegia; Dejerine-Roussy syndrome of posterior thalamic infarct
Doppler, Christian Andreas	Austrian physicist and mathematician	Doppler effect
Edinger, Ludwig	German Neuroanatomist and Clinical Neurologist	Edinger-Westphal nucleus is the parasympathetic component of the oculomotor nucleus
Erb, Wilhelm Heinrich	German neurologist	Erb's paralysis
Fleischer, Bruno	German Ophthalmologist	Kayser-Fleischer ring in Wilson's disease
Forel, Auguste Henri	Swiss Neuropsychiatrist	Fibre bundles in the subthalamus, known as the fields of Forel; and ventral tegmental decussation in the midbrain
Foville, Achille-Louis-François	French Physician	Paramedian tegmental pontine syndrome of Foville
Frey, Lucja	Polish Neurologist	Gustatory hyperhidrosis
Galen, Claudius	Roman Physician	Great cerebral vein
Gasser, Johann Laurentius	Austrian Anatomist	Sensory ganglion of the trigeminal nerve was named for him by one of his students, A.B.R. Hirsch
Gennari, Francesco	Italian Physician	White line in the visual cortex (stria of Gennari)
Golgi, Camillo	Italian Histologist	Type I and type II neurons; Golgi tendon organ; and Golgi apparatus
Goll, Friedrich	Swiss Neuroanatomist	Fasciculus gracilis (tract of Goll)
Gubler, Adolphe-Marie	French Physician	Ventral pontine syndrome of Millard-Gubler
Herophilus	Greek Physician	Confluence of the dural venous sinuses at the internal occipital protuberance is known as the torcular Herophili
Heschl, Richard	Austrian Anatomist And Pathologist	Transverse temporal gyri (Heschl's convolutions), for the auditory area of the cerebral cortex.
Heubner, Johann Otto Leonhard	German Pediatrician	Recurrent branch of the anterior cerebral artery
Hilton, John	British surgeon and anatomist	Hilton's law
Hirschsprung, Harald	Danish Physician	Congenital aganglionic megacolon
Horner, Johann Friedrich	Swiss Ophthalmologist	Horner's syndrome, caused by interruption of the sympathetic innervation of the eye
Huntington, George Sumner	American General Medical Practitioner	Huntington's chorea resulting from neuronal degeneration in the corpus striatum
Kayser, Bernhard	German Ophthalmologist	Kayser-Fleischer ring in Wilson's disease
Kellie, George	Scottish physician	Monro-Kellie doctrine
Kleine, Willi	German psychiatrist	Kleine-Levin syndrome
Klumpke, Augusta	French neurologist	Klumpke's paralysis- Paralysis of lower trunk of brachial plexus
Klüver, Heinrich	American Psychologist	Klüver-Bucy syndrome caused by bilateral lesions of the temporal lobes
Korsakoff, Sergei Sergeievich	Russian Psychiatrist	Korsakoff's psychosis, in chronic alcoholism, includes a memory defect, and fabrication of ideas
Krause, Wilhelm Johann Friedrich	German Anatomist	Sensory endings in the skin, the end bulbs of Krause
Labbé, Charles	French surgeon	Inferior anastomotic vein of Labbé

Name of the scientist / discoverer	Nationality	Anatomical structure named after
Levin, Max	American neurologist	Kleine-Levin syndrome
Lissauer, Heinrich	German Clinical Neurologist	Dorsolateral tract of spinal cord (Lissauer's tract)
Luschka, Hubert von	German Anatomist	Lateral foramina of the IV ventricle (of Luschka)
Luys, Jules Bernard	French Clinical Neurologist	Subthalamic nucleus (nucleus of Luys)
Magendie, François	French Physiologist	Bell-Magendie law; and median aperture of the fourth ventricle (foramen of Magendie)
Martinotti, Giovanni	Italian Physician	Cells of Martinotti in the cerebral cortex
Meckel, Johann Friedrich	German Anatomist	Trigeminal ganglion is situated in Meckel's cave
Meissner, Georg	German Anatomist and Physiologist	Touch corpuscles in the dermis; and the submucous nerve plexus of the gastrointestinal tract
Merkel, Friedrich Siegmund	German Anatomist	Tactile endings in the epidermis (Merkel's disks)
Meyer, Adolph	American Psychiatrist	The fibres of the geniculocalcarine tract that loop forward in the temporal lobe constitute Meyer's loop
Meynert, Theodor Hermann	Austrian Neuropsychiatrist	Habenulointerpeduncular fasciculus (fasciculus retroflexus of Meynert); dorsal tegmental decussation of Meynert in the midbrain; and nucleus basalis of Meynert is in the substantia innominata
Millard, Auguste Louis Jules	French Physician	Ventral pontine syndrome of Millard-Gubler
Monro, Alexander, II	Scottish Anatomist	Interventricular foramen between the lateral and third ventricles is known as the foramen of Monro; Monro-Kellie doctrine
Müller, Heinrich	German anatomist	Müller's muscle
Nissl, Franz	German Neuropsychiatrist	Staining grey matter with cationic dyes to show the basophil material (Nissl bodies) of nerve cells
Pacini, Filippo	Italian Anatomist and Histologist	Sensory endings known as the Pacinian corpuscles
Papez, John Wenceslas	American Anatomist	Circuitry of the limbic system
Parinaud, Henri	French Ophthalmologist	Paralysis of upward gaze is due to a lesion of the midbrain, due to pressure from a pineal tumor
Parkinson, James	English Physician, Surgeon, and Paleontologist	"Shaking palsy" or paralysis agitans, which is more frequently called Parkinson's disease
Purkinje, Johannes (Jan) Evangelista	Bohemian Physiologist	Purkinje cells of the cerebellar cortex and Purkinje fibres in the heart
Ranvier, Louis-Antoine	French Histologist	Nodes of Ranvier in the myelin sheaths
Raymond, Fulgence	French Neurologist	Paramedian basal pontine syndrome of Raymond
Raynaud, Maurice	French Physician	Vasospasm, due to cold, decreases blood supply to limbs
Reil, Johann Christian	German Physician	Insula, or the island of Reil
Renshaw, Birdsey	American Neurophysiologist	Interneurons in the spinal cord are called Renshaw cells
Rexed, Bror	Swedish Neuroanatomist	Grey matter of the spinal cord into laminae of Rexed
Rinne, Heinrich Adolf	German ENT surgeon	Rinne's test
Robin, Charles Philippe	French Anatomist	Perivascular spaces of the brain (Virchow-Robin spaces)
Rolando, Luigi	Italian Anatomist	Central sulcus of the cerebral hemisphere; and the substantia gelatinosa of the spinal cord

Name of the scientist / discoverer	Nationality	Anatomical structure named after
Romberg, Moritz Heinrich	German Clinical Neurologist	Romberg's sign of impaired proprioceptive conduction in the spinal cord
Rosenthal, Friedrich Christian	German Anatomist	Basal vein of Rosenthal
Roussy, Gustave	Swiss-French neuropathologist	Dejerine-Roussy syndrome of posterior thalamic infarct
Ruffini, Angelo	Italian Anatomist	Sensory endings, known as the end bulbs of Ruffini
Schultze, Max Johann	German Histologist and Zoologist	Comma tract or fasciculus interfascicularis of the spinal cord
Schütz, H	German Anatomist	Dorsal longitudinal fasciculus of the brain stem
Schwann, Theodor	German Anatomist	Neurolemmal (Schwann cells) of peripheral nerves
Sherrington, Sir Charles Scott	English Neurophysiologist	Reflexes; decerebrate rigidity; reciprocal innervation; and the synapse
Sydenham, Thomas	English Physician	Sydenham's chorea
Sylvius, Francis De La Boe	French Anatomist	Lateral sulcus of the cerebral hemisphere
Sylvius, Jacobus	French Anatomist	Cerebral aqueduct of the midbrain (of Sylvius)
Trolard, Paulin	French Anatomist	Inferior anastomotic vein of Trolard
Vicq d'Azyr, Felix	French Anatomist	Mammillothalamic fasciculus
Virchow, Rudolph Ludwig Karl	German Pathologist	Perivascular spaces of the brain (Virchow-Robin spaces)
Wallenberg, Adolf	German Physician	Lateral medullary syndrome
Waller, Augustus Volney	English Physician and Physiologist	Degenerative changes in the distal portion of a sectioned peripheral nerve, known as wallerian degeneration
Weber, Ernst Heinrich	German Physician	Weber test
Weber, Sir Hermann David	English Physician	Midbrain lesion causing hemiparesis and ocular paralysis
Wernicke, Carl	German Neuropsychiatrist	Wernicke's sensory language area and Wernicke's aphasia are named for him
Westphal, Karl Friedrich Otto	German Clinical Neurologist	Edinger-Westphal nucleus in the oculomotor complex
Willis, Thomas	English Physician	Arterial circle of Willis
Wilson, Samuel Alexander Kinnier	British Clinical Neurologist	Hepatolenticular degeneration (Wilson's disease)
Wrisberg, Heinrich August	German Anatomist	Sensory root of the facial nerve (nervus intermedius of Wrisberg)

Index

Page numbers followed by *f* refer to figure, *fc* refer to flow chart, and *t* refer to table.